THE HUMAN SIDE OF HEALTH ADMINISTRATION

A Guide for Hospital, Nursing, and Public Health Administrators

ROBERT L. VENINGA

*School of Public Health,
University of Minnesota*

PRENTICE-HALL, INC., Englewood Cliffs, New Jersey 07632

Library of Congress Cataloging in Publication Data

Veninga, Robert L.
    The human side of health administration.

    Includes bibliographies and index.
        1. Health facilities—Administration.
2. Health services administration.   I. Title.
RA971.V38   362.1′068   81–19930
ISBN   0-13-447821-5   AACR2
ISBN   0-13-447813-4 (pbk.)

362.1068
V461h

DEDICATED TO NORMAN A. CRAIG,
MY PUBLIC HEALTH MENTOR,
WHOSE WISDOM AND FRIENDSHIP
I WILL ALWAYS VALUE

Editorial/production supervision and interior design
    by Zita de Schauensee
Cover design by Ray Lundgren, Tony Ferrara Studio
Manufacturing buyer: John Hall

Printed in the United States of America

10 9 8 7 6 5 4 3 2

ISBN 0-13-447821-5
ISBN 0-13-447813-4 {pbk.}

Prentice-Hall International, Inc., *London*
Prentice-Hall of Australia Pty. Limited, *Sydney*
Prentice-Hall of Canada, Ltd., *Toronto*
Prentice-Hall of India Private Limited, *New Delhi*
Prentice-Hall of Japan, Inc., *Tokyo*
Prentice-Hall of Southeast Asia Pte. Ltd., *Singapore*
Whitehall Books Limited, *Wellington, New Zealand*

Contents

71593

3 COMPETENCY: MANAGING YOUR TIME AND YOUR WORK   55

4 COMPETENCY: COMMUNICATING EFFECTIVELY   81

5 COMPETENCY: SELECTING, MOTIVATING, AND EVALUATING PERSONNEL   105

     AND JOB BURNOUT   290

     The nature of stress   291
        Stress defined   292
        Eustress versus distress   293
        Personality factors and stress   294
     Determinants of stress: Occupational factors   297
        Factors intrinsic to a job   297
        Role in the organization   300
        Career development   301
        Relationships at work   302
        Organizational structure and climate   302
     Determinants of stress: Psychological factors   303
     The stress response: Occupational burnout   306
        Stages of burnout   309
           Stage 1: Job contentment   309
           Stage 2: Job disappointment   310
           Stage 3: Job disillusionment   311
           Stage 4: Job despair   313
           Stage 5: Work redefined   313
     Strategies for preventing occupational burnout   314
        Becoming conscious of the consequences of work
             stress   314
        Developing space from work   317
        Setting challenging yet realistic goals   319
        Developing social support   320
        Practicing relaxation techniques   321
           Planning ahead   321
           Relaxing at work   321
           Taking a vacation   322
           Meditating   323
        Knowing when a job is hopeless   323
        Addressing the problems associated with shift work   326
        Adopt flexible working schedules   327
        Building a healthier organization   328
        Maintain your vitality   330

     Index   333

To the Reader

The purpose of this book is to assist you in becoming a *competent* health administrator. A basic premise of each chapter is that administrative competencies can be *learned* and that, once mastered, these competencies will form the basis for your future success.

I would like to give you a brief sketch of this book and also tell you some of my personal goals in writing it. The first chapter is designed to give you a *framework for understanding the concept of administrative competence.* In this chapter we will examine four levels of effectiveness ranging from unconscious incompetence to conscious competence. One of the primary goals of this chapter is to describe the characteristics of health administrators who are able to create productive and healthy organizations.

Each of the following chapters will identify a single administrative competency. In Chapter 2 we will present a method by which to examine an organization's *culture.* We will show how an institution's culture is reflected in the way it is formally organized and, equally important, in the way in which power is used and misused. The underlying theme is that the effectiveness of a hospital, nursing, or public health administrator is dependent upon an understanding of the tacit rules of behavior that govern all institutions.

In Chapter 3 we will examine the competency of *time management.* Time is a resource that is often mismanaged, leading to frustration and work dissatisfaction. Administrators who want to make maximum use of their time must define challenging, demanding, and performance-related objectives.

They must also learn how to delegate responsibility and authority to ensure that work is completed in an efficient manner.

Effective interpersonal communication is the basis for trust in contemporary organizations. In Chapter 4 we will examine the differences between disagreements, misinformation, and misunderstandings, as well as the barriers to effective communication. We will then turn to some of the most provocative writings of Carl Rogers in order to understand the hidden variables that influence our relationships with colleagues and friends.

One of the most critical skills that we will be exploring is the ability to create a *productive work environment.* In Chapter 5 we will discuss methods of locating and selecting prospective employees, and ways to evaluate their performance. We will also examine current motivational theory and highlight six principles of human motivation that lead to high productivity in human service organizations.

Most health administrators find themselves spending an enormous amount of time in *committee meetings.* In Chapter 6 we will examine the strengths and limitations of committees and discuss ways to maximize their effectiveness.

Because a significant portion of administrative energy is spent in *responding to change* and *managing conflict,* a major portion of the book is devoted to the subject of conflict resolution. In Chapter 7 we will define several major causes of conflict within health organizations. Chapter 8 will examine strategies through which interpersonal, intradepartmental, and interagency conflicts can be addressed. Chapter 9 will focus on the types of changes impinging upon health organizations and how *strategies of planned change* can be used in better responding to the needs of clients *and* the needs of employees.

The final competency discussed in this book is the ability to *manage occupational stress and job burnout.* Health organizations—particularly hospitals—produce stressful work environments. When the stresses of work become unreasonable, staff productivity and morale decline while absenteeism and employee turnover markedly increase. One of the most formidable challenges of a health administrator is to create a working environment where morale is high and where people feel good about their accomplishments. Upon completing the final chapter you will be able to identify the most common causes of debilitating organizational stress and define specific administrative actions that create a productive and humane work environment.

Let me now turn to some of the major considerations that went into the writing of this book. My first goal was to write a book on *health* administration. During the past ten years there has been a virtual explosion of information in the field of management, communication, and organizational behavior. Fortunately we now have theory, based upon research data, about what administrators can do to build productive organizations. However, not all of that theory and research has direct application to *health* organizations—

particularly those health organizations that exist in the public sector. Winnowing the many studies and scholarly works in the general field of management and finding those which have particular relevance to health delivery systems was one of the major objectives I had in the writing of each chapter.

My second goal was to write a *practical* book—one that has direct relevance to the actual work that hospital, nursing, and public health administrators undertake. To that end I have sought to use many examples of situations, problems, and issues that confront contemporary health administrators. An effort is made in each chapter to identify several administrative concepts, explain the rationale of each, and then demonstrate how these concepts apply to the real-world work of human service administration.

Above my typewriter I have sketched in large letters Kurt Lewin's observation that "there isn't anything as practical as a good theory." I believe this to be true and have attempted to reflect the practicality of sound administrative theory in each chapter.

A third goal was to define *specific learning end points* so that you, the reader, will have a clear understanding of the material to be mastered. Therefore, at the beginning of each chapter you will find an overview to serve as a type of road map indicating the knowledge you should obtain. In addition, each chapter contains a concise summary noting the critical areas of study covered in the previous pages.

Finally, it is important not to leave the impression that the nine competencies discussed in this book are the only ones needed to ensure effective health administration practices. Others are equally important. However the competencies that have been identified in these pages represent some of the most basic interpersonal skills that are needed in mastering the complex environments in which health administrators are employed.

I hope you find the book readable, helpful, and challenging.

ACKNOWLEDGMENTS

I want to acknowledge the organizations and people who have made a special contribution to my learning. I want to specifically thank the Hennepin County Medical Center, Minneapolis, Minnesota, for their interest in scholarly research and the New England Hospital Assembly for permitting me to learn about the real-life problems confronting health administrators. I am appreciative of Les Block's encouragement to write this book and of Ray Carlaw's friendship and support which enabled me to complete the manuscript. I will always be indebted to William Howell for his guidance and to George Shapiro who helped me see the interface between communication theory and health administration practice. A special thanks goes to Roger Fredrikson who helped me understand the power that exists in creative ideas, to Marilyn Eells who kept me organized, and to Karen Spiczka and Mary Potter who saw to it that the final manuscript was typed with speed and accuracy. I am grateful for Lee Stauffer's influence on my life and for the many enjoyable hours we have spent working together. And I am particularly grateful for two special people, Barbara Walton Spradley and James Spradley, who taught me the joy of writing and the meaning of friendship. Then too, there was the staff at Prentice-Hall, Inc., who contributed to the book. I am grateful to Dudley Kay whose insight and ideas were greatly appreciated, to Diane Spina who kept our communication links intact, and to Zita de Schauensee who gave competent technical assistance. I want to thank a very special little friend, Brent Karl Veninga, for his love and support. Finally, I want to thank my wife, Karen Smit Veninga, who gives purpose, perspective, and joy to all that I do.

St. Paul, Minnesota   Robert L. Veninga

A book is the only place in which you can examine a fragile thought without breaking it, or explore an explosive idea without fear that it will go off in your face. It is one of the few sources of information left that is served up without the silent black noise of a headline, the doomy hulabaloo of a commercial; it's one of the few havens remaining where a person's mind can get both provocation and privacy.
—Edward P. Morgan

1 The Pursuit of Excellence in Health Administration

The endurance of organizations depends upon the quality of leadership.—Chester Bernard

OVERVIEW   The purpose of this chapter is to describe characteristics of consciously competent health administrators. Upon completion of this chapter the reader will be able to:

- Differentiate four levels of administrative competence

- Describe defense mechanisms utilized by incompetent administrators

- List changes in American society that are impacting on health organizations

- Describe three salient skills utilized by consciously competent administrators

It is a truism of recent vintage that the health system is undergoing a revolution. This truism, however, is as outdated as it is imprecise. It is more accurate to state that the health system, like the society it reflects, is undergoing a series of revolutions and that these revolutions relate directly to the quality of life of every citizen.

The revolutions in health have been brought on by rising consumer expectations, new generations of technology, a shift in interest from communicable diseases to the diseases brought on by our life-styles, and a bewilderment about how much all of this costs. As with any revolutionary happening, battle lines are drawn between providers and consumers, those in power and those who want power, those who wish change and those who hold out for the values of the present.

The net result of this ferment is that a key domestic issue of the 1980s relates to the quality of our lives and the health delivery system which is to support that quality.

Health administrators, by virtue of their central role within the health delivery system, will increasingly confront a multitude of pressures, criticisms, and challenges. Hospital administrators will continue to be the target of a variety of self-interest groups who are becoming increasingly sophisticated in mobilizing pressure to enhance their political and economic power. Nurses, laboratory technicians, paraprofessionals, secretaries, and custodial employees will heighten their demand for an ever-increasing salary and fringe benefit base. Medical staff will demand a large share of responsibility in governing the total institution. Hospital trustees, in response to the deafening criticisms relative to costs, will put the burden for reducing costs at the door of the chief executive officer.

Public health administrators will not be immune to the pressures experienced by their counterparts in the private sector. In the period immediately after World War II local and state health departments and the U.S. Public Health Service grew and flourished as the guardians of the people's health. Unfortunately, in the last thirty years public health agencies have lost much of their momentum. The once strong U.S. Public Health Service has disappeared and its replacements have often been transitory both in terms of leadership and composition. The net result is considerable confusion and pessimism about the future role of city, county, and state health departments.[1]

There is a strong need for public health administrators to regain their leadership role in protecting the health of the public. However, if credibility is to be regained, public health officials must clearly define their organization's mission and purpose. As Charles Harper and Donald Smith incisively note, "It's time for them [public health officials] to set concrete objectives and per-

---

[1] M. Terris, "The Epidemiologic Revolution, National Health Insurance and the Role of Health Departments," *American Journal of Public Health,* 66 (December 1976), 1155.

formance criteria based on the mission and purpose they define. It is time for them to structure their organizations, not only on external funding sources but on efficiency and effectiveness. And it is time for them to focus on the critical dimensions of organizational management."[2]

The challenges to those entering nursing administration are equally formidable. Nursing administrators will increasingly find themselves in the vortex of societal changes. Transforming the perception of nursing as a profession of handmaidens to one that fully understands, appreciates, and utilizes the skills of the baccalaureate, master, and doctorally prepared nurse will take great political skill. In her study on the job satisfaction of nurses, Marjorie A. Godfrey points out that many nurses feel that the real reason nursing is not valued and respected is due to the "old devil," sex discrimination. "Too many people, including nurses, still think of nursing as 'women's work,' and until the profession has its consciousness raised there will never be substantive changes."[3] A New Jersey nurse stated: "We perform one of the most essential roles in society. We're there when people are born, when overwhelming crisis strikes them, and when they die. Yet I make less money than my uncle who's a garbage collector."[4] The concern about nursing wages, now ranked as the number one cause of nursing dissatisfaction, is bound to be a volatile issue throughout the 1980s.[5]

While the issue of nursing salaries will demand much attention, nursing administrators will be confronted with other, equally pressing challenges. The concepts of "prevention" and "wellness" require objective analysis from a nursing perspective and the cost-benefit ratios of such programs need to be validated. As nursing becomes more specialized and adept at using advanced technology, there will be an increased need for nursing administrators to communicate the competencies and independent decision-making capabilities of nurses to those unfamiliar with or threatened by these developments.

In summary, when an individual chooses a career in health administration, it means living in an environment of conflict, change, and crisis. The word "crisis" has been defined as the decisive moment, or as indicated in Chinese script, as the time of opportunity. If health administrators are to seize the opportunity in creating more productive health organizations, competent patterns of administration will need to be practiced at all levels within the organization.

[2] Charles Harper and Donald Smith, "Declining Public Health Organizations—Will Management Make A Difference?" *Health Care Management Review,* 4, no. 4 (Fall 1979), 31.

[3] Marjorie A. Godfrey and the *Nursing 78* staff, "Job Satisfaction—Or Should That Be Dissatisfaction?" *Nursing 78,* April 1978, p. 91.

[4] Ibid., p. 91.

[5] Mabel A. Wandelt, Patricia M. Pierce, and Robert R.Widdowson, "Why Nurses Leave Nursing and What Can Be Done About It," *American Journal of Nursing,* 81, no. 1 (January 1981), 73.

CONSCIOUS COMPETENCE: THE BASIC CHALLENGE

John Gardner tells of a time when he asked a highly regarded music teacher to explain the secret of his extraordinary success with students. The teacher's response: "First I teach them that it is better to do it well than to do it badly. Many have never been taught the pleasure and pride in setting standards and then living up to them."[6]

The pursuit of excellence in one's occupation represents one of the most important of all human pilgrimages. To be uncommon in terms of skill and commitment represents a significant departure in an age of commonness. Gardner states: "We must face the fact that there are a good many things in our character . . . which are inimical to standards—laziness, complacency, the desire for a fast buck, the American fondness for short cuts, reluctance to criticize slackness, to name only a few. Every thinking American knows in his heart that we must sooner or later come to terms with these failings."[7]

Standards! That is a word that should be printed in bold type on a plaque sitting on the desk of every health administrator. If the past decade represented the emergence of consumer consciousness related to medical malpractice, the current decade may be the era when consumers understand and are determined to do something about administrative incompetence. Accountability will be demanded by a diverse number of groups including public officials, trustees, governing boards, professional organizations, accrediting bodies, employees, and consumers. Paradoxically, while such groups will demand administrative accountability, each will probably have its own evaluative criteria. Such criteria will probably conflict with and contradict one another. It therefore becomes essential for administrators to articulate the rationale and logic supporting administrative actions and, in so doing, to demonstrate that competent administrative practices are being implemented.

As one examines contemporary administrative practices, four levels of administrative competence are evident:

1. Unconscious incompetence
2. Conscious incompetence
3. Unconscious competence
4. Conscious competence[8]

We want to now define these levels and examine the characteristics of each.

[6] John W. Gardner, *Excellence* (New York: Harper & Row, 1961), p. 158.
[7] Ibid., pp. 158–59.
[8] Ernest G. Bormann, William S. Howell, Ralph G. Nichols, and George L. Shapiro, *Interpersonal Communication in the Modern Organization* (Englewood Cliffs, N.J.: Prentice-Hall, Inc., 1969), pp. 131–36. The author is indebted to Dr. George Shapiro for the description of the competence-incompetence methodology originally applied to the study of interpersonal communication processes.

Unconscious Incompetence

Administrators who are unconsciously incompetent are unaware of how their incompetence is negatively influencing the organization. They can blithely walk through a day oblivious of the fact that the organization is lacking in sound administrative policies, procedures, and leadership. Well-defined goals and objectives are usually not in existence; consequently, it is unlikely that there will be any formal review of employee performance. Responsibility and authority will not be formally delegated, although, given the leadership vacuum, staff members may usurp such authority. The unconsciously incompetent individual will probably ignore or be unaware of the discontent of employees even though the warning signals of administrative ineffectiveness are dramatically evident in high rates of employee absenteeism and turnover.

Why do contemporary organizations tolerate incompetent administrative practices? At times the incompetence is not immediately observable, particularly if the institution is financially solvent and is not in a competitive market. In some organizations employee longevity is often rewarded and may be the single most important reason why an incompetent administrator is not dismissed. In other organizations friendships become more important than productivity, thus ensuring that the incompetent individual's employment will continue.

Can unconsciously incompetent administrative practices be changed? No generalized answer can be given although, for those who respond favorably to personal change, there is the possibility of learning new administrative skills. However, even if there is a desire to change, the unconsciously incompetent individual will need a closely supervised tutorial experience. The fact that this administrator does not know how to change generally means that a sizable investment of time in training must be made if new administrative attitudes and behaviors are to be learned.

Conscious Incompetence

Some administrators have a keen understanding of their administrative shortcomings. Hardly a working day passes but something occurs that vividly reminds them that they do not possess credible administrative skills. When criticisms from clients mount and subordinates become vocal about "the lack of leadership," consciously incompetent administrators become painfully aware of their shortcomings. When administrators perceive that others do not respect their judgment or when administrators begin to feel that they have been left out of the communication system by supervisors, peers, and subordinates, feelings of administrative inadequacy become acute.

As the day-to-day frustrations brought on by ineptness engulf the administrator several coping mechanisms are employed. One such mechanism is to run from the situation believing it to be impossible to ever master the new tasks. This coping mechanism is frequently observed in individuals who have been promoted from a staff to a management position. Once they realize that the technical skills that served well in a staff capacity do not necessarily help in an administrative position, such individuals may panic. The first thought that comes to mind is to resign and return to the area where they *know* they are competent.

For example, a physical therapist known for her clinical competence was promoted to a managerial position in a large metropolitan hospital. Unfortunately, the skills she demonstrated in working with patients did not transfer to her new role as supervisor of nine therapists. When the administrative pressures became too great she confided to a friend: "I'm just not cut out for all the political pressure that goes with the job. And I don't know the first thing about budgets and grievances and all the things we talk about in the Executive Council. I really would rather be a skilled physical therapist." Four months after taking her new job she resigned and resumed her clinical responsibilities.

For some individuals, returning to a staff position is in their best interest and in the best interests of the institution. For others such a coping mechanism is self-defeating. If the new administrator has a trusted mentor who can help in mastering new roles, the feelings of failure and the painful withdrawal that often occur after resigning can be avoided. If newly employed administrators who have not had the benefit of formal management training can recognize their limitations, learn from trial and error as well as from the expertise of others, and seek to overcome administrative weaknesses, professional and personal growth will invariably follow.

Another coping strategy utilized by consciously incompetent administrators is rationalization. This involves the giving of desirable reason for one's behavior rather than the real reason. For example, the director of an environmental health department rationalized the ineffectiveness of his department by saying, "You can't run a major environmental program with only two sanitarians." In reality the problem was caused by inadequacy of the supervision of the two sanitarians rather than by a shortage of workers.

Projection occurs when there is a failure and blame is ascribed to someone who is not the direct cause of the problem. Consider the request of a rural Health Systems Agency (HSA) for "full designation status" which was rejected by the State Health Coordinating Council (SHCC). Instead of blaming himself or his agency, the executive director of the HSA vented his anger on the membership of the State Health Coordinating Council: "Look at the membership of the Council. Most of them are city residents. What do they know about our rural health problems? They probably have never even seen a farm. All they care about is that they get good health services in the city." Such projections seek to absolve the executive director of responsibility for the failure to obtain full designation. Since most of us find it helpful to periodically scapegoat, this defense mechanism is frequently employed in all organizational settings.

Compensation is frequently used by individuals promoted to leadership positions but who have difficulty mastering the tasks that go with the position. Such individuals frequently ignore their new responsibilities and continue to do the work associated with their old job. An administrator who is compensating may say, "Move over. Let me show you how that's supposed to be done." Compensators will eagerly do the work of subordinates because they know that they can do the job well—work that they enjoyed in the "good old days" before assuming their leadership position.

Unfortunately compensation is self-defeating behavior. When leaders spend energy doing tasks of subordinates their own work goes undone. It is also self-defeating for subordinates because it takes away their sense of control over their own work.

Rationalizing, projecting, or compensating are not healthy ways of reacting to the frustrating situations. The hostility that is aroused in staff members when these mechanisms are employed usually accentuates the problems confronting the administrator and the organization.

Can consciously incompetent administrators change their behavior? Yes, providing they *desire* to learn new patterns of administrations. Yes, providing that their supervisors and peer groups will be patient so that new concepts and skills can be practiced and mastered.

Unconscious Competence

Individuals who are unconsciously competent are effective without being aware of the reasons for their success. An example of unconscious competence might be seen in a state health commissioner who is very effective in the political arena. Due to the commissioner's skills, health-related bills are always on the agenda in the state legislature. If you were to ask the commissioner to articulate the reasons behind his success he might chuckle and say: "Well, I really don't know how we get all this legislation passed. I guess it is just plain old-fashioned luck." But it is not "luck." There are definite, identifiable reasons for the commissioner's success; the only problem is that the commissioner is not cognizant of those reasons.

How can administrators achieve success without knowing the reasons for their achievements? One answer is that many individuals have become successful through simple trial and error. Over a period of years they have discovered strategies that produce success and have discarded strategies that result in failure. A dietary supervisor, for example, who has never had a great deal of formal training in management might be quite successful in matching difficult patients to the unique personalities and skills of the dietitians she supervises. The dietary supervisor may never have heard of McGregor's Theory X and Theory Y or of Blake and Mouton's managerial grid. Yet over the years a valuable education has taken place that has produced patterns of success.

Is there any reason why the unconsciously competent individual should seek to become consciously competent? After all, one may argue, isn't success the ultimate criteria of administrative effectiveness? There are two important reasons why this type of administrator should become *consciously* competent.

First, most administrators spend a great deal of time teaching others how to perform tasks. In fact, one of the most important administrative functions is the carrying out of teaching responsibilities. When administrators are asked to recall conversations with employees, it is quickly apparent that they spend a great deal of their time instructing staff on how to undertake particular assignments. If administrators are not aware of the rationale and logic behind their instruction, it will be difficult to teach others effectively. If instructions to others are to be credible, it is imperative that instructors be able to justify their counsel with supporting evidence and logic.

A second reason why health administrators should strive for conscious competence is that many management problems are not routine and must be addressed from perspectives different from the one with which the administrator feels most comfortable. The administrator who realizes that a given approach has worked nine consecutive times, but who alters the approach the next time around because of some variance in the situation, will be more effective than the administrator who does not have the insight to note and respond to the variance. Understanding the logic and rationale behind different administrative strategies permits competent administrators to modify their approach dependent upon the circumstances. This is a valuable skill that is needed when confronting complex problems that defy pat solutions.

Conscious Competence

If there is one word that best summarizes the consciously competent administrator, it is the term "responsive." The consciously competent administrator is responsive to two audiences: the community in which the institution resides and the community of employees within the organization. We now want to turn our attention to the dynamic forces operating within these communities and, on the basis of that analysis, learn about the issues, problems, and opportunities confronting contemporary health administrators.

During the past two decades Americans have become increasingly critical of our basic institutions: the church, the schools, and the health industry. As Robert Blake and Jane Mouton note: "Sharp challenges that often end in wrenchings and upheavals are frequent occurrences in families, neighborhoods, schools, and communities. Traditions, precedents, and past practices that have long ordered, regulated, and stabilized many social institutions are under attack."[9]

[9] Robert Blake and Jane Mouton, *Building a Dynamic Corporation through Grid Development* (Reading, Mass.: Addison-Wesley, 1969), p. 1.

Sharp challenges that often end in wrenchings and upheavals directly influence the practice of health administration. Our traditions and precedents concerning health economics are under attack. There is a growing feeling that "something has to be done" about the rapid growth in *health expenditures*. In 1970 the nation paid about $85 billion for health care, or 7.6 percent of the gross national product (GNP). In 1979, the nation's health tab was approximately $212 billion or 9 percent of GNP. Per capita expenditures for health care soared from $359 to $943 during the same period. Business spent $63 billion on health insurance premiums in 1980, an increase of $20 billion over 1978.[10]

In response to the rapid growth in health expenditures, new policies are frequently proposed. Between 1978 and 1982, we saw political leaders calling for a "cap" on hospital expenditures so that they could not rise above a specified percentage. In that same time period national health planning legislation was altered by Congress so that more responsibility for controlling costs could be delegated to state and local planning agencies. We also saw an increased interest in Health Maintenance Organizations as an alternative method of delivering less expensive medical care.

Health administrators are directly affected by changes in national health policy as well as by the rules, regulations, and guidelines that accompany the policy. The administrator of a fifteen-bed long-term care facility in a rural community can be faced with the choice of shutting the place down or raising the monthly bill of residents (who exist on fixed incomes) in order to pay for the renovations required by the Occupational Health and Safety Act (OSHA). The state health officer, confronted with a 5 percent across-the-board reduction in the financial allocations to state agencies is faced with seemingly untenable choices about which public health services to reduce or abolish.

New technology is also creating change. Most physicians who have been trained in the United States during the past twenty years have completed three years of post-M.D. specialty training. The care that they give to patients makes maximum use of high-technology instruments, procedures, and personnel. Increasingly physician reimbursement schedules "reward prestigious, intrusive medical care and provide disincentives for diagnosis and treatment of the common ailments that are addressed by primary care practitioners.[11] Because the payback to physicians in using high technology is high in terms of increased prestige and economic benefits, hospital administrators will continue to be the target of assertive physicians demanding "the very best equipment."

[10] "Health: What the Fuss Is All About," *Metro Monitor,* St. Paul, Minnesota, January 1981, p. 5A.
[11] Fred H. Mitchell and Cheryl C. Mitchell, "Entering the 1980's: The Health Care System and Primary Care," *Family and Community Health,* 3, no. 2 (August 1980), 107.

Public health administrators will also hear the same plea for new technology. Environmental health personnel want the latest laboratory equipment to detect and monitor toxic elements in our environment. Biometricians argue for better data processing technology while nutritionists increasingly advocate the purchase of sophisticated computer technology through which the nutritional status of clients can be measured.

The changing nature of the *work force* is also creating ferment. The number of college graduates has risen from 286,000 in 1955 to more than 900,000 in 1977. In 1940 only one out of every 220 employees had graduated from college. Today one in four workers holds a college degree.[12]

As the number of college-educated individuals in the work force has increased, so have their expectations about what they hope to achieve in their careers. Among the top five job priorities in a *Pscyhology Today* survey of 23,000 people were "a chance to learn new things," "opportunity to develop your skills and abilities," and "the amount of freedom you have."[13] Today's health professionals want to implement their knowledge; they do not want to be stuck with the historical stereotypes of their profession. The term "ancillary personnel," which often denotes a second-class status, is increasingly abhorred by individuals who have invested years of study to become proficient in their profession.

One of the most important changes in the work force is that women, who have historically occupied less desirable jobs, are increasingly resentful of their second-class citizenship. In 1979 the National Commission on Working Women reported that 80 percent of all employed women are "undervalued, underpaid and underappreciated."[14] In 1965 women's salaries were only 60 percent of those of white men; in 1976, after ten years of effort to improve the work status of women, their earnings had actually declined to 59 percent of what white males earn. In a survey undertaken by the American Management Association only 4.5 percent of the women earned between $15,000 and $25,000. Six times as many men took home these higher salaries. Fewer than 0.5 percent of women earn $25,000 or more, while twenty times as many men earn that amount or higher.[15]

In response to these economic injustices, professions dominated by women employees will be entering into collective bargaining agreements in larger numbers. There will undoubtedly be less tolerance for those who do not understand the magnitude of the economic problems facing women and who

[12] Eli Ginzberg, "The Professionalization of the U.S. Labor Force," *Scientific American*, 240, no. 3 (March 1979), 49.

[13] Patricia A. Renwick, Edward E. Lawler, and the *Psychology Today* staff, "What You Really Want from Your Job," *Psychology Today,* May 1978, p. 56.

[14] *National Survey of Working Women: Perceptions, Problems, Prospects* (Washington, D.C.: Center for Women and Work, June 28, 1979), p. ii.

[15] Martha Burrow, *Developing Woman Managers: What Needs to Be Done* (New York: AMACOM, 1978), p. 2.

are not committed to achieving equal employment and advancement opportunities.

Finally there is an insurgent mood of *conservatism* on the part of many citizens and political leaders. There is a perception that federal government has grown too large and that more responsibility and authority for managing human service programs should be delegated to state and local government. There is a feeling that Medicare and Medicaid expenditures are too high and that individuals need to take more responsibility for their own lives—including the payment of a reasonable portion of their medical expenses. And there is growing belief that competitive marketplace economics may be more effective than government regulation in controlling health expenditures and in ensuring that the system is delivering quality care.

In response to this ever-changing environment the consciously competent health administrator will need to employ three salient skills. *First, consciously competent administrators must be innovators.* The organization that will survive in this rapidly changing environment is the organization that clearly excels and stands apart from its competitors.

Organizations—even those in the public arena—exist within a competitive environment. There is always someone seeking to build a better mousetrap or a more fuel-efficient car, or a more effective health delivery system. When the better mousetrap or car or delivery system is constructed, the rewards invariably are redirected to the innovator.

The consciously competent administrator understands that organizations, like human organisms, have a life cycle. In the United States more than 350,000 out of approximately 2,500,000 organizations discontinue their existence each year. As Haynes and Massie point out, "Many of these departures must be attributed to failure to estimate correctly, in advance, what opportunities the environment might provide. Others reflect failures to adapt to declines in markets. Even the largest corporations are subject to rise of decay and failure, whereas others successfully employ the new developments in markets and technology."[16]

All organizations are susceptible to decay as well as to growth. It is of more than passing interest to management theorists that General Motors, which did not exist in 1909, became the fifth largest U.S. corporation by 1919, and the second largest in the period subsequent to 1919. At the same time, however, the Central Leather Company, which was seventh largest in 1909, fell to thirty-seventh in 1919, and has since disappeared altogether.[17]

Competent administrators do not rest on past accomplishments. Rather, they constantly scan the environment seeking to adapt to new economic,

[16] W. Warren Haynes and Joseph L. Massie, *Management, Analysis, Concepts and Cases* (Englewood Cliffs, N. J.: Prentice-Hall, Inc., 1969), p. 253. These estimates on discontinued businesses are taken from an unpublished manuscript by John D. Glover entitled, "Strategic Guidance of Corporations—A System of Concepts and Analysis."

[17] Haynes and Massie, *Management,* p. 253.

political, and ideological realities. In the process of innovating they know that mistakes will be made, yet they can be comforted by Peter Drucker's observation that "the man to distrust . . . is the man who never makes a mistake, never commits a blunder, never fails in what he tries to do. He is either a phony, or he stays with the safe, the tired, and the trivial. The better a man is the more mistakes he will make for the more new things he will try.[18]

*A second characteristic of consciously competent administrators is that they think in terms of the interests and needs of consumers.*There is a tendency for organizations to think of themselves as producers and sellers of particular goods and services rather than as creators of products to meet consumer needs. Theodore Levitt makes the interesting observation that the decline of the railroads was in large part due to their failure to see the fundamental need for transportation services.[19] The railroad enterprise, unfortunately, was "railroad oriented" rather than "transportation oriented" and therefore missed opportunities created by changes in particular modes of transportation. If the chief executive officers of the major railroads had decided at the turn of the century that the railroad industry was in the "people moving" business, instead of in the passenger, hardware, or real estate business, the industry would own airlines, automobiles, or even bicycle companies today.[20]

If human service organizations are not only to survive but also to be credible in terms of the quality of services they offer, they must continually ask the question, How can we better meet the needs of people who utilize our services? This approach to marketing implies both a short-term and long-term analysis and commitment.

In the short term, the organization that is credible will be adjusting its day-to-day operations so that it can more directly meet the needs of the people it serves. Employing a hospital receptionist who is bilingual may be the small modification that could have significant effects in building the bridges of credibility to the Chicano community. Publishing a list of services for community residents may help to make the organization's mission statement understandable. Having open hearings where consumers and administrators can talk to one another can do much for bolstering institutional credibility within the community.

If the organization is to be credible in the long term it must monitor the ongoing changes in our society. Inflation should probably be counted on as a long-term reality even though there may be periods of abatement. Prevention services, now mostly rhetoric, will become a reality as cost-benefit ratios

[18] Peter Drucker, *Management: Tasks, Responsibilities and Policies.* (New York: Harper E Row, 1975), p. 456–57.

[19] Theodore Levitt, "Marketing Myopia," *Harvard Business Review,* July-August 1960, pp. 45–56.

[20] Peter Drucker, *The Chief Executive Office and Its Responsibilities* (New York: AMACOM, 1970), p. 82.

become known.[21] Issues relative to the quality of life of senior citizens will become greater in magnitude. Some form of government-sponsored insurance plan to deal with catastrophic health costs will continue to be debated by legislators and probably will engender much controversy. Any health organization that is not consciously thinking about the future in terms of prevention, inflation, gerontology, and cost consciousness is undoubtedly slipping in its competitive position. At best, status quo organizations that have lost their focus in meeting the human needs of their constituents will certainly be delegated to a secondary role within the health care system; at worst, they will not survive. For the modern organization, the lesson is clear: "Given the facts of rapid, unplanned change, a status organization cannot survive. Yesterday's success means very little in a world of rapidly changing markets, consumers, products, values, life-styles, and so forth. In order to survive, modern organizations must devise means of continuous self-renewal. They must be able to recognize when it is necessary to change, and, above all, they must possess the competency to bring about change when it is required."[22]

The third characteristic of consciously competent administrators is that they are able to create a productive and humane work environment. Creating a work environment that is stable and where employees needs for security, belonging, respect, and achievement can be realized might be the single greatest challenge confronting health administrators. There is growing evidence in a broad spectrum of industries, including hospitals and public health organizations, that workers are dissatisfied with their working environments.[23]

The shift in attitudes among American workers is aptly summarized in a report undertaken for the Department of Health, Education and Welfare, entitled *Work in America.* Job discontent, according to the report, is evident in all segments of society including blue collar workers, white collar workers, managers, young persons, old persons, women, and racial minorities. The authors suggest that the negative attitudes individuals have about their work are not so much due to the fact that jobs have changed, but rather that workers have changed in terms of their expectations concerning the role of work in their lives.[24]

It would appear that a growing number of individuals have come to understand the poignant meaning behind the words of Albert Camus:

[21] Ken Wakershauser, "Staying Well Pays Off," *Minnesota Business Journal,* January 1981, pp. 21–32.

[22] Newton Margulies and John Wallace, *Organizational Change: Techniques and Applications* (Englewood Cliffs, N.J.: Prentice-Hall, Inc., 1973), p. 418.

[23] See, for example, Gary L. Calhoun, "Hospitals Are High Stress Employers," *Hospitals,* June 16, 1980, p. 171–73; and Ayala Pines and Ditsa Kafry, "Occupational Tedium in the Social Services," *Social Work,* 23, no. 6 (November 1978), 499–507.

[24] *Work in America, Report of a Special Task Force to the Secretary of Health, Education and Welfare* (Cambridge, Mass.: M.I.T. Press, 1973), pp. 13–17.

"Without work all life goes rotten. But when work is soulless, life stifles and dies."[25] A soulless work environment is usually easy to detect. The people who work there feel used; they believe they could quit, walk out, and never be missed. They put in their time, returning home each evening with little sense of accomplishment or pride concerning the day's happenings. Soulless jobs evolve when the working atmosphere causes employees to negate their sense of individuality and creativity; they come about when individuals are asked to blandly blend into a faceless working group. As Fidencio Moren, a steel-worker, put it: "I should have quit long ago. Now my dad, he ran a bar. When he'd come home us kids would run to him and say, 'How'd it go?' My dad always had pride in his work. He'd talk about all the things the customers would say and do. Me, I go home, they don't understand a damn thing. All I do is dump a little coal into an oven. Why would my wife or kids be interested in that?"[26]

When work is not meaningful a pervasive and overpowering feeling of *atonie* can pervade the thinking and behavior of the worker. The term *atonie* refers to a condition of deracination or a feeling of rootlessness, lifelessness, and dissociation. It comes from a Greek word that was used to describe a slack string that did not vibrate.[27]

The feelings of "rootlessness, lifelessness, and dissociation" within the context of work were well summarized by a nurse: "We're overworked, underpaid, and get very little professional respect. Yet we're supposed to enjoy our work because we are helping people. I'm angry when people justify these untenable conditions with the statement, 'But you're a nurse.' People look aghast when I remind them it's only a job. How many other professions demand this much from their workers for so little compensation?"[28]

A sense of being alienated from the very organization that puts bread on our table is not confined to any organizational level. The physician who resents the increased government financing and control of health services can eloquently remember the "good old days" when the chief concern of physicians was the well-being of their patients. The medical records librarian can and does resent health professionals who have the librarian stereotyped as a clerk or filing secretary.

Can health administrators exert positive influence in helping to create a better environment within their organizations? Consider, as an example, some of the causes of nursing dissatisfaction.

UNSAFE PRACTICES
Dangerous understaffing
Toleration and retention of incompetent nurses

[25] Cited in *Work in America,* p. xx.
[26] "The Job Blahs: Who Wants to Work?" *Newsweek,* November 26, 1973, p. 79.
[27] *Work in America,* p. 5.
[28] Godfrey, "Job Satisfaction," p. 95.

Alcoholic doctors "practicing" medicine
Patients stacked in hospital halls like so many sausages

POOR LEADERSHIP
Head nurses who use scheduling as a weapon
Inflexible supervisors determined to preserve the status quo
Nursing directors who haven't laid a hand on a patient in 20 years
Authoritarian administrators concerned only with cutting costs—at any price

COMMUNICATION BREAKDOWN
Learning about vital changes in the hospital—from the newspapers
Being transferred to a different unit without being forewarned
Going through channels to relay important messages and getting no
    response whatsoever
Having supervisors verbally promise something (more help, a raise), then
    having them "forget" the conversation entirely[29]

There are few, if any items, in the above listing of job dissatisfiers that
cannot be positively influenced by competent administrative policies, procedures, and practices.[30] To be certain, employees have to take responsibility
for their own well-being and there are variables (such as relationships outside
of the working environment) that may influence perceptions about work
which administrators cannot control. Nevertheless administrators—regardless
of the level at which they practice—are in a key position to create a humane
and productive work environment.

To repeat: An important challenge confronting health administrators
relates to their ability to create a working environment in which the needs of
employees for security, belonging, respect, and achievement can be satisfactorily realized. The ability to build a stable organization that can meet the
complex needs of employees will separate the truly competent administrators
from those who, to use the steelworker's words, are "just dumping a little
coal into the oven."

What then characterizes consciously competent health administrators? It
is their responsiveness to two audiences: the community in which the institution resides and the community of employees within the organization. As
Joseph Massie and John Douglas have noted: "Managing a contemporary
world means living with uncertainty and differences. You also live with one
eye on the internal parts of the organization and one eye on the external environment. If you only integrate (put the parts together), you may miss opportunities to grow and develop. If you only innovate, you may overstimulate the

[29] Ibid., p. 91.
[30] Paula L. Stamps and Gretchen Ramirez-Sosa, "Dealing with Nurse Dissatisfaction:
A Management Tool That Works," *Health Services Manager,* 13, no. 12 (December
1980), 3-6.

organization to a point of exhaustion. Balance is essential. You must be ready to consciously adapt if you are to manage in the contemporary world.[31]

SUMMARY

This chapter has sought to examine four levels of administrative competence. It was noted that the basic challenge to health administrators is to develop patterns of administration that are consciously competent. Consciously competent patterns of administration reflect an ability to meet the changing health needs of the community through an innovative, yet stable working environment. The remaining chapters of this book will focus on specific competencies, each of which can assist in the pursuit of excellence in health administration.

STUDY QUESTIONS

1. What societal changes do you foresee that are going to have an impact on health organizations? Which of the changes listed in this chapter will be most important in the next five years?

2. Think of an organization in which you have been employed. Is it productive? Do individuals enjoy their work? How do you explain your answer?

3. Have you ever worked with an "incompetent" administrator? How did you cope? Did you stay in the job very long? Can incompetent bosses become competent?

4. Have you ever worked with a "competent" administrator? List his or her characteristics. How did you know the administrator was competent?

ADDITIONAL READING RESOURCES

BORST, DIANE, and PATRICK J. MONTANA, eds., *Managing Non-Profit Organizations.* New York: AMACOM, 1977.

BURROW, MARTHA, *Developing Women Managers: What Needs to be Done.* New York: AMACOM, 1978.

FLEXNER, WILLIAM A., and ERIC N. BERKOWITZ, "Marketing Research in Health Services Planning: A Model," *Public Health Reports,* 94, no. 6 (November-December 1979), 503–13.

---

[31] Joseph L. Massie and John Douglas, *Managing* (Englewood Cliffs, N.J.: Prentice-Hall, Inc., 1977), p. 541.

FORD, LORETTA C., "Nursing at the Cutting Edge of Health Services Reform," *American Journal of Nursing,* August 1980, pp. 1476–79.

HARPER, CHARLES L., and DONALD S. SMITH, "Declining Public Health Organizations: Will Management Make a Difference?" *Health Care Management Review,* 4, no. 4 (Fall 1979), 31–39.

MITCHELL, FRED H., and CHERYL C. MITCHELL, "Entering the 1980's: The Health Care System and Primary Care," *Family and Community Health,* 3, no. 2 (August 1980), 105–13.

SNOW, CHARLES C., and LAWRENCE G. HREBINAK, "Strategy, Distinctive Competence and Organizational Performance," *Administrative Science Quarterly,* 25, no. 2 (June 1980), 317–36.

WALSH, DIANA CHAPAN, and RICHARD H. EGDAHL, eds., *Women, Work and Health: Challenges to Corporate Policy.* New York: Springer-Verlag, 1980.

2 Competency: Understanding the Culture of an Organization

Take away our factories, take away our trade, our avenues of transportation, our money. Leave us nothing but our organization and in four years we shall have reestablished ourselves.—Andrew Carnegie

OVERVIEW The purpose of this chapter is to define a methodology by which the culture of an organization can be examined. The reader, upon completing the chapter, will be able to:

- Define three elements commonly found in organizational mission statements

- Describe the characteristics of vertical, horizontal, and matrix organizations

- Delineate the positive and negative effects of the informal organization

- Describe five types of power found in organizations

- Examine the financial culture of an organization by analyzing budgetary concepts

- Describe evolutionary, revolutionary, and systematic development processes within organizations

Before you can competently manage an organization you must understand it. Every organization has a history, a set of traditions, and a social structure that supports its activities. It also has a set of values, rituals, and rules. When we use the expression "organizational culture" we are referring to the cumulative banking of knowledge, experience, meanings, beliefs, values, attitudes, power, and wealth that is acquired by an organization.

Organizational cultures are often taken for granted much like the goldfish who considers the water in his fish tank to be the natural state of affairs. Unfortunately, as Daniel Wren has noted, many individuals only examine present organizations, read contemporary authors, and have little appreciation for the background of our technologies, political bodies, and arrangements for the allocation of scarce resources.[1] Yet management "did not develop in a cultural vacuum; managers have always found their jobs affected by the existing culture. To study modern management, the past must be examined to see how our communal heritage was established."[2]

The purpose of this chapter is to present a method by which the culture of an organization can be examined. We will be considering selected variables, each of which will give us some insight into the "meanings, beliefs, values, attitudes, power, and wealth" of the organization. Each variable, when studied in isolation, gives us a portrait of one aspect of the organization. Taken together they constitute a cultural mosaic that is unique to the organization being studied.

At the outset one may properly ask why it is important to examine an organization's culture. One reason is to learn about the *traditions* that have influenced the philosophy, goals, and objectives of the institution. Organizations have many kinds of philosophical, political, and economic traditions. There are traditions of strong governing boards and of weak governing boards and traditions of competent and of incompetent patterns of administration. There are traditions of strong union activity and traditions in which there has never been collective bargaining. There are traditions that reflect widely different approaches to organizational change and traditions of organizational conflict, cooperation, and harmony.

What an administrator is able to accomplish will be circumscribed by such traditions. If you choose to work in a public health agency you will be influenced by the values of prevention, early intervention, health education, and working with large populations. If you are employed in an organization where the board of trustees has traditionally valued a particular administrative style, your mode of operation will probably be influenced by the board's expectations. If your institution has a religious affiliation there may be theological and moral perspectives that may influence your base of funding.

An examination of the organization's culture also enables you to under-

[1] Daniel A. Wren, *The Evolution of Management Thought* (New York: John Wiley, 1979), p. 5.
[2] Ibid., p. 6.

stand the *values* that philosophically support its activities. You will be able to examine the original values that brought the organization into existence as well as determine how those values have changed over the years.

Peter Drucker has observed that we live in an "age of discontinuity" in which fast-moving changes in politics and technology threaten the once-stable cultural fabric of the organization.[3] As one examines cultural variables it becomes apparent that the values that once ordered and gave a sense of stability to an organization have often been rendered impotent by new values that seem to better address contemporary realities. The hospital board of trustees, for example, could once order expensive equipment, renovate buildings, and build structures without asking permission from any governmental agency. Today a certificate of need must usually be obtained necessitating an immense amount of justification of the proposed expenditures. In previous generations physicians could charge what they wanted for their services with the only restriction being the demand of the marketplace. Today physician billings come under the scrutiny of peers and third-party payers. Historically the core values of public health professionals were to conquer infectious disease. In the 1980s the public is demanding protection from toxic contaminants and reassurance that a Three Mile Island accident will not be repeated.

An examination of the culture of an organization not only informs you about the traditions and values that support the enterprise, but will also help you understand the *implicit variables* that influence management and operations.

An anthropological concept that is basic to understanding organizationan structure is the differentiation between "explicit" and "implicit" cultures. According to anthropologists James Spradley and David McCurdy "the cultural knowledge that people discuss, explain, and talk about is called explicit culture."[4] Explicit cultural information is exemplified in the actions of an administrator who informs staff members as to the proper ways to respond to an issue. In so doing the administrator is outlining expected subordinate behaviors. Culture becomes explicit when employees inform one another about technical advances or shortcuts that minimize the time a given procedure usually takes to complete. Perhaps the best example of explicit culture is the organization's personnel policies. The policies give explicit instructions to employees about expected norms of conduct and the consequences that accrue if there is deviance from these norms.

In every organization, however, employees obtain cultural knowledge that is not verbally communicated. Implicit culture, sometimes referred to as tacit culture, is the shared knowledge that people do not discuss.[5] Informal

[3] Cited in Wren, *Evolution of Management Thought,* p. 555.

[4] James P. Spradley and David W. McCurdy, *Anthropology: The Cultural Perspective* (New York: John Wiley, 1975), p. 31.

[5] Ibid., p. 32.

rules that permit workers to start their work day five or ten minutes late, or stretch their coffee break from fifteen to twenty minutes represent examples of implicit cultural norms of conduct. When an administrator does not dismiss an incompetent employee even though there are ample explicit grounds for the dismissal, the justification might be an implicit understanding in the organization that no one gets fired if they have worked in the organization for fifteen or twenty years.

To understand an organization it is important to examine both the explicit and the implicit cultures. It is important to understand the formally written policies, rules, expectations, and ways of doing things. It is equally important to understand the rituals, values, and informal understandings that are only on the fringes of awareness but that exert a powerful influence on day-to-day operations.

If you agree with the premise that the pursuit of excellence in administration begins with an understanding of an organization's culture, then we must be prepared to systematically study that culture. To do that it is necessary to have a framework by which organizational culture can be examined.

Figure 2–1 represents one method by which the critical culture elements of an organization can be identified. Initially, one must focus on the mission of the organization, for the *mission statement* explicitly outlines the organization's philosophy, values, and goals. The organization's success in producing goods and services valued by the public is contingent upon the effectiveness of four organizational structures: (a) the *formal structure* which outlines the hierarchical responsibilities of departments and individuals, (b) the *informal structure* which includes the networks of relationships supported by tacit values that control the quality and quantity of the work, (c) the *political structure* which has vested within it power that is used in support or defiance of explicit organizational goals; and (d) the *financial structure* which supports the organization's activities. Finally, organizations are culturally different from one another depending upon how they interface with their *environment*.

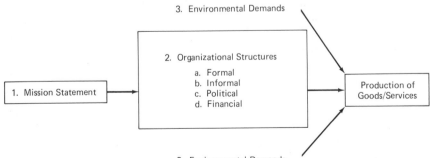

Figure 2–1 Organizational culture: An analytic framework.

THE MISSION OF THE ORGANIZATION

The best place to begin to understand an organization's culture is the organization's mission statement. Sometimes referred to as a statement of philosophy or goals and objectives, the mission statement delineates the key ideals that undergird the enterprise. Mission statements usually include (1) a statement of the *history* of the organization, (2) an expression of the *values* to which the organization adheres, and (3) a statement that outlines the basic *purposes* of the organization.

Every organization has a *history* that helps explain its contemporary priorities. A reading of the history helps you identify the societal factors that influenced the birth, growth, and development of the organization. The history often identifies noteworthy individuals who charted a course for the institution. It may describe periods of growth, stability, turmoil, and possibly entropy as the organization sought to adjust to the financial and political forces impinging upon it. It will also document that the organization had watershed years in which important decisions influenced its growth and development.

The history of an organization is often punctuated with interesting and unplanned happenings that shaped its future. In that sense an organization's history reads like a novel filled with intriguing characters, plots, and subplots. Patients who come to the University of Minnesota Hospitals, for example, learn through patient education materials that the hospital had very humble beginnings. In fact, the hospital was started in a fraternity house on campus. Gradually the hospital grew in terms of the diseases it was prepared to treat. Organizations such as the Veterans of Foreign Wars and the Masons of Minnesota contributed funding so that the University of Minnesota Hospitals could grow and be more responsive to the needs of its clients. As medical practices became more sophisticated new programs were implemented and new buildings were constructed; but all of this came about because a small group of individuals were willing to invest in a small hospital located in a fraternity house.

Mission statements often contain a section that delineates the *values* that support the institution. This is true both in religious and secular institutions although religious organizations may seek to highlight those values more explicitly than their secular counterparts.

To exemplify what is meant by a statement of values, consider the following information:

> University Hospitals' first priority is quality health care for our patients. Our total mission, however, is somewhat different from most private or county hospitals. As part of the University of Minnesota Health Sciences Center the Hospitals share the Health Sciences goal of developing programs to meet the health care needs of the state. To carry out this mission, health professionals within the Hospitals continually work together to improve patient care, educa-

tion, and research. Because of this, our patients can benefit from the most up-to-date medical practices available. While you are here you will meet many health care professionals. They all work with each other to form the "Health Care Team," a treatment designed to give you the most comprehensive care possible.[6]

A reading of this statement will make explicit some of the values of this hospital. As a *state institution,* it *serves a regional clientele.* The hospital undertakes *research* and *education* in addition to clinical care. It emphasizes the *application of recent knowledge* to medical problems and offers *comprehensive care* to patients. Finally, the hospital *practices a team approach* in meeting the needs of patients.

In reading a mission statement it is important to determine the degree to which the institution is striving to incorporate contemporary concepts and values. For example, some mission statements will define "wellness" not simply as the absence of disease, but as the optimal level of health an individual can obtain. An organization that defines wellness in such a way strives to be congruent with the current thinking that hospitals should do more than treat disease. If the mission statement contains phrases such as "comprehensive care," "cost effective treatment programs," "patient education programs," and "preventive care" it is probable that administrators are trying to incorporate contemporary research, theory, and issues within the cultural fabric of the institution.

Mission statements usually outline the *priorities* of the organization. Sometimes these priorities will be interwoven within the section on values. Other times there will be a specific statement that delineates the goals that the organization is seeking to achieve.

A statement of goals provides an important clue to resource allocation. We would expect that substantial resources will be given to those departments that have the responsibility for achieving the main goals. If one of the priorities of a state health department is to protect the public from toxic wastes, it is likely that the environmental health program will have one of the largest staffs. On the other hand, if the priority is to educate the citizens concerning accident prevention, the health education department will probably have substantial resources allocated to it.

Mission statements vary in the precision with which they specify goals. If there is a precise statement of goals, it is likely that someone in the organization has done a great deal of thinking about the organization's purpose. On the other hand, if the mission statement lacks a statement of purpose, and if no one can tell you the goals of the enterprise, a leadership vacuum probably exists. If, in fact, there is a leadership vacuum, you have learned something important about the culture of that organization.

Finally, it is helpful to determine whether the mission statement has anything to say about the employees of the organization. While some

[6] University of Minnesota Hospitals, Patient Information.

organizations take employees for granted, others will highlight the fact that the organization is a community within itself—one that seeks to treat employees fairly, responsibly, and with a sense of concern for their well-being.

While the words in a mission statement may or may not be reflected in daily transactions, the words do give you insight into the culture of the institution. The history, values, and stated purposes represent the beginning point in examining the cultural mosaic.

THE STRUCTURE OF THE ORGANIZATION

The organization's mission statement resembles an architectural blueprint. It gives the reader a picture of what the enterprise should look like and the foundation on which it rests. However, mission statements and blueprints don't do much good until someone acts upon them. Work must be carried out if mission statements are to become a reality. To understand how work is carried out it is necessary to examine the formal, informal, political, and financial structures of the organization.

The Formal Structure

An essential part of an institution's culture is the formal arrangement of departments, programs, and personnel. The organizing of resources is essential whether the enterprise is small or large. The 35-bed long-term care facility may have fewer than a dozen employees; nevertheless, if that organization is to be effective, all employees will need to understand their particular role in the facility. Likewise, in a large bureaucracy, such as a 750-bed hospital, employees will need to understand how their responsibilities interface with the objectives of the department.

William Newman states that the primary objectives in any organization are to (1) divide and group the work that should be completed into individual jobs, and (2) define the established relationships between individuals filling these jobs.[7] Such a division of labor is usually portrayed on an organization chart. An organization chart illustrates the five major aspects of an organization's structure:

1. *The division of work.* Each box represents an individual or subunit responsible for a given part of an organization's work load.
2. *Managers and subordinates.* The solid lines indicate the chain of command (who reports to whom).

[7] William Newman, *Administrative Action* (Englewood Cliffs, N.J.: Prentice-Hall, Inc., 1963), p. 144.

3. *The type of work being performed.* Labels or descriptions for the bosses indicate the organization's different work tasks or areas of responsibility.
4. *The grouping of work segments.* The entire chart indicates on what basis the organization's activities have been divided—on a functional or regional basis, for example.
5. *The levels of management.* A chart indicates not only individual managers and subordinates but also the entire management hierarchy. All persons who report to the same individual are on the same management level, regardless of where they may appear on the chart.[8]

There are three systems of organizing with which you should be familiar. These are reflected in the vertical, horizontal, and matrix organizational structures depicted in Figures 2-2, 2-3, 2-4.

Vertical structures, sometimes referred to as "tall" organizational charts, are commonly found in large, bureaucratic institutions. Such organizations emphasize three management principles in order to control the quality of work that is to be performed: (1) chain of command, (2) unity of command, and (3) span of control.

The chain-of-command principle is based upon the premise that all individuals from bottom to top should have a supervisor to whom they are accountable. Most organizations, whether they be military, governmental, religious, or economic organizations, have learned that there is value in having an unbroken chain of command from the lowest-level private, citizen, parishoner, or worker to the most elevated general, president, bishop, or ex-

[8] James A. F. Stoner, *Management* (Englewood Cliffs, N.J.: Prentice-Hall, Inc., 1978), p. 225.

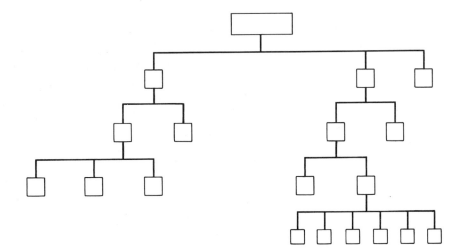

Figure 2-2 A vertical ("tall") structure.

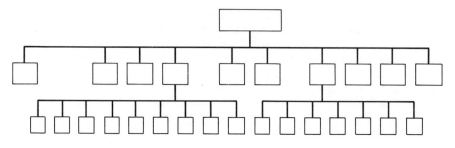

Figure 2-3 A horizontal ("flat") structure.

ecutive.[9] Figure 2–5 illustrates the chain-of-command principle. Note that everyone is accountable to someone. By emphasizing accountability, unproductive behavior is discouraged.

The chain-of-command principle is deeply ingrained in the consciousness of most American workers. Most have learned that it is not in one's self-interest to violate the chain of command. The head nurse (H) would be offended if a staff nurse (L) took her complaint directly to the executive vice-president (C). As Webber states, "Most superiors expect subordinates to com-

[9] Ross A. Webber, *Management: Basic Elements of Managing Organizations* (Homewood, Ill.: Richard D. Irwin, 1979), p. 355.

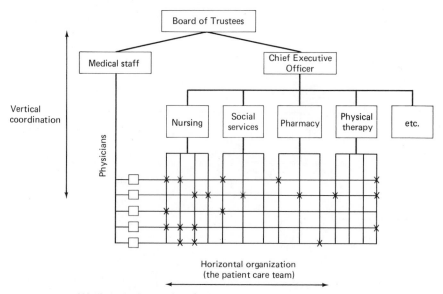

X indicates both a member of a department and a patient care team.

Figure 2-4 A matrix structure.

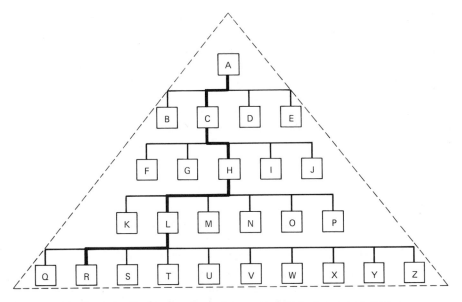

Figure 2-5 Chain of command in organizational pyramid. [From Ross A. Webber, *Management: Basic Elements of Managing Organizations* (Homewood, Ill.: Richard D. Irwin, Inc., 1979), p. 354.]

municate through them as a common courtesy, and they violate this expectation at their peril.''[10]

There may be times, however, when the chain-of-command principle must be violated. This often occurs when a subordinate becomes aware of incidents that threaten the effectiveness of the department. When the subordinate has called such incidents to the attention of the superior and has not found the grievance to be successfully adjudicated it may be necessary to "jump" the chain of command and talk directly to the superior's superior.

As indicated earlier, subordinates who violate the chain of command do so at their own risk. The prudent subordinate can diminish the punitive reprisals by first informing the superior of the intent *and the motivations behind the intent* to discuss a situation with someone else. Sometimes the threat of taking an issue to someone other than the supervisor may, in itself, be powerful enough to obtain needed redress of a grievance. If not, the subordinate's forthright approach will usually gain the respect, if not the approval, of the one to whom the grievance is eventually brought.

The unity-of-command principle states that each person in the chain of command should have only one direct supervisor to whom he or she is accountable. There are few organizational principles older than this one.

In practice this principle is often bent—sometimes beyond recognition. The more complex the working environment, the more likely that the worker

[10] Ibid., p. 357.

will receive instructions from multiple sources. A health educator working in a city health department may be requested to initiate education programs from the directors of the public health nursing department, the environmental health department, and the nutrition department. A hospital personnel officer may receive instructions from a variety of vice-presidents within any given day.

To overcome problems that develop when multiple individuals are giving instructions to a single employee, most organizations clearly define one supervisor who will evaluate the work of the subordinate. In so doing the integrity of the unity-of-command principle remains intact. Employees recognize that they are accountable to one individual even though they may respond to the directives of many.

The span-of-control principle defines the number of people who will report to a common supervisor. In Figure 2-6, A has a span of control of only two individuals, B of seven, and C of sixteen.

Much has been written about what is the appropriate span of control. At one time the number seven was suggested since it was thought that this was the maximum number of subordinates that a supervisor could effectively manage.[11] Today it is generally agreed that the nature of the work should be the guiding factor in determining an effective span of control. When subordinates are assigned simple, repetitive, programmed, and easily measured tasks, a large span of control—even up to forty or fifty individuals—may be appropriate. However, in those units with unpredictable work loads, where subordinates are given considerable autonomy in determining how to accomplish the work, where there is less ability to measure results, or where there is great task interdependence, it is usually desirable to have a smaller number of individuals reporting to one superior. By narrowing the span of control the administrator can supervise workers more closely and can more effectively coordinate the work of the department.

Horizontal structures, sometimes referred to as "flat" organization charts, also emphasize the chain and unity-of-command concepts. They are differentiated from vertical structures by the relatively few administrative

[11] G. A. Miller, "The Magical Number Seven, Plus or Minus Two: Some Limits on Our Capacity for Processing Information," *Psychological Review,* 63 (March 1956), 39–47.

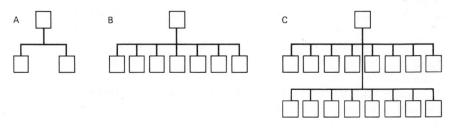

Figure 2-6 Span of control.

layers that exist between management and the employees of the organization.

Flat organization charts usually reflect a "decentralized" approach to management. The objectives of decentralizing are (1) to permit workers to organize the work in the most efficient and effective manner, (2) to eliminate costly middle-management positions, and (3) to permit relatively few upper-level managers to supervise a large number of departments within an organization. The main intention of decentralizing is not to democratize the organization but to gain greater control at the operating level. The key distinction that differentiates flat from tall structures is the intent to have workers *themselves* control the quality of work rather than having control rest in the hands of a number of middle- and lower-level managers.

During the past decade a new form of organization has developed that reflects the growing sophistication of many health and human service organizations. The key characteristic of *matrix organizations* is that individuals are assigned to two or more units and experience supervision from several sources.[12] Matrix organizations emphasize the existence of both hierarchical (vertical) coordination through departmentalization and the formal chain of command and simultaneously lateral (horizontal) coordination across departments.[13]

An example of a matrix organization is a city health department. Most cities with a population of more than 100,000 residents will have a health department whose responsibility it is to protect the community's health. The health department will have a health officer who is administratively responsible for the agency and will have on its staff public health dentists, environmental specialists, health educators, nutritionists, nurses, physicians, and social workers. Each of these professionals will have his or her specific responsibilities, yet each will interrelate with other professionals on projects designed to improve the health of the community.

The agency itself will relate to many organizations. It is likely that the health officer will report to the city commissioners, yet also be accountable to federal officials for the allocation of federal funds (Figure 2–7). The various professionals on the staff will relate to state and county officials in planning new programs and responding to new legislation. Professional staff will also relate to professional organizations such as the medical, dental, and nursing societies. In addition, most staff members will be interacting with various health coalitions made up of citizens.

A matrix chart of a city health department would plot the complex relationships with federal, state, county, and city agencies, professional organizations, and citizen groups. In all likelihood the chart would be a maze of dotted lines connecting to scores of institutions.

[12] Alan C. Filley, Robert J. House, and Steven Keer, *Managerial Processes and Organizational Behavior* (Glenview, Ill.: Scott, Foresman, 1976), p. 368.

[13] Jonathan S. Rakich and Kurt Darr, *Hospital Organization and Management: Text and Readings* (New York: Spectrum Publications, 1978), p. 37.

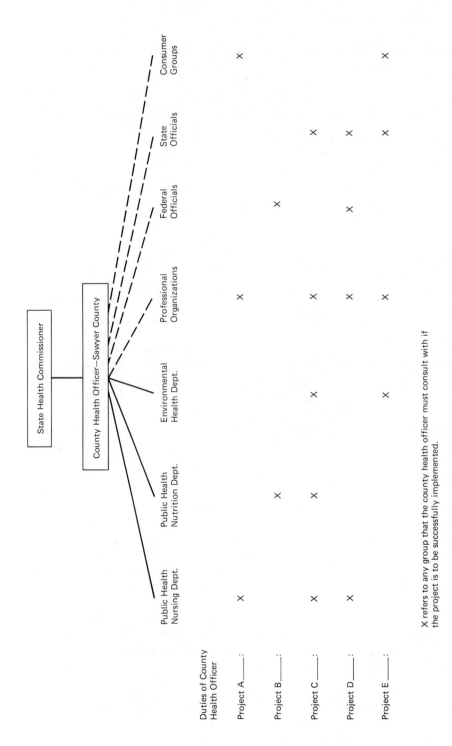

Figure 2-7 Matrix organization—county health officer.

Duties of County Health Officer	Public Health Nursing Dept.	Public Health Nutrition Dept.	Environmental Health Dept.	Professional Organizations	Federal Officials	State Officials	Consumer Groups
Project A ____:	X			X			X
Project B ____:		X			X		
Project C ____:	X	X	X	X		X	
Project D ____:	X			X	X	X	
Project E ____:			X	X		X	X

X refers to any group that the county health officer must consult with if the project is to be successfully implemented.

In summary, by examining an organization chart you are able to see at a glance the total system. You can determine how work is organized by looking at the departments and subunits of those departments. You usually can determine the major functions of each department and see how the formal communication networks are prescribed to operate. A fairly typical organization chart for a medium-sized hospital can be seen in Figure 2-8. If your career goal is to work in a public agency, you should examine Figure 2-9 which is an organization chart of a large state health department.

The organization chart also helps you understand certain aspects of the organization's culture. Vertical structures usually signify that there will be close supervision of employees in order to minimize errors and to ensure quality products or services. Horizontal structures often indicate that employees have more freedom to do the job in their own way than their counter-

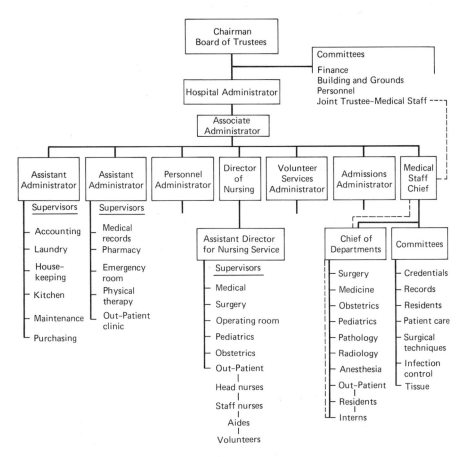

Figure 2-8 Organization of a 450-bed hospital. [Adapted from Ross A. Webber, *Management: Basic Elements of Managing Organizations* (Homewood, Ill.: Richard D. Irwin, Inc., 1979), p. 416.]

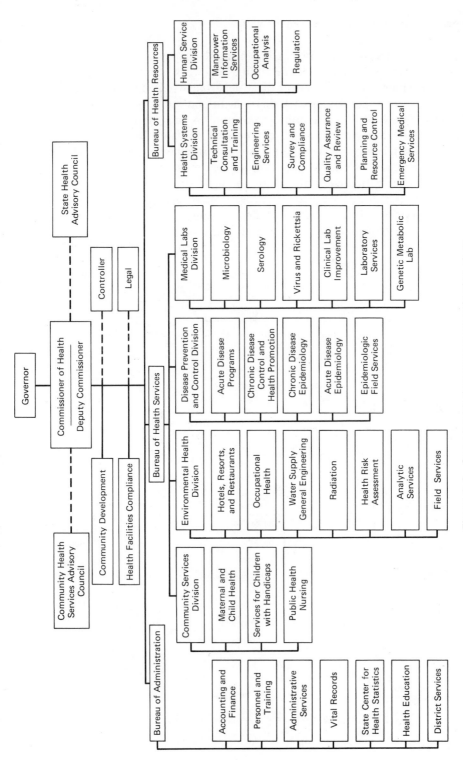

Figure 2-9 State health department organization chart.

parts who work in vertical systems.[14] Horizontal structures often reflect less social stratification among employees and are more in accord with an equalitarian political and social philosophy.[15] Matrix organizations signify that professionals are expected to function in an interdisciplinary mode with other professionals.

As a postscript, we should note that one form of organization is not inherently more effective than another. Each form of organization had its place, depending upon the task(s) that need to be accomplished.

The Informal Structure

Ever since three Western Electric studies were completed in the 1930s there has been widespread interest in the social fabric of an organization. The Western Electric studies demonstrated the presence of an informal organization consisting of a network of "personal and social relations not established or required by formal authority but arising spontaneously as people associate with one another."[16] Keith Davis has described the informal organization as follows:

> Beneath the cloak of formal relationships in every institution exists a more complex system of social relationships consisting of many informal organizations. Although there are many different informal groups, we may refer to them collectively as the informal organization. It is a powerful influence upon productivity and job satisfaction. Both the formal and the informal systems are necessary for group activity, just as two blades are essential to make a pair of scissors workable. Together, formal and informal organizations constitute the social system of work groups.[17]

Many administrators would be pleased if they could work strictly with the formal organization. Consider Joyce Kraemer, a newly appointed director of a public health nursing department in a community health department. Kraemer is responsible for supervising six public health nurses. The six nurses have worked with one another for the past four years and have learned to support one another as supervisors have come and gone.

Kraemer discovered early in her employment that the staff nurses would become defensive when any new initiative was proposed. When she suggested that the case load be increased, each objected vehemently. They maintained that if the case load was increased it would diminish the quality of care. When

---

[14] Robert Sutermeister, *People and Productivity* (New York: McGraw-Hill, 1969), pp. 203–17.

[15] Ibid., p. 217.

[16] Henry H. Albers, *Principles of Management: A Modern Approach* (New York: John Wiley, 1974), p.69.

[17] Keith Davis, *Human Behavior at Work* (New York: McGraw-Hill, 1977), p. 272.

it was suggested that the department develop collaborative relationships with nurses in a neighboring hospital she was informed that "We've tried that before and they will never cooperate." When a complex issue emerged concerning one of their patients the nurses would consult with a physician in the maternal and child health department. Seldom did they ask for advice from their new supervisor. One of the things that Kraemer found particularly irritating was that the staff nurses always went to lunch together but never invited her to be with them.

The frustrations that Joyce Kraemer experienced were a direct result of the tightly knit informal organization of the public health nursing department. She learned quickly that the informal organization was a powerful influence upon productivity, morale, and her own job satisfaction.

The informal organization functions every day in every organization. It is seen when employees consult with one another even if they do not formally report to one another. It is apparent when a rumor is passed through the grapevine about an impending administrative directive. It is functioning when a group of subordinates have coffee with one another in the hospital lunch room and discuss how they are going to "handle" the new supervisor.

Problems caused by the informal structure   The informal organization can undermine both productivity and morale. Keith Davis has suggested that there are four ways that the informal system can thwart the effectiveness of the organization.[18]

First, the informal organization can prevent meaningful change from taking place. Each work group develops, over a period of time, established ways of going about their work. They cultivate comfortable routines. They determine how hard they are going to work and how they will help one another.

The six public health nurses that Joyce Kraemer supervised had determined that they would make five home visits per day and that all of the home visits would be completed in the morning. After the home visits they met at a restaurant across from the health department for lunch. Often the lunch break would extend into the afternoon.

Several supervisors had attempted to change this situation. One supervisor discharged one of the nurses for insubordination. When the other five nurses heard about the action they came to the defense of the staff nurse by threatening to resign as a group. They even said they would take their case to the editor of the community newspaper. The supervisor, not wanting adverse publicity, backed down. The informal organization had flexed its corporate muscle and had won.

To repeat, one of the chief functions of the informal organization is to

[18] Ibid., p. 271.

guard against change that upsets comfortable working patterns. The informal organization will resist change that is perceived to upset the status quo and that will make unwarranted demands on workers' time. Therefore, most workers are on guard whenever a new supervisor is appointed. They will carefully watch the actions of the new boss to see if comfortable routines are threatened. When supervisors take actions that workers do not perceive to be in their best interests, they will fight overtly or covertly. When Joyce Kraemer insisted that each staff nurse maintain a case load of eight patients per day they complied. Six months later, however, when Kraemer was checking the medical assistance payments to patients, she inadvertently discovered that the staff had returned to a case load of five per day.

Second, conflicts between the formal and informal organizations can create difficult working conditions for employees. Most employees want to meet the requirements of their job *and* the expectations of their peer group. However, when a supervisor wants one thing and the peer group another, an employee may feel caught in the middle—often unable to meet conflicting expectations. Consider Betty Janzen, one of the six public health staff nurses. She would be willing to have a larger case load and to make home visits in both the morning and the afternoon. She does not think that her supervisor is making an unreasonable request. Yet she has never spoken in defense of Kraemer. The reason is simple, yet powerful: Being in good standing with her peers is a stronger motivator than being in good standing with her supervisor. Each day, however, she feels that she is in the middle of a tug of war. While she is angry at herself for being manipulated by the group, she nevertheless remains silent. The fear of being sanctioned by the work group is a powerful deterrent to change.

Third, the informal organization undermines the formal structure when it carries messages that are not accurate. According to Keith Davis, the term "grapevine" arose during the Civil War. Telegraph lines bringing valuable intelligence to the home base were strung loosely from tree to tree in the manner of a grapevine. Often the messages from the telegraph lines were garbled, incorrect, and confusing. Therefore, any rumor was said to be from the grapevine.[19] Today the term refers to all informal communication in an organization.

The grapevine does not always undermine the formal structure. In fact, there are times that the grapevine complements the formal communication system. The grapevine has the capacity to translate formal management policy into language and operational patterns that employees can understand. The grapevine has the capacity to transmit information rapidly. One study of Canadian government engineers, for example, found that 32 percent of the engineers who were to be transferred first learned about the transfer through

[19] Ibid., p. 278.

the grapevine.[20] The grapevine also has the ability to transmit large quantities of information. If all the information that was passed orally in a given work day had to be transcribed it would run into volumes of pages. Finally, it should be remembered that valuable information is often sent *up* through the grapevine to management. Such messages are valuable for they often contain information about employees, the quality of their work, and problems that may be developing that normally would not be put in writing.

While the informal network of communication can assist management it also may have a negative effect. Usually this takes place when rumors run rampant in an organization. A "rumor" might be defined as grapevine information that is communicated without secure standards of evidence being present. By chance it could be correct, but generally it is in error.[21]

Rumors often contain incomplete and, at times, inaccurate information. Unfortunately, when a rumor is circulating, those who receive the information often read their own meanings into the rumor *and then behave as if it were a fact.* Consider, for example, a worker who thinks he overhears a manager say that everyone will be receiving an 8 percent raise in salary. At lunch he mentions this to his best friend. Soon the message that "everybody is going to receive an 8 percent raise" spreads through the department and then into other units of the organization.

Let's examine that rumor. As is usually the case, rumors contain accurate and inaccurate information. In this case the accurate information is that an 8 percent raise will be given. However, not everyone will receive that raise, for the 8 percent figure represents the average raise that employees will receive. Some may receive 12 percent while others receive 4 percent. As you can imagine, those who finally learn that their salary increase will only be 4 percent will probably feel hostile at management who, they perceive, has not lived up to their expectations.

Unfortunately, when erroneous yet important rumors flow through an organization, much management effort may be needed to correct the situation. Often managers may find themselves in a position where they must either substantiate or deny the validity of the rumor. If the rumor is correct but contains information that was not to have been released until a later point in time, the manager will then have to deal with the consequences of premature release.

While many rumors are inconsequential, those that threaten the productivity of the organization must be confronted. The best way to deny a rumor is in a face-to-face meeting in which the facts of the situation are released. However, it is important to release the facts immediately without first mentioning the rumor. Whenever a rumor is repeated, particularly by a credible

[20] Ronald J. Burke, "Quality of Organizational Life: The Effects of Personnel Job Transfers," in *Proceedings of the Academy of Management,* ed. Vance F. Mitchell et al. (Vancouver: University of British Columbia, 1973), p. 242.

[21] Davis, *Human Behavior,* p. 283.

source, it is likely that the workers will hear it instead of the refutation. They will then assume that the rumor has been confirmed.[22]

The fourth way that informal organizations can undermine the formal structure is by creating conformity in employees. All work groups must determine their informal working relationships. These informal discussions influence the quantity and the quality of the work that is to be performed. There will be informal understandings as to how the workers will assist one another, how they will respond to the directives of their supervisor, how much effort they should put into the job, and what constitutes acceptable standards of quality.

Such informal understandings create a sense of cohesiveness among workers; however, the cohesiveness also creates conformity. Once a pattern has been established as to how workers go about their tasks and once the norms of group behavior are determined, there is a reluctance to innovate. Innovations are perceived as creating change and often conflict between members of the group. You may recall that Betty Janzen was unable to become more productive because the norms of her work group reinforced conformity. Whenever conformity becomes the most important norm to which the work group adheres, it is likely that there will be little creativity.

Benefits of the informal structure   While the informal organization can undermine the formal structure, it is also true that informal systems have a number of benefits. *First, the informal organization has the capacity to cut through bureaucratic policies and red tape in order to complete a task.* As Robert Dubin states, "informal relations in the organization serve to preserve the organization from the self-destruction that would result from literal obedience to the formal policies, rules, regulations, and procedures."[23]

Examples of how the informal organization benefits the formal structure are numerous and can be observed in most work settings. The nurse, physical therapist, and dietitian may not have any formal relationship portrayed on an organization chart, yet they often meet to discuss the treatment program of a stroke victim. When the personnel department has some unexpected demands placed upon them it is not uncommon for staff members to divide the work among themselves in order to complete the task. They may even agree to work overtime to see that a report is completed. If a snowstorm leaves drifts in the driveway to the emergency room, employees in the maintenance department may forego their lunch in order to clear a path for incoming emergency vehicles.

The extent to which employees will informally agree to help one another is determined, in part, by their loyalty to the organization. If they are committed to the general purposes of the organization and if they perceive that others

[22] Ibid., p. 285.
[23] Robert Dubin, *Human Relations in Administration* (Englewood Cliffs, N.J.: Prentice-Hall, Inc., 1951), p. 68.

would assist them if they needed help, it is likely that they will undertake responsibilities that are not explicitly required in order to complete a task.

A second benefit of the informal organization is that it provides a structure for meaningful relationships at work. The informal organization often operates as a safety valve for employee frustrations. Oftentimes employees relieve emotional pressures by talking with a colleague about their problems. Joyce Kraemer began having lunch with other department heads shortly after she had commenced her employment in the health department. Soon she was sharing with them her frustrations and, more importantly, was able to find new ideas as to how to work with the six members on her staff. She looked forward to these informal lunch meetings and often felt renewed after talking with her colleagues—many of whom had problems similar to her own.

Sometimes workers will agree to difficult working conditions because they enjoy the people with whom they are associated. If one of the norms of the informal group is that "we stick together" no matter how difficult the working conditions may be, there is a strong reason to continue to do the work even if it is emotionally depleting. Any nurse who has worked in an oncology department or has treated terminally ill children knows how important it is to have peers who support one another.

A third benefit of the informal organization is that it has the capacity to be creative. While we noted that there are strong pressures to conform, it is possible for the informal work group to innovate. This often takes place when there is a threat to the informal structure.

The resistance that Joyce Kraemer felt existed between herself and the six public health nurses began to dissipate when a federal grant that supported the department was unexpectedly terminated. Unless new support could be generated, three of the staff positions would be abolished. Joyce Kraemer called a day-long staff meeting in which the seven of them began to look for solutions to their problem. Soon the seven-member work group had identified half a dozen alternative ways of finding financial support. Responsibilities for pursuing the various options were assigned to each of the staff members. The energy of the group was no longer directed at undermining the supervisor. Rather it was now being spent on finding creative solutions to their problems.

While an external threat may be a frequent motivator to action, some informal groups will continually look for new and better ways of doing their work. Usually this takes place when employees are so committed to their tasks that they are constantly searching for new methods that will benefit others as well as themselves. A group of dietitians in a long-term care facility were concerned about the constant complaining of residents about their meals. In response to this problem they formed a committee composed of residents who would help them plan the daily menus. Soon the complaining about the meals stopped and, when the dietitians undertook a nutritional assessment, it was found that the residents were eating a well-balanced diet. Everyone had benefited from this "informal consultation."

Finally, the informal organization validates the meaning of an employee's work. Friends and relatives are usually not in a position to know whether we are effective in our work. However, when a colleague says, "Thank you for the work you did on that difficult task," or "That was the best patient care I have seen anyone give in a long time," it helps to validate the meaning of what we do. Word spreads quickly in an organization when an employee is competent and credible. Such positive reinforcement is needed and motivates workers to continue to work at a high level of performance.

In summary, the informal organization is one aspect of an organization's culture that merits examination if one is to understand the complexities of an enterprise. The informal organization is a powerful influence on productivity and morale. To ignore it would be to miss one of the most vital determinates of whether the organization will achieve its mission.

The Political Structure

Stephen P. Robbins has observed that "It has only been in the last ten years that organizational behavior researchers have come to acknowledge and accept what practitioners have long known: Organizations are political systems."[24] As Clayton Reeser and Marvin Loper note, "Whatever else organizations may be (problem solving instruments, sociotechnical systems, reward systems, and so on) they are political structures."[25] This means that organizations operate by setting goals, distributing authority, and setting a stage for the exercise of power.[26]

The concept of power has been described by Bertrand Russell as "the fundamental concept in social science . . . in the same sense in which energy is the fundamental concept in physics."[27] Yet, even though the concept of power is an important one to master, it is difficult for most people to deal with it objectively. Many have ambivalent feelings about power. Leaders are often instructed to "walk softly yet carry a big stick"—a prescription that tries to meld two seemingly incongruent axioms. We admire power in others, yet we resent it if it is utilized against us in a capricious manner. We know that if we are to meet our own goals we must possess power, yet most would be reluctant to tell others that their goal is to possess power.

Power simply defined is "the ability to affect and control anything that is of value to others."[28] *Politics* is the "complex of intuitive and deliberative

[24] Stephen P. Robbins, *Organizational Behavior: Concepts and Controversies* (Englewood Cliffs, N.J.: Prentice-Hall, Inc., 1979), p. 402.

[25] Clayton Reeser and Marvin Loper, *Management* (Glenview, Ill.: Scott, Foresman, 1978), p. 179.

[26] Ibid.

[27] Bertrand Russell, *Power: A New Social Analysis* (London: Allen & Unwin, 1938), p. 12.

[28] Robbins, *Organizational Behavior*, p. 263.

strategies through which power is acquired and manipulated."[29] There are five types of power found in organizations: legitimate power, expert power, coercive power, rewards power, and referent power.[30]

Legitimate power is the power that is bestowed in a given position within the organization. Such power represents the "formal rights one receives as a result of his or her authoritative position or role in the organization."[31] Individuals who hold management or supervisory positions have a certain amount of legitimate authority bestowed on them by virtue of their role in the institution.

Expert power is seen in workers who have particular knowledge or skill that is valued by others. Knowledge is power and is one of the most potent sources of influence in an organization although it is not necessarily correlated with organizational position. An assistant health commissioner who has been at his job for many years may have more knowledge about the health department than anyone else—including the health commissioner. Over time, legislators, politicians, and employees within the organization may have learned that, "If you want the straight scoop, go straight to Jim. He knows how this place works." The more the assistant commissioner is relied upon because of his base of information, the more power he will accrue.

Coercive power is perhaps most poignantly summarized by Al Capone who said, "You can get much farther with a kind word and a gun than you can with a kind word alone."[32] One reacts to coercive power out of a fear of negative consequences. Sanctions such as being deprived of the rewards of the organization, being excluded from peer groups, or even losing one's job are examples of the use of such power.

Reward power is associated with those individuals who give out things that we value, including money, recognition, and a sense of belonging. Rewards may include favorable performance appraisals, interesting work assignments, the giving of adequate resources to do the job, and periodic promotions.

Reference or personal power is seen when one worker identifies with another because of personal traits or characteristics. "I just trust him" is a common response when people are asked why they consulted with another person. Such an individual has strong referent power.

To understand the cultural fabric of an organization you will want not only to understand the concept of power but to answer three specific questions:

[29] Reeser and Loper, *Management,* p. 177.
[30] John R. P. French and Bertram Raven, "The Basis of Social Power," in *Studies in Social Power,* ed. Dorwin Cartwright (Ann Arbor: University of Michigan, 1959), pp. 150—67.
[31] Robbins, *Organizational Behavior,* p. 266.
[32] Ibid., p. 262.

Who has power?
Who wants power?
How is power being used?

The power brokers   A broker is one who uses resources to obtain additional resources. In this context a power broker in an organization is one who has power, uses it, and obtains additional power. An important fact of organizational life is that power obtains additional power. In *Men and Women of the Corporation,* a penetrating inquiry into organizational politics and power, Rosabeth Moss Kanter writes:

> Power begets power. People who are thought to have power already and to be well placed in hierarchies of prestige and status may also be more influential and more effective in getting the people around them to do things and feel satisfied about it. In a laboratory experiment, subordinates were more likely to cooperate with and to inhibit aggression and negativity toward leaders of higher rather than lower status. In a field study of professionals, people who came into a group with higher external status tended to be better liked, talked more often, and received more communications. The less powerful, who usually talked less, were often accused of talking *too much*. There was a real consensus in such groups about who was powerful, and people were more likely to accept direct attempts to influence them from people they defined as among the powerful. Average group members, whether men or women, tended to engage in deferential, approval-seeking behavior toward those seen as higher in power. Thus, people who look like they can bring something that is valued from outside the group, who seem to have access to the inner circles that make the decisions affecting the fate of individuals in organizations, may also be more effective as leaders of those around them—and be better liked in the process.[33]

A power broker is one who is perceived to have influence "outward and upward" in the system. Power brokers are perceived to be able to get for a group, for subordinates, or followers a favorable share of the resources, opportunities, and rewards that exist within the organization. This has less to do with how they relate to followers than it does with their ability to successfully interact with other power brokers. It has less to do with the quality of superior-subordinate relationships than with the power broker's ability to obtain coveted resources. The implications of this are fairly important. Early organizational theorists assumed that subordinates would have high morale if the quality of their relationship with their supervisor was high. But what appears to be more valid is that the quality of leader-follower relationships is dependent upon whether their leader has the ability to influence others in the wider system. In other words, do they have influence on their own superiors and on decisions made in the larger system? When the leader has good human

[33] Rosabeth Moss Kanter, *Men and Women of the Corporation* (New York: Basic Books, 1977), pp. 168–69.

relations *and* power there are positive effects on workers' morale. However, when leaders have good human relation skills but are perceived to have little power there are negative effects on morale. "What good," asks Kanter, "is praise or a promise if the leader can't deliver?"[34] There is good scientific evidence that workers will attach more importance to having a competent boss rather than a nice boss—they want someone who can get things done.[35]

In order to obtain the coveted resources of others, individuals will rely on one of the five types of power that we have discussed. Some will utilize their position power and will send directives demanding a particular response. Others will use their coercive power and threaten punishment. Some will persuade through knowledge that only they have. Others will hold out the possibility that rewards will be bestowed if certain behaviors take place.

To identify the holders of power you will want to examine the organization chart (the formal structure) which will tell you who has position power. But you will probably need to look into the informal structure as well, since organizational power is often wielded through the informal networks of communication. For example, you may learn that the vice-president for nursing services may have the most comprehensive understanding of what is happening in the hospital at any given point in time (expert power). That knowledge is due partly to her position in the organization, but it is also due to the fact that she has access to almost all of the communication networks within a hospital hierarchy. You may learn that a physician who has served the hospital for fifteen years as chief of staff is the most trusted confidant (referent power). You may find that the high absenteeism and turnover in a particular department is due to the autocratic and capricious ways of the department head (coercive power). And, you may learn that the assistant hospital administrator is invited to weekly social gatherings because employees know that he makes yearly recommendations to his boss concerning merit salary increases (reward power).

In identifying people who can influence others, it is important to recognize that power is usually diffused in large organizations. One should resist the point of view that power is usually in the hands of only a few individuals. Every department has some power. Even in those departments that are perceived to have less power than others, there will be a power hierarchy. Learning who has power, even in those units that are relatively powerless, is an important step in understanding that unit.

The coveters of power   Some individuals within organizations are not satisfied with the amount of power they possess. They desire more influence and the ability to obtain additional rewards, favors, and resources of others.

The most predominant method of obtaining additional power in

[34] Ibid., p. 168.
[35] Ibid.

organizations is to form alliances. Such alliances are often formed on two levels. On the one level we see individuals linking their interests with a more powerful person and, in so doing, expanding their scope of influence. On the other level we see departments uniting with other departments. By conglomerating their resources they are able to expand their base of power and influence.

On an individual level, workers often obtain additional power by finding a sponsor. Many seasoned veterans can point to an individual who gave them a boost in their career. Research by Margaret Henning and Anne Jardim on women in top management positions in U.S. corporations dramatically showed how important sponsors were to those who eventually were promoted to top level leadership positions.[36] A study undertaken in Britain demonstrated that "office uncles" were important because they offered suggestions to aspiring individuals so that they could advance in their career. The office uncles often would fight so that the promotions of the one they were sponsoring would take place.[37]

A sponsor is usually thought of as a seasoned teacher who "knows the ropes" and who can give a younger person valuable insights into "how things are done." They help the individual understand the system which, in the context of our discussion, enables them to discern the culture of the organization. Sometimes sponsors will cut red tape so that the individual can realize career goals. Other times they may give the individual "inside information" that will help them get ahead. Still others will actually "go to bat" for a younger employee with their own boss if a position becomes vacated.

Identifying the sponsors of others is an important factor in learning who is likely to have control of power in the future. Most organizations will have the "office uncles" who take pride in helping subordinates on their career paths. They open the doors and prepare the subordinate to walk through the doors. They too are brokers of power whose uniqueness is that they use their power to help others obtain influence. Of course, as Machiavelli points out, they are not doing it totally out of altruistic motivations. The more favors one dispenses, the more IOU's one has nestled away that can be cashed in at a later point in time.

Alliances between departments is also a way of enhancing the power of various groups. Powerless groups sometimes enter into a formal or informal arrangement with other groups in order to enhance their own prestige and power. Usually this takes place when a group is threatened from an external source. For example, if a small department within a hospital is threatened with a reduction in funding or outright extinction, there will usually be a search for a more powerful department that will serve as a faithful ally. An

[36] Margaret Henning and Anne Jardim, *The Managerial Woman* (New York: Pocket Books, 1967), p. 155–56.

[37] Michael Fogarty, A. I. Allen, Isabel Allen, and Patricia Walters, *Women in Top Jobs: Four Studies in Achievement* (London: Allen & Unwin, 1971), p. 217.

administrator who is bent on eliminating a department may have second thoughts if it is suddenly clear that other departments (alliances) would fight the change.

Sometimes organizational productivity is adversely affected when alliances fight other alliances. When this happens the energy of workers is often directed to the fight rather than to achieving organizational objectives. It is interesting to note, however, that when you examine the disputes between alliances, they may appear to relate to legitimate organizational issues. Most of the time, however, the etiology of such conflict is rooted in a basic issue: Who is going to gain power and who is going to lose power if a proposed action takes place.

The faces of power   To understand the political structure it is not only important to learn who has power and who is seeking to obtain it, but one must examine how existing power is being used. David McClelland has suggested that there are two faces of power—a negative face and a positive face.[38] The negative face is usually expressed in terms of dominance versus submission: "I will win and you will lose." This type of perspective on power implies that every organizational dispute will result in winners and losers. Someone will gain power and someone will lose power. In such a system leadership views people "as little more than pawns to be used or sacrificed as the need arises. Such an approach to power is self-defeating since people who feel they are pawns tend either to resist leadership or to become overly passive. In either case their value to the manager is severely limited."[39]

The positive face of power is seen when a leader has a concern for group goals and is committed to helping individuals design, implement, and evaluate such goals. The key factor of positive power is that it exerts influence *on behalf of* rather than *over* others. It is portrayed in the actions of a health officer who consults with the head of the nutrition department prior to making a policy on a food contamination issue. It is seen when the director of a health education department asks the director of the public health nursing program whether she would like to collaborate on an anti-smoking program. It is reflected in the actions of a hospital personnel officer who consults with the nursing division as well as the chief executive officer before proposing a salary structure for nursing personnel.

In summary, for an organization to be effective, power must be utilized. Power does influence performance and individual satisfaction. However, power per se is neither negative nor positive. It is how power is used (or misused) in an organization that will determine whether one should ascribe positive or negative values to it. If we examine the five types of power

[38] David C. McClelland, "The Two Faces of Power," *Journal of International Affairs,* 24, no. 1 (1970), 29–47.

[39] Ibid., p. 31.

previously discussed we see that certain types are more effective than others. Expert power demonstrates the most consistent relationship with high performance while referent power is the second strongest, especially among professional workers. While legitimate power can be effective in positively influencing workers' attitudes and behaviors, reward and coercive power are generally negatively related to performance.[40]

The Financial Structure

When anthropologists study the culture of a group such as a primitive tribe they will examine the resources that sustain the group. They want to learn whether the tribe is wealthy or poor, whether resources such as water and grain are predictable, and the process by which the wealth is distributed to the group's members.

In studying an organization's culture it is equally important to examine the financial health of the enterprise. You will want to know the magnitude of the organization's resources, the predictability and stability of those resources, and the process by which budgets are established.

One way to examine the financial culture of an organization is to analyze the master budget, the operating budget, and the process by which allocations are made to departments. It is also important to determine how financial adjustments are made if unforeseen events necessitate a change.

The master budget The simplest way of assessing the financial strength of an organization is to examine the *master budget,* sometimes referred to as the *balance sheet budget.* The balance sheet budget is a "forecast of expected financial status as of the last day of the budget period, usually the close of the fiscal year."[41] The forecast will show whether the organization is making a profit, breaking even, or incurring a deficit.

If the organization is in a profit or surplus position, and if this occurs on a yearly basis, it is important to know how such surpluses are expended. Some institutions will place their surpluses in a high-interest-earning bank account that is specifically designed for future operating needs. Such an account is much like an "emergency" or "rainy day" account that many families have to help pay for unpredictable bills. Sometimes institutions will place surpluses in an endowment fund. The interest from an endowment account is frequently targeted for special needs of the organization. While the interest of an endowment fund is often spent, most organizations will not liquidate the principal except in the most unusual circumstances. Still other institutions will designate surpluses for the systematic upgrading of equipment and buildings. Equipment has a limited life-span which means that every piece of equipment will

[40] Stoner, *Management,* pp. 270—71.
[41] Henry L. Sisk, *Management and Organization* (Cincinnati, Ohio: Southwestern Publishing Co., 1977), p. 499.

eventually need to be replaced. If an institution has a yearly profit, some percentage may be designated for the purchase of new instruments or the remodeling of outdated buildings.

In public institutions there is often an established procedure for the disbursement of surpluses. Sometimes the surplus will be returned to the state, county, or city. If an administrator wishes to carry over the funds for use in a new fiscal year, a request is made to public officials outlining how the monies will be spent. Sometimes the state may request that charges to consumers be lowered so that a surplus will not recur in subsequent years. In private institutions, profits may be distributed to shareholders as well as designated for emergency, endowment, or equipment replacement accounts.

With high rates of inflation, organizations often have difficulty in balancing the budget at the end of a fiscal year. When this happens the *accounts receivable* (income) are less than the *accounts payable* (expenditures). Most organizations are able to meet periodic deficits by utilizing surpluses that accrued in more profitable years. At some point, if there is a recurring drain on such funds, they will be exhausted and the total expenditures will have to be reduced. The reduction of departmental budgets is usually translated into a reduction of programs and staff.

Whether an organization is able to achieve its mission is predicated, in part, by the strength of its financial resources. An organization that can meet its financial obligations is a healthier organization than one that has a recurring deficit. An organization that has a stable and predictable source of income that exceeds expenditures will be able to initiate new programs and meet the changing needs of consumers. On the other hand, an organization that yearly reduces services is one that is gravely ill. If new financial capital cannot be found, the prognosis for returning to optimal organizational health is not good.

The operating budget   The *revenue and expense budget,* usually referred to as the *operating budget,* will give you information on labor costs (salary and fringe benefits), material and supply costs, and indirect costs (such as utilities, maintenance, and insurance). As the name implies, operating budgets describe how the operations of the organization are financially supported. The operating budget identifies precisely the amount of money allocated to each department and the name of the person who is responsible for managing departmental resources.

The budget design process   Before discussing the budgeting process, it might be helpful to make several comments concerning the term "budgeting." For many people the concept of budgeting has negative connotations. Sometimes this is due to the fact that individuals do not understand financial management and are somewhat intimidated by computer printouts and the jargon of individuals trained in financial affairs. Some have had negative experiences with administrators who use their budget power to capriciously reward and punish individuals. Still others may look upon budgeting as a "necessary evil" if the "real objectives" of the organization (such as patient care, or giving services) are to be realized.

While budgeting has the potential to control individuals in negative ways, it also has the potential to help organizations and their members reach their goals. V. Bruce Irvine has described some of the potentially helpful aspects of budgets.[42]

Budgets can have a positive impact on motivation and morale. A basic human need is to belong and to be accepted by one's work group. Budgets can help to meet this motivational need by creating the feeling that everyone is working toward a common financial goal.

Budgets make it possible to coordinate the work of the entire group. By examining the budget it is possible to determine how resources are being allocated and spent in each unit of the organization.

Budgets can be used as a signaling device for taking corrective action. An organization must have points of control to ensure that it is meeting its goals. When there is a deviation the appropriate organization members need to be alerted that a standard has not been met. Budgets are feedback systems that help to monitor performance.

The budget system helps people learn from past experience. There is an old axiom that we learn from our mistakes. By examining past budgets managers can analyze what occurred, specify errors that took place, and take corrective action to ensure that the errors are not repeated.

Budgets improve communication. When requesting financial support managers must communicate their priorities and objectives to others. Budgeting requires managers to precisely define what it is that they are requesting and why they are requesting it.

Budgets let new people see where the organization is going. As we have seen, the operating budget clearly identifies the amount of resources given to each department. An examination of operating budgets helps a new manager determine the priorities of the organization.

The budgeting process is usually carried out through a budget officer, sometimes referred to as the comptroller or the financial officer. Usually the *financial officer* has a staff of individuals who are trained in financial

---

[42] Stoner, *Management,* p. 609. Adapted from V. Bruce Irvine, "Budgeting: Functional Analysis and Behavioral Implications," *Cost and Management* (March-April 1970), pp. 6–16.

management. In addition to preparing the payroll, they are responsible for keeping a detailed accounting of all revenues and expenditures.

The financial officer usually occupies a powerful position within an organization. Therefore, it is important to learn all you can about this office. You will want to know the extent to which the office provides timely reports concerning the financial affairs of the organization. You will want to know the types of information the office has on file and how accessible that information is to other departments when they have need of it. It is important to learn the extent to which the budget officer assists managers in preparing budgets as well as to determine the financial officer's veto power. In brief, you will want to know the explicit and implicit authority that rests within that office.

It is particularly important to learn the role that the financial officer has in the preparation of budgets. Some organizations utilize a centralized approach to budgeting in which a few top-level executives (including the financial officer) determine the budget for all departments. Subordinates may be given an opportunity to comment and offer counter proposals, but these may or may not be accepted. The objective of a centralized approach to budgeting is to maintain control not only of the budget but of the activities of departments.

Most organizations utilize a decentralized approach in preparing budgets.[43] The key characteristic of this process is that budgets are prepared, at least initially, by those who implement them. Once prepared, the budgets are sent up the hierarchy and approved by the appropriate administrator. James Stoner states that this type of "bottom up" financial management has five distinct virtues:

1. Supervisors and department heads at the lower levels of responsibility have a more intimate view of their needs than those at the top.
2. Lower level managers can provide more realistic breakdowns to support their proposals.
3. Managers are less likely to overlook some vital ingredient or hidden flaw that might subsequently impede implementation efforts if they develop the budgets for their own units.
4. Managers will be more strongly motivated to accept and meet budgets that they have had a hand in shaping.
5. Morale and satisfaction are usually higher when individuals participate actively in making decisions that affect them.[44]

Finally, it is important to learn how budgets can be changed. Most financial officers resist changing budgets once they have been established. The reason for this is that it is difficult, if not impossible, to balance the budget at

[43] Stoner, *Management,* p. 597.
[44] Ibid., p. 597.

the end of the fiscal year if departments are spending more then what was originally allocated to them.

Nevertheless, unplanned events do take place and may result in requests for additional funding. For example, equipment may break down, supplies may become more expensive to purchase, or a new federal requirement might mean employing additional personnel. To deal with unanticipated situations, some organizations will have a *cash reserve* that can be utilized to meet emergency expenses. Others will request department heads to periodically update their budgets. When this is done on a regularly scheduled basis some departmental budgets will increase while others may decrease.

In summary, one aspect of an organization's culture is the financial strength of the enterprise. The master and operating budgets will inform you about the total resources of the institution and the operating budget will inform you of how the funds are distributed. An examination of the budget-setting process will help you understand the role of the financial officer and whether the enterprise has a centralized or a decentralized approach to financial administration.

ENVIRONMENTAL DEMANDS

Cultural anthropologists have identified tribes who were so enamored with tradition that they found it difficult to adapt to new realities. Even though their environment changed dramatically, these tribes clung to cherished values in an effort to preserve the past.

The adherence to past values often extracted a high cost to such tribes. In some cases intratribe warfare took place between the village elders who were determined to preserve the status quo and younger tribe members who were equally determined to adopt new values. In some cases, intratribe fighting became so destructive that it led to the tribe's extinction.[45]

By contrast, anthropologists can identify other tribes who quickly adopted new values without contemplating what they stood to lose when old traditions were cast aside. The interest of many Americans in understanding their historical roots reflects a desire to retain or recapture some of the values of previous generations. For some there is a belief that cherished ethnic traditions have been lost as they have become a part of American culture.

Contemporary organizations respond to their environments in similar ways. Some resist all efforts to change existing values, objectives, formal procedures, and informal ways of doing the work. A hospital administrator who believes that the government has little right to intervene in the proposed construction of a new hospital may resist the efforts of government planners to

---

[45] Robert F. Allen, "The Ik in the Office," *Organizational Dynamics,* Winter 1980, pp. 26–41.

obtain census data. The personnel director in a state health department may
delay the processing of affirmative action reports if she believes that another
agency does not have rights to certain kinds of hiring information.

Other organizations adopt new philosophies, objectives, and modes of
operation if they see it to be in their immediate self-interest. The leadership in
such organizations will monitor the environment to see what internal changes
should be adopted in order to respond to external pressures. When it became
apparent, for example, that hospitals could be sued for significant sums of
money for malpractice, there was an increased interest in making "incident
reporting" a priority for all staff members.

While it is helpful to understand the forces of change impinging upon an
organization, it is equally important to determine the *process* by which the
leadership responds to emerging political and economic realities. The environment in which an organization operates is constantly changing. Embryonic
political opinions that are casually discussed in legislative halls can blossom
into the force of law. The economy staggers through periods of prosperity and
recession. To understand the cultural fabric is to determine whether there are
internal mechanisms by which the organization responds to external pressures.

Robert Blake and Jane Mouton suggest that there are three modalities
that organizations utilize in responding to their environments.[46] *Evolutionary
approaches* to change are seen in organizations that want to preserve the past
and who view major internal changes as a threat to the stability of the enterprise.

> Evolutionary accommodation rarely violates the tradition or customary practices
> of those involved in it or accepted by it. An underlying assumption is that pro-
> gress is possible if each problem is dealt with as it arises. Changes are usually
> piecemeal, taking place one by one. Because they are adjustments within the
> status quo, they seldom promote great enthusiasms, arouse deep resistance, or
> have dramatic results. Solutions that prove sound are repeated and reinforced.
> Those that are unsound simply disappear.[47]

There are a number of limitations inherent within evolutionary approaches to change. Only those problems that force themselves to be considered are addressed. Often such problems are not the most critical ones in
terms of the organization's health. Since there is very little planning for the
future, you do not sense an enthusiasm about what the organization will be as
a future entity. Since status quo values are constantly reinforced there are real
barriers to progress. At times the historical values are so entrenched that there
are strong sanctions imposed on those who would question them. In addition,
evolutionary processes are usually so slow that even though change is occur-

[46] Robert Blake and Jane Mouton, "Change by Design, not by Default," *Advanced
Management Journal,* April 1979, pp. 29–34.
[47] Ibid., p. 32.

ring, its tempo does not prevent the organization from falling behind competitors who are examining environmental realities.

Perhaps the fatal flaw in this *laissez-faire* approach to change is that the leadership of the organization does not recognize that all systems have a life cycle. In the first stage of the life cycle the organization gets started and expands its scope of influence. In the second stage the organization becomes stabilized, determines what it does best, and determines its priorities. Two possibilities confront the organization in the third stage. If the organization does not adapt to its environment, it may die a slow death. On the other hand, if it innovates with new ideas, programs, and services, a period of growth may be imminent.[48]

Organizational cancer begins in a small way. It is often located in a philosophical perspective that the organization can continue doing what it has in the past and can ignore those who are demanding reform and change. By ignoring legitimate needs, the organization allows the cancer to spread, making it less and less able to creatively respond to the needs of constituents. In its weakened state it may recognize that it should have been addressing the changing environment. Unfortunately, it may be too late to respond, particularly if other organizations have exerted leadership in meeting consumer needs.

The quickest way of determining whether an administrator understands that organizations have a life cycle is to ask one penetrating question: Where will this organization be five years from now? If that question cannot be answered or if it is not even being addressed, the probability is great that an evolutionary approach to change is being practiced.

A second way that organizations change is by initiating a *revolution*.[49] The primary goal of a revolution is to change the status quo. This usually takes place when it has been concluded that the existing leadership is so corrupt, decayed, or ineffective that the organization can no longer tolerate the existing order.

The primary objective of revolutionary change is to clean house of old policies, old patterns of reward and punishment, and those who hold powerful positions. One of the first acts of revolutionaries is to render existing leadership impotent. When the revolution took place in Iran, the Shah's generals were executed; when revolutionaries took over the government of Liberia, the president was killed. On an organizational level, the new guard will "eliminate" the existing leaders by terminating their employment or by assigning them a benign role.

One of the major purposes of revolutionary change is to establish a new order as quickly as possible. To do this, edicts are backed with force. Revolu-

---

[48] Joseph L. Massie and John Douglas, *Managing* (Englewood Cliffs, N.J.: Prentice-Hall, Inc., 1977), p. 17.
[49] Blake and Mouton, "Change by Design," p. 31.

tionaries usually defend strong-arm tactics by pointing to the incompetence and misdeeds of the old leadership. Their rhetoric seeks to convince others that the new leaders had no choice but to overthrow the previous structure.[50]

The changes that take place through revolutionary tactics are dramatic and may result in either positive or negative results. On the positive side long-standing problems might be resolved. If the old leadership was incompetent there is the possibility that the new will be effective. The directions chartered by revolutionaries often engender a sense of pride and a commitment to make certain that new values will be established.

Unfortunately, negative effects may outweigh the positive benefits. Often the end result of a revolution is merely to shift old powers to new leaders rather than to make the enterprise more responsive to an altruistic goal. Sometimes revolutionaries have difficulty separating out what is good for the enterprise from what is good for them personally. Their personal ambitions become so enmeshed in new organizational priorities that they find it difficult to objectively analyze what needs to be done.

Revolutions also create disagreements and divisions within an enterprise. There are always individuals who benefit from the status quo and who receive rewards through the existing power structure. They will not welcome revolutionary changes and often fight back in attempting to sabotage the efforts of the new leadership. If they have been stripped of their power they may simply agree to "go along" without any sense of commitment to the new order. In brief, it is difficult not to have long periods of intrasystem conflict after a revolution has taken place. This is true whether the system is the Iranian government which suppresses the rebellion of separatists in Kurdistan, or an American organization in which those who suddenly have grasped new power have to fight or placate those who disagree with their tactics and policies.

A third process by which organizations respond to their changing environment is through *systematic development* which Robert Blake and Jane Mouton call "the new scientific way to change." There are three philosophical premises that are central to systematic development theory.

The first premise is that organizations do, in fact, exist within an environment that is constantly changing. As such, the organization that ignores emerging needs of clients will gradually lose its competitive position to those who meaningfully address political and economic realities.

The second premise is that organizations must have formalized mechanisms by which the environmental forces can be interpreted and through which new organizational priorities can be determined. John Gardner, for example, has noted that organizations should have at least one "department of continuous renewal that could view the whole organization as a system in need of continuing innovation.[51] Implicit in that judgment is that organizations reach

[50] Robert Veninga, "The Role of Symbols in Legend Construction: Some Exploratory Comments," *Central States Speech Journal,* Fall 1971, pp. 66–71.
[51] John Gardner, *Self-Renewal* (New York: Harper & Row, 1963), p. 76.

a point in their development in which they either wither and die or enter into a new period of growth, innovation, and stability.

The third premise is that organizations should change systematically. Not by chance. Not by evolution. Not through revolution. This means that organizations must stipulate what the "ideal" model of the organization should be in the future and take specific steps to ensure that such an ideal can be practically achieved.[52]

There are many models by which systematic development can take place. In Chapter 9 we will delineate one such model which approaches change through a scientific methodology. While there are many models of organization development, all share a common philosophical perspective: "In a world buffeted by change, faced daily with new threats to its safety, the only way to conserve is by innovation.[53]

In the preceding paragraphs we have seen that organizations change through evolution, revolution, or systematic development. One important aspect of the cultural fabric is the identification of the method the organization most frequently utilizes in meeting emerging issues, problems, and challenges. What the organization will accomplish in the future is largely dependent upon the method of change that is practiced in the present.

SUMMARY

The thesis of this chapter is that if one is to understand an organization it is necessary to examine its culture. The basic purpose of an organization is to produce goods or services that are valued by a constituency. To accomplish organizational goals, work must be performed through formal, informal, political, and financial structures. The extent to which organizations are successful in meeting the demands of the environment is dependent upon whether evolutionary, revolutionary, or systematic development philosophies of change are present. The ultimate goal of understanding the culture of an enterprise is to determine those factors that are influencing the productivity of the organization.

STUDY QUESTIONS

1. Identify an organization in which you have been employed. Analyze its culture according to the organizational structures discussed in this chapter.

[52] Blake and Mouton, "Change by Design," p. 31.
[53] From Peter Drucker, *Landmarks of Tomorrow,* as quoted in Gardner, *Self-Renewal,* p. 7.

2. How does one obtain power in complex bureaucratic organizations?

3. Is the most powerful department within an organization invariably the one which has the greatest financial resources?

4. Identify an organization that is undergoing rapid change. Make an analysis of the organization by identifying (a) the forces for change that are impinging upon the organization, (b) the reasons why employees are advocating or resisting proposed changes, and (c) the consequences the changes are having on employee productivity and morale.

ADDITIONAL READING RESOURCES

BACHARACH, SAMUEL B., and EDWARD J. LAWLER, *Power and Politics in Organizations.* San Francisco: Jossey-Bass, 1981.

McNEIL, KENNETH, "Understanding Organizational Power: Building on the Weberian Legacy," *Administrative Science Quarterly,* 23 (March 1978), 44–78.

MINTZBERG, HENRY, *The Structuring of Organizations: A Synthesis of Research.* Englewood Cliffs, N.J.: Prentice-Hall, Inc., 1978.

NATHANSON, CONSTANCE A., and LAURA L. MORLOCK, "Control Structure, Values, and Innovation: A Comparative Study of Hospitals," *Journal of Health and Social Behavior,* 21, no. 4 (December 1980), 315—33.

REYNOLDS, JAMES, and ANNE STUDDEN, "The Organization of Not For Profit Hospital Systems, *"Health Care Management Review,* 3, no. 3 (Summer 1978), 23–36.

3 Competency: Managing Your Time and Your Work

Any task worth doing, was worth doing yesterday.—Anonymous

OVERVIEW   The purpose of this chapter is to examine methods that administrators can use to manage their time and their work more effectively and efficiently. Upon completion of the chapter the reader will be able to:

- Define the causes of time mismanagement including wasted effort, unproductive meetings, and crisis-oriented management

- Specify procedures by which the resource of time can be effectively utilized

- Define the characteristics of a well-written performance objective

- Differentiate the concepts of "managing" and "operating"

- Define six principles implicit in the delegating process

E. B. Osborn said, "If your aim is control, it must be self-control first. If your aim is management, it must be self-management first."[1] Few have stated the issue more succinctly. Before you can competently manage the complex human and financial resources of an organization it is necessary to develop disciplined patterns of work.

The purpose of this chapter is to examine the most effective ways by which you can manage your time and your work. We will learn that the self-management process consists of three factors:

1. The ability to recognize that *time* is a unique resource that must be skillfully managed
2. The ability to define *objectives* that will serve as a blueprint for the work that must be accomplished
3. The ability to *delegate* specific tasks in order to ensure that the organization is achieving its mission

MANAGING YOUR TIME

The first step in the self-management process is to recognize that time is a valuable resource. Whatever you may accomplish as an administrator is predicated on whether you can use this resource effectively and efficiently.

It is not uncommon to hear managers state that they "simply do not have enough time to do the job." Alec Mackenzie noted that of the thousands of managers whom he surveyed—from board chairmen and chief executives to first-line supervisors—only one in a hundred stated that they had enough time to meet the demands that are made of them. When Mackenzie asked how much more time they would need to do the job they would like to do, one out of ten stated that they needed 10 percent more, four said 25 percent, and the remaining half felt they needed 50 percent more time.[2]

The feeling that "there isn't enough time" is a reflection of a stark fact: Time is not elastic. It cannot be expanded. It must be spent. As the late Walter Williams, Dean of the University of Missouri School of Journalism, told his students, "There's one thing each of you has in exactly the same amount, and that is time."[3] Time per se is not the problem. Rather, the problem of not having enough time lies within ourselves. It is not how much we have but rather what we do with the time we have—how we use it. As Peter Drucker has stated, "Time is the scarcest resource and unless it is managed nothing can be managed."[4]

---

[1] Cited in R. Alec Mackenzie, *The Time Trap* (New York: AMACOM, a division of American Management Associations, 1972), p. 61. All rights reserved.
[2] Ibid., p. 1.
[3] Ibid., pp. 1–2.
[4] Peter F. Drucker, "How to Be an Effective Executive," *Nation's Business*, April 1961, p. 47.

Causes of Time Mismanagement

Effective time management begins with an understanding of how this resource is misused. The primary causes are wasted effort, unproductive meetings, and a crisis orientation.

Wasted effort   The demands on our time increase as we receive additional administrative responsibility. Unfortunately, many requests for attention have little, if any, productive return. A colleague telephones "just to say hello." Most of the conversation is about the weather, last week's ski trip, or the local election. A middle manager drops by to ask the policy on overtime pay. Even though the answer is in the policy manual, most administrators would patiently respond to the inquiry. Some administrators feel compelled to attend staff functions even if their presence is not needed. Soon their calendars are filled with meetings that have little productive return.

Every executive can identify certain activities that waste valuable time. Peter Drucker observed that a large part of time is wasted on things that, though they apparently have to be done, contribute little to the effectiveness of the organization.[5] The day is spent in unproductive thirty-minute conferences. Meetings without carefully planned agendas are routinely held. Travel between meetings consumes valuable psychological energy. Gradually the executive has little time to think, plan, and work on major organizational issues.

One example of wasted effort is seen in the writing of reports. A well-designed report will usually take six or seven hours to write.[6] Some administrators will spend a half hour a day on the task until it is completed. There will be many false starts and probably many moments of staring at a blank piece of paper. As the days pass with little accomplished there will be a nagging feeling that "I've just got to get this thing done." When the report is finally completed it may read like it was written "on the run." Far better if the administrator would close the door to his or her office, have the secretary screen incoming telephone calls, and wrestle with the report for five or six hours without interruption.[7] Such a strategy will usually result in a quality product that engenders pride in the author.

Many judgmental mistakes occur when administrators do not have adequate time to think about an issue prior to acting. Someone suggests developing a new policy, a new subcommittee, or implementing new objectives. In the rush of getting on to other tasks there may be nods of agreement with little critical thinking. The administrator makes a decision and puts it into effect.

[5] Peter F. Drucker, *The Effective Executive* (New York: Harper & Row, 1966), p. 36.
[6] Ibid., p. 29.
[7] Ibid.

When it becomes apparent that the decision was not a good one, it will take valuable time to correct resulting problems.

One of the major reasons that administrative time is not productively used is a reluctance to delegate work to subordinates. Some administrators assume that they should do all the work themselves. They may feel that subordinates cannot accomplish the task as well as themselves; they may feel uneasy giving subordinates authority to complete a project. Administrators who are reluctant to delegate must not only determine the priorities for the organization but must actually be involved in doing the work themselves. As we will see later, the distinction between "managing" and "operating" becomes blurred. Soon the administrator is into everything—often producing work that is not of high quality simply because there are not enough hours in the day to accomplish all that needs to be accomplished.

How do you eliminate tasks that waste valuable time? The most elementary and yet perhaps the most profound question you can ask is simply, "What would happen if I did not do this task at all?" If your answer is that nothing would happen, then you have identified a task that can be eliminated.[8] But if you discover that the task should be done, a second question follows: "Who is the most appropriate person to whom the task should be assigned?" As stated earlier, time is not elastic. Time spent on one project is not available for other responsibilities. Far better to spend time on the tasks that will make a positive difference to the organization than on tasks that have few productive outcomes.

It is also helpful to reserve large blocks of time for important projects. The more critical the task, the more carefully you should allocate sufficient time in order to complete the project. Consider, for example, the recruitment of personnel. There are few administrative functions as important to the organization as hiring the best applicant for a vacant position. The person selected will probably influence the organization for years to come. Far better to reserve time to adequately think through the personnel issues than to rush to a premature judgment. Alfred P. Sloan, the former head of General Motors, usually made a tentative judgment on personnel after several hours of deliberative thinking. Then he would delay making a decision for several days or even weeks. Often he would delay the decision again. Only when the name came up after two or three times would he make his final decision. When he was once asked what his secret was for picking outstanding subordinates he replied, "No secret—I simply accepted that the first name I come up with is likely to be the wrong name—and I therefore retrace the whole process of thought and analysis a few times before I act."[9]

---

[8] Ibid., p. 36.
[9] Ibid., p. 32.

Unproductive meetings   In a recent survey of executives from nine nations including the United States, "meetings" were cited as the biggest time waster of all.[10] The other time wasters cited were telephone interruptions, drop-in visitors, and ineffective delegation. The fact that executives consider meetings the single greatest contributor to ineffective management appears rather startling, particularly when you consider that 69 percent of executive time is spent in meetings with two or more people.[11]

We live in a meeting-prone culture. We have ad hoc committees, standing committees, informational meetings, advisory meetings, and problem-solving conferences. We even have a committee whose purpose it is to find members for other committees. As you might expect, it is called the "committee on committees."

When administrators find themselves rushing from one meeting to another rather than working on issues that have particular importance to them, they often become frustrated, tense, and angry. "I feel powerless to call a stop to all this committee nonsense," said one hospital administrator. An examination of his calendar shows that he attended sixteen different formal committee meetings during the previous week, which consumed 75 percent of his time. A hospital chaplain said: "I'm burned out on meetings. You never have time to do the things that really count."

Organizational theorists have long suspected that meetings can contribute to ineffectiveness and inefficiency. Recently researchers have confirmed that fact: A high frequency of meetings is strongly correlated with negative and dehumanized attitudes towards work.[12] Such negative attitudes arise because the individual believes that meetings are consuming valuable time that could be better utilized on other tasks.

There are various explanations for the high frequency of meetings in contemporary organizations. A major reason is that power is shared in complex systems. Administrators have formal authority that is inherent within their position, yet the informal organization also yields considerable power. Typically, before any significant decision is made, those who have the formal power must consult with those who possess the informal power. If those who have the informal power are not consulted, they will be in a position to sabotage administrative actions unilaterally taken.

Meetings are also scheduled in order to obtain accurate information from subordinates. Health organizations have become so complex that it is impossible for most executives to have complete information on all the topics

---

[10] Herbert E. Meyer, "The Meeting-Goer's Lament," *Fortune,* October 22, 1979, p. 95.

[11] Ibid.

[12] Ayala Pines and Christina Maslach, "Characteristics of Staff Burnout in Mental Health Settings," Hospital and Community Psychiatry, 29 (April 1978), 235.

they must address. To make good decisions it is often necessary to bring together specialists who have an in-depth knowledge about a given area. By pooling information administrators are in a better position to arrive at high-quality decisions.

Government regulations and political pressures also contribute to a high frequency of meetings.[13] The number of government regulations that impinge on health facilities has exploded during the past two decades. We now have audit, affirmative action, health planning, and cost-containment committees. Since important issues are discussed in these meetings, most administrators make certain that they, or a trusted subordinate, are participating. Even when the agenda contains only issues of minor importance, most administrators will make a point to attend. Sometimes the conversations held in the corridors before or after the meeting are as important as the meeting itself.

The amount of time executives spend in standing committees (those that are regularly scheduled) and ad hoc meetings (those that are scheduled when an issue arises) is staggering. What compounds the time investment is that many of these committees are divided into subcommittees. A state health coordinating council, whose purpose is to coordinate regional health planning, may have a number of subcommittees. These may include a subcommittee to review the health systems plan of the health service agencies, another to review the annual implementation plan of the same agencies, and still another to take testimony from providers and consumers about the impact of the health planning process. It is not uncommon to find members of a major committee appointed to several subcommittees. Instead of attending perhaps one major committee meeting a month, the individual may be expected to attend frequent subcommittee meetings.

Meetings are a fact of life for all administrators. They are needed to gain support for administrative policies, to obtain information from staff members, and to solve emerging problems. What does not need to be a fact of life, however, is meetings that are unproductive. Committees can be administered effectively and efficiently. As Herbert E. Meyer has noted, "What most executives fail to realize is that the purpose of the meeting—in a sense, the only purpose of a meeting—is to save time.[14] In Chapter 6 we will define strategies that will assist in ensuring the committee meetings are contributing to, rather than eroding, the productivity of your organization.

Crisis orientation   Some administrators enjoy putting out organizational "fires"—that is, solving problems one at a time. Since they are ultimately responsible for the enterprise, they often feel an obligation to address issues that threaten the well-being of the organization.

There are many reasons why managers develop a crisis orientation to

[13] "Meyer, "Meeting-Goer's Lament," p. 96.
[14] Ibid.

their work. Some find the process of defining, implementing, and evaluating organizational objectives to be so time consuming and mentally demanding that they prefer to answer the mail, respond to telephone calls, and resolve emerging problems. Others prefer to work on specific problems simply because uncertainty about the future makes planning difficult. Winston Churchill made this point when he stated that it is difficult to look farther ahead than you can see.[15] Still others find fire fighting an innately rewarding managerial function. If you can resolve a festering problem and do it in a way that incurs the gratitude of others, you cannot help but feel that "something worthwhile has been accomplished."

Unfortunately, fighting fires has little to do with fire prevention. A crisis orientation usually has two negative effects on an organization. First, long-range planning is abandoned, or at the very least, receives a low priority. Planning, for most crisis-oriented administrators, is perceived to be a luxury, not a necessity. Second, crisis-oriented administrators often do not go through established administrative channels in solving difficult issues. In their eagerness to bring closure to issues they may ignore the staff member who is in the best position to solve the problem. When subordinates are bypassed, their authority is cut from underneath them. If this happens repeatedly, it will undermine their morale and likely trigger a series of conflicts between the administrator and the subordinates.

One way of determining whether an administrator has a crisis orientation is to examine the appointment calendar. If 80 percent of the day is spent in planned activities and 20 percent left to respond to emerging issues, it is likely that the administrator is making good use of time.[16] If, on the other hand, the administrator cannot tell you what is to be accomplished in a given day or week, it suggests a crisis orientation.

Charles Hummel aptly summarizes the need to move away from crisis orientation:

> The important task rarely must be done today, or even this week. The urgent task calls for instant action. The momentary approach of these tasks seems irresistible and they devour our energy. But in the light of time's perspective their deceptive prominence fades. With a sense of loss we recall the important tasks pushed aside. We realize we've become slaves to the tyranny of the urgent.[17]

Strategies for Managing Your Time

In a Daniel Howard Survey of 179 chief executives, 83 percent stated that they didn't have time to keep up with the reading that was essential to their field, and 72 percent stated that they didn't have time to think or to

[15] Mackenzie, *The Time Trap,* p. 40.

[16] Ibid., p. 44.

[17] Cited in Mackenzie, *The Time Trap,* p. 43.

plan.[18] Obviously, if you don't keep up in your profession you will fall behind. Likewise, if you don't plan, the future will be decided by fate rather than rational thinking.

To reverse this situation you must take firm control of your schedule. Such control cannot be accomplished, however, until there is a philosophical belief that it is possible to manage time. Consider the following statements:

Example 1: "I never know what kind of problems I will have to handle until I look at the mail or see how many phone calls I have to return."

Example 2: "The phone never stops ringing. It's impossible to get things done."

Example 3: "I have an open door policy—it's the best way to get to know employees."

Each example reflects an administrative priority. In Examples 1 and 2 the mail and the telephone dictate how the work day will be spent. The Charles Dartnell Institute for Business research found that in a typical day an executive will spend two to three hours reading and answering mail. In addition, nine out of ten executives will spend at least an hour on the phone, while four of the ten will spend at least two hours on the phone.[19]

In Example 3 the administrative day is spent conversing with employees who "drop by." If the welcome is genuine, the administrator will soon see the day eroded with social chit chat. At the end of the day little will have been accomplished with the possible exception of a compilation of a long list of problems "that I didn't have time to get to."

Instead of scheduling their time wisely, many executives become victims of external events. Peter Drucker has stated that if you were to define an executive by his activities you "would have to define him as a captive of the organization. Everyone can move in on his time, and everyone does."[20] In order to help administrators gain control over their schedules, Drucker produced a film entitled *Managing Time.* In the film Drucker visits with a company president who is committing virtually all the errors that administrators typically commit in not managing their schedules. When audiences watch this film they quickly identify with the pressures confronting the corporate president, but they also are able to quickly differentiate externally motivated time wasters from internal, or self-generating time wasters. For example, note the two lists of time wasters in Figure 3-1. List A of commonly thought of time wasters was composed by forty chief executives before they saw the Drucker

[18] Cited in Mackenzie, *The Time Trap,* p. 45.
[19] Cited in Mackenzie, *The Time Trap,* pp. 72, 93.
[20] Drucker, *The Effective Executive,* p. 10.

	List A		List B
1.	Incomplete information presented for solutions to problems	1.	Attempting too much at once
2.	Employees with problems	2.	Unrealistic time estimates
3.	Lack of delegation	3.	Procrastinating
4.	Telephone	4.	Lack of organization
5.	Routine tasks	5.	Failure to listen
6.	Lunch	6.	Doing it myself
7.	Interruptions	7.	Unable to say no
8.	Meetings	8.	Refusal to let others do the job
9.	Lack of priorities	9.	Delegating responsibility without authority
10.	Management by crises	10.	Involving everyone
11.	Personal attention to people	11.	Bypassing the chain of command
12.	Outside activities	12.	Snap decisions
13.	Poor communication	13.	Blaming others
14.	Mistakes	14.	Personal and outside activities

© R. Alec Mackenzie

Figure 3-1 Perceived causes of time mismanagement. [Reprinted by permission of the author of *The Time Trap,* R. Alec Mackenzie, AMACOM, a division of American Management Associations, 1972, p. 6. All rights reserved.]

film. List B was composed after they had seen it. The different items in List B reflect how the executives had begun to realize that effective time management is the responsibility of the administrator.[21] The first step, therefore, in exercising effective time management is to understand that you and you alone are responsible for how your time will be spent. As Mackenzie observes, "While most books on management talk about managing the work of others as well as those through whom the work is performed, one can really be certain of managing only himself."[22]

A corollary step in exercising effective time management is to determine what you will and will not be doing in a given day. Some administrators find it helpful to set aside at least an hour at the beginning of the day to think, to set priorities, and to outline a plan for the day. Others find it useful to take the last hour of the day to prioritize the following day's activities. Whatever the method, adequate time should be allocated to set forth a plan of action for each workday.

One way of defining such a plan of action is to identify "posteriorities"; that is, determine the tasks that one will *not* do, and then stick with that deci-

[21] Mackenzie, *The Time Trap,* p. 6.
[22] Ibid., p. 15.

sion. Deciding what *not* to do is a difficult process. However, keeping many balls in the air is a circus stunt. Even professional jugglers will do it for only ten minutes or so. If they did it longer all the balls would soon be dropped.[23]

A good example of an executive who understands the importance of determining posteriorities is the president of a large suburban hospital. In an address to the hospital's board of trustees he stated, "We will not try to do everything, for that requires little judgment. I would suggest that by May 15th we jointly evaluate each of our services and determine those which should remain a priority for the next five years."

Learning to say no is a difficult concept for many administrators to implement. Every project that comes across the administrator's desk usually has advocates who argue that the project should be a priority. As Theodore Levitt noted,

> Relentless pressure is beamed at the President from his lieutenants in each department, each constantly telling him that his direct personal support is needed immediately lest the enterprise suffer irreparable harm. The chief's sympathetic and undeviating attention is demanded for production, finance, personnel, community relations, R and D, and, of course, marketing. If the poor man responded fully, he would scarcely have time to be president.[24]

Learning to say no is, however, a critical prerequisite to being a good manager of your time. "Over the years," says Robert Updegraff, "I have listened to people complain about not having time for the things they ought to do or would like to do and I have discovered that many of them suffer from a common trouble: They are timid about using the greatest time saving word in the English language, the little two-letter word 'NO.' "[25] Parkinson's Second Law states that we tend to devote time and effort to tasks in inverse relation to their importance. The ability to consciously decide what it is that we will and will not do prevents Parkinson's Law from becoming a reality.

Finally, the gaining of control over your schedule is facilitated by undertaking a self-inventory of how you actually spend your time. The recording of how time is spent is one of the oldest of all managerial concepts. It was made popular at the turn of the century by Frederick Taylor and has become known as Scientific Management. It reflects a commonsense truth: You must know how your time is spent before you are in a position to determine whether it is being used effectively.

There are several common methods of recording your time. Some executives keep a time log, writing down at half-hour intervals what it is they are doing. Others will ask their secretary to keep a record. Others will write down the length of every conversation and make an assessment as to whether the

[23] Drucker, *The Effective Executive,* p. 101.
[24] Cited in Mackenzie, *The Time Trap,* p. 56.
[25] Quoted ibid.

time was used wisely. Whatever the method, the basic point is that a time log should be periodically kept and that the time log should be based upon "real" time—that is, a recording at the time of the event itself, not from your distant memory hours later.[26]

The net result of making a time log is to show you the degree to which your time may be mismanaged. Do not be surprised if you learn that a lot of your time is wasted on activities that have little productive return. It has been found that most executives, regardless of rank of their position, can usually consign a quarter of the demands on their time to the wastepaper basket without anybody's noticing their disappearance.[27]

Time *is* a unique resource. It is a resource that must be spent. It cannot be stored, saved, or put to use at a later time. Because of its uniqueness it must be carefully managed. It is one of the most basic elements that supports consciously competent patterns of administration.[28]

DEFINING WRITTEN OBJECTIVES

The second step in the self-management process is to write explicit objectives that reflect those tasks that merit attention. The writing of objectives assists in separating the essential work roles from those that have little, if any, productive return.

Defining objectives, utilizing such objectives in the management process, and measuring individual and organizational performance against these objectives has become known as "management by objectives" (MBO). MBO has one basic purpose: to improve the performance of the organization.

An objective might be defined as "the end point or goal toward which management directs its efforts."[29] There are four benefits that accrue to an organization when precise objectives are defined and achieved.

First, objectives provide *a sense of direction*. By examining objectives it is possible to see the end results that are to be achieved. The objectives provide a type of organizational road map that leads to a predetermined destination.

Second, objectives *serve as motivators*. The most ideal work environment is one where workers recognize the importance of their objectives and are strongly committed to achieving them by a predetermined date. When workers believe in the importance of their objectives they are motivated to do the best possible job.

Third, objectives are *standards of performance*. Objectives define expectations for the organization, its departments, and its members. Objectives

---

[26] Drucker, *The Effective Executive,* p. 35.

[27] Mackenzie, *The Time Trap,* p. 37.

[28] Drucker, *The Effective Executive,* p. 26.

[29] Henry L. Sisk, *Management and Organization* (Cincinnati: Southwestern Publication Co., 1977), p. 45.

build teamwork as employees learn that they can accomplish more col-
laboratively than they could if they were working in isolation from one
another.[30]

Finally, objectives *reflect the organization's desired image.* Objectives,
particularly those stated by the chief administrators, can describe how the
organization wants to be perceived by external observers. Sometimes it may be
difficult to achieve the desired image. Nevertheless, if objectives are articulated and if consistent efforts are made to reach the desired end result, the
organization will be driven closer to its ideal than if the objectives were never
defined.[31]

The basic process for formulating objectives can be found in Figure 3-2.
The typical approach is for managers to meet periodically with subordinates
to evaluate past performance and to design new objectives. Each subordinate
should have an opportunity to shape the objectives while learning how these
objectives interface with the goals of the department and the entire organization. Such an understanding helps the worker see how his or her sphere of action contributes to the larger purposes of the organization.

Out of this initial discussion between manager and subordinate will

[30] Ibid., p. 46.
[31] Clayton Reeser and Marvin Loper, *Management* (Glenview, Ill.: Scott, Foresman, 1978), p. 61.

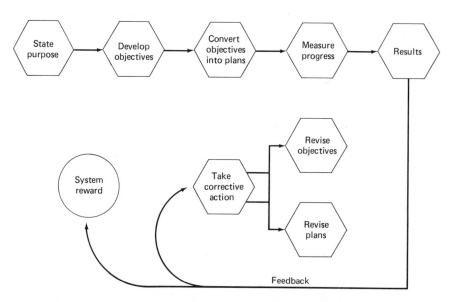

Figure 3-2 The objective-setting process. [From Joseph L. Massie
and John Douglas, *Managing: A Contemporary Introduction,* 3rd ed.
(Englewood Cliffs, N.J.: Prentice-Hall, Inc., 1981), p. 252. Copyright ©
1981. Reprinted by permission of the publisher.]

come "preliminary" or "draft form" objectives. The subordinate should be encouraged to reflect on the objectives, rewrite them if needed, and then submit them to the supervisor for final approval. The objectives should have the following characteristics:

> *The objectives should be measurable.* The more precise the objective the easier it is to determine whether the objective has been successfully achieved. An objective that states that "the health department's continuing education department will become more actively involved in the community" leaves doubt as to how to proceed. On the other hand, if the objective reads as follows, there will be little doubt whether or not it has been achieved: "The number of home visits conducted by public health nurses will increase by 5 percent per annum through 1985 in order to enroll 1,400 community residents."

> *The objective should be clear.* If you have to read an objective more than once in order to comprehend it, then you know that you have failed in writing a clearly worded statement.

> *The objective should make sense.* After reading an objective you should be able to say, "Yes, that states precisely what it is that I intend to do." In other words, the objective should be a motivator to action.

> *The objective should be realistic and obtainable.* The supervisor and subordinate should agree that the objective can be achieved in a given period of time.

Once objectives have been agreed upon, a decision should be made as to how often progress reports should be given to the manager. The decision is influenced by the amount of confidence the manager has in the subordinate and in the nature of the objectives. A subordinate who has a long history of competent work will probably need little supervision and will probably not need to prepare frequent interim reports. On the other hand, if the objective is critical to the success of the organization, the manager may want progress reports at regularly scheduled intervals.

At a predetermined date the manager and the subordinate should meet to discuss the completed project. As noted in Figure 3–2, feedback is to be given. If the objective was completed in a competent and timely manner, recognition should be given. If it wasn't, corrective action should take place either in revising the objective or in revising the plans by which the objective was to be achieved.

For MBO to have a positive impact on the organization, everyone from the chief executive officer to the head of the building and grounds department should be responsible for designing, implementing, and evaluating their own objectives. The objective-writing process must be carefully coordinated so that there is a resulting hierarchy of objectives. As Joseph Massie and Paul

Douglas note, "At the top the entire organization aims in a given direction; each department in turn directs its efforts toward its own objectives; each division of each department has its own meaningful aims; and finally, each individual position can be assigned definite objectives which can clarify the role of the person that fills that position."[32]

While most organizations have had good results with MBO, some have not. Usually when results have not been equal to expectations it has been due to a misunderstanding of the MBO process. Sometimes organizations will define objectives that are not realistic or attainable. This results in employee frustration. Sometimes individuals become so involved in the mechanics of writing the objectives that they miss the point for which the objectives are written. Problems also develop when objectives cannot be operationalized or if they are merely platitudes that maintain the status quo.

One of the ways to avoid such negative repercussions is to define objectives according to three categories: routine objectives, problem solving objectives, and innovative objectives.

> For each of these categories there should be an agreement on three levels of achievement: pessimistic (absolute minimum), realistic (normally expected), and optimistic (ideal). This structure helps both parties, since it gives the superior targets that he can support while it gives the subordinate a framework by which he can check himself on a day-by-day basis.[33]

Of the three categories, the most important may be the innovative objectives. John Gardner has vividly noted the tendency of organizations as they grow older to cease to be the innovative and idealistic enterprises that they once were:

> When organizations and societies are young, they are flexible, fluid, not yet paralyzed by rigid specialization, and willing to try anything once. As the organization or society ages, vitality diminishes, flexibility gives way to rigidity, creativity fades, and there is a loss of capacity to meet challenges from unexpected directions. Call to mind the adaptability of youth, and the way in which that adaptability diminishes with the years. Call to mind the vigor and recklessness of some new organizations and societies—our own frontier settlements, for example—and reflect on how frequently these qualities are buried under the weight of tradition and history.[34]

One way to avoid being "buried under the weight of tradition and history" is to ask yourself and members of your staff to write at least one

---

[32] Joseph L. Massie and John Douglas, *Managing* (Englewood Cliffs, N.J.: Prentice-Hall, Inc., 1977), p. 277.

[33] Ibid., p. 282.

[34] John Gardner, *Self-Renewal* (New York: Harper & Row, 1964), p. 3.

creative objective that addresses a future need or opportunity. Such instructions prevent staff members from focusing only on immediate problems and keep them oriented to issues that will influence the future of the organization.

In summary, MBO is not a panacea by which unproductive individuals are suddenly transformed into productive workers. Nevertheless, in the twenty-five years MBO has formally been taught to executives, administrators in both public and private settings have seen their organizations strengthened through the objective-setting process. When employees at all levels focus their energy on specific assignments, the entire organization benefits from such single-mindedness of purpose.

DELEGATING FOR RESULTS

The first step in the self-management process is to manage your time. The second step is to write precise objectives that reflect what it is that you intend to accomplish. The third step is to delegate responsibility and authority. This ensures that issues that you choose not to address are, nevertheless, receiving an appropriate forum from members of the staff.

Dale D. McConkey has stated that probably no part of the management process is more misunderstood than the concept of delegation.[35] Yet, delegation is the lifeblood of an organization and as such is a concept with which every administrator must be thoroughly familiar.[36]

If objectives are to be effectively and efficiently met, the flow of work will have to be carefully assigned to staff members. The members of the staff will need a precise definition of what it is they are expected to accomplish and the date by which the task should be completed. They will need to learn who will evaluate their work and the process that will be followed in assessing the quality of the product or service. They will also need to understand how their work interfaces with the work of others. And, they will need to know to whom they can turn for assistance if they have difficulty in achieving the desired end result.

The concept of delegation is popularly defined as "getting things done through people." It has its origin in the overworked manager who cannot keep up with all the demands that are made on his or her time and who therefore hires someone to give some assistance.[37] The definition that we will use and that outlines the key factors in the successful delegation of responsibilities is as follows:

[35] Dale D. McConkey, *No-Nonsense Delegation* (New York: AMACOM, a division of American Management Associations, 1964), p. v.

[36] Theo Haimann, *Supervisory Management for Health Care Institutions* (St. Louis: Catholic Hospital Association, 1973), p. 119.

[37] Ross A. Webber, *Management: Basic Elements of Managing Organizations* (Homewood, Ill.: Richard D. Irwin, 1979), p. 358.

Delegation is the achievement by a manager of definite, specified results, results previously determined on the basis of a priority of needs, by empowering and motivating subordinates to accomplish all or part of the specific results for which the manager has final accountability. The specific results for which the subordinates are accountable are clearly delineated in advance in terms of output required and time allowed and the subordinate's progress is monitored continuously during the time period.[38]

Most administrators readily agree that delegation is one of the critical components in the management process. Yet, as Henry Albers points out, "practice does not always reflect preachments."

The management literature is replete with double talk about delegation. Greater delegation or decentralization has been lauded by many executives, but practice does not always reflect preachments. Executives are often more reluctant to delegate than they themselves will admit. Perhaps the most common problem in this respect is the failure to delegate responsibility over relatively minor matters. Far too many executives clutter their desks and minds with details that could be handled by a literate office boy. Some of them are so concerned with the position of the sheet music on the stand that they fail to conduct the orchestra. They frequently disrupt the work of subordinates to neglecting to develop a systematic approach to delegation.[39]

William Newman lists the following behavioral factors as obstacles to effective delegation:

REASONS FOR RELUCTANCE TO DELEGATE
1. Some executives get trapped in the "I can do it better myself" fallacy.
2. Lack of ability to direct.
3. Lack of confidence in subordinates.
4. Absence of selective controls to warn of impending difficulties.
5. A temperamental aversion to taking a chance.

WHY SUBORDINATES AVOID RESPONSIBILITY
1. Often the subordinate finds it easier to ask the boss than to decide for himself how to deal with a problem.
2. The fear of criticism for mistakes.
3. Lack of necessary information and resources to do a good job.
4. The subordinate may already have more work than he can do.
5. Lack of self-confidence.
6. Positive incentives may be inadequate.[40]

[38] McConkey, *No-Nonsense Delegation,* p. 4.

[39] Henry Albers, *Principles of Management: A Modern Approach* (New York: John Wiley, 1974), p. 245.

[40] William Newman, "Overcoming Obstacles to Effective Delegation," *Management Review,* January 1956, pp. 36–41.

One of the most important reasons why administrators do not delegate is their confusion in distinguishing between the concepts of "managing" and "operating." Managing is the process of defining, implementing, and evaluating administrative policies. It involves supervising others to ensure that work is completed in a timely manner. Operating is the actual carrying out of the work.

For example, a public health nurse who is a department head must determine the number of case visits the nursing staff will be making in a given period of time. That is a policy issue and reflects the management process. If, however, the public health nurse's supervisor decides to make some of the home visits herself, she is then participating in the operations of the department.

Most administrative positions have elements of operations woven within them. Figure 3–3 indicates the relative percentage of time that administrators spend in managing and operating.

As long as there is a conscious distinction in the mind of the administrator as to when she is managing and when she is operating, few problems will result. The staff will have a clear understanding that the administrator is primarily a manager and when operations are undertaken, it is to complement the work of the staff rather than to do the work for them.

Problems arise when the concepts of managing and operating become blurred. Consider the case of a mechanic who had great skill in diagnosing mechanical problems in cars. He had endless patience in correcting them and

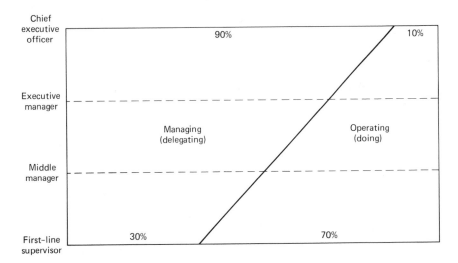

Figure 3-3 Proportions of managing and operating work at various management levels. [Reprinted by permission of the publisher of *The Fundamentals of Top Management* by Ralph C. Davis (New York: Harper Publishers, 1951).

was very successful in solving problems. As is often the case, because he was an outstanding mechanic, he was promoted to shop foreman. Suddenly he was the manager. Unfortunately, he had difficulty in acting like a manager. He wanted to continue being a mechanic. Often he would become involved in the daily operations rather than ensuring that the work was being undertaken by others. When a car was brought to the shop he would look into it no matter how busy he was, often stating that "I'll work it in somehow." He never let a piece of work go out of the shop until he was fully satisfied with it. He spent little time at his desk because he usually was up to his elbows in dismantled motors while subordinates who should have been doing the work were standing around waiting for instructions. The result was that the repair shop was always in a state of confusion.[41]

When staff members are promoted to managerial positions they may have difficulty giving up the operational aspects of their former position. The newly promoted head nurse may, for example, continue to spend most of the workday giving patient care rather than planning for the future of the nursing station. If the head nurse enjoys patient care and receives positive reinforcement from the medical staff, other nurses, and the patients, she may prefer doing the work rather than managing the work. This is an understandable, yet lamentable, position for the head nurse to take. While she may wish to exercise her clinical skills, once a management position has been taken, management work should be the primary focus of her work. This means delegating tasks to others to ensure that the nursing staff is working in an optimally productive manner.

In Figure 3–4 you will note a list of statements that reflect either "managing" or "operating." To ensure that you have mastered this concept, indicate whether each statement is a management function or whether it reflects the carrying out of operations. You can correct this exercise by referring to the key—but don't look at it until you have completed the task!

The actual process of delegating begins with a review of your objectives. Some of the objectives will necessitate work that you, and only you, are in a position to carry out. Other objectives can be delegated in whole, or in part, to staff members. Six principles should guide the delegation process.[42]

First, understand the content of the work that you intend to delegate. This implies that you must be reasonably familiar with the work itself. You should have an understanding of the complexity of the work and its importance to the organization. If the work had been previously delegated and the results were not equal to a desired standard, you should be aware of the constraining forces that influenced the quality of the work. You should have a good understanding of the time frame in which the work will be completed.

[41] Mackenzie, *The Time Trap,* pp. 124–25.
[42] Adapted from McConkey, *No-Nonsense Delegation,* pp. 90-99.

	Managing	Operating
1. Deciding whether to engage in a capital improvement program	———	———
2. Deciding whether to add a new staff position in the housekeeping department	———	———
3. Informing a subordinate why a raise is being given	———	———
4. Going with a subordinate to a meeting with consumers	———	———
5. Deciding whether a staff member should be able to attend a continuing education conference	———	———
6. Attending a conference to learn the latest technical information in your field	———	———
7. Meeting with a consultant to determine a strategy for negotiations with a union	———	———
8. Calling the maintenance department and asking one of the workers why the snow hasn't been removed from the parking lot	———	———

Key: (1) Managing—you are determining the future of the organization. (2) Managing—you are developing the organizational structure. (3) Managing—you are creating the work conditions for positive motivation. (4) Operating—it may be desirable to attend the meeting to show your interest, but you are not obtaining results through others. (5) Managing—if you are the person to whom the staff member reports; operating—if you are meddling in the responsibilities of the staff member's supervisor. (6) Operating—if the stated intent is to learn the latest technical developments it is unlikely that your attendance will help you manage the organization. Better to send the person who needs the latest knowledge and have them brief you. (7) Managing—you are engaged in the planning process. (8) Operating—you should be talking to the head of the maintenance department. It is his responsibility to determine why the snow hasn't been removed.

Figure 3-4 Statements that reflect "managing" and "operating."

You should be able to project the minimum amount of time a subordinate should spend on the task, as well as the maximum amount of time that can be allocated. It is also necessary to have a sound understanding of the human and financial resources available to the subordinate in completing the task. Finally, your instructions should state the degree to which you want to be kept informed concerning work progress.

Second, determine the competencies of staff members. Dale McConkey has noted that the selection of the right person is perhaps the most important factor in maximizing the benefits of delegation:

Delegating to an incompetent who cannot grow and mature constitutes delegating for the sake of delegating rather than for its benefits. Additionally, the

existence of an incompetent in the chain of command imposes an absolute block
to delegation: no delegation can be made to him and he, in turn, can't delegate to
those below him.[43]

Tasks that are vitally important to the organization should be assigned
to the most talented and skillful staff member. The more critical the task the
more you will want to delegate to a subordinate's strength. This implies that
you have made an assessment of your staff members' backgrounds, work experience, and skills. Tasks that have far-reaching consequences should be
assigned to individuals who have a tested, proven track record.

There is danger, however, in always delegating to the same people. As
Theo Haimann has noted:

If too much reliance is placed on one or a few persons, the department will be in a
bad spot if they are absent or if they should leave the employment of the enterprise. Thus, it is always a good idea to have a sufficient number of available
employees who have been trained in the department's most difficult tasks. And
the supervisor's problems of assigning various duties will become simpler as he
builds up the strength and experience of his employees.[44]

Building up the strength and experience of employees is an important
managerial function. An administrator should not put the organization in a
position where everything would be in a state of confusion and disarray if one
or two key staff members resigned. It is far better to assist subordinates in
learning new tasks, new ways of thinking, and in performing new responsibilities so that they can move into expanded roles. Ralph J. Cordiner, the
former President of General Electric, stated the issue well when he noted that
"The Chief Executive Officer, if he is discharging his responsibilities . . . should, within a period of not longer than three years after he has accepted his assignment, have at least three officers equal to or better than
himself who could succeed in his position."[45]

Third, consult with subordinates prior to delegating tasks to them. One
of the major aspects of the delegation process is to have subordinates assume
responsibility for completing the assigned tasks. Responsibility is the obligation of a subordinate to complete a task. Without the assumption of responsibility the entire process of delegation would not be complete.

It is important to recognize that while you can delegate authority, you
cannot delegate responsibility. Responsibility is something that the subordinate does or does not accept. You can assign a task and delegate authority

[43] McConkey, *No-Nonsense Delegation,* pp. 80–81.
[44] Haimann, *Supervisory Management,* pp. 120–21.
[45] Cited in Peter F. Drucker, *The Practice of Management* (New York: Harper & Row,
1954), p. 170.

to perform a specific job, but unless the subordinate assumes responsibility, the task will not be satisfactorily completed.

How do you obtain a commitment from a subordinate to assume responsibility? As we learned earlier, obtaining a good interface between the work that needs to be completed and the interests and skills of a worker will influence the outcomes of the delegation process. A second factor is whether adequate lead time is given so that the subordinate can study the newly assigned tasks, obtain necessary counsel from others, and act in a deliberative and productive manner.

It is also important to delegate in advance. Dale McConkey has noted that a frequent method of delegation is to wait for a problem to rise and then delegate its handling at that time.[46] If an administrator can examine the issues, problems, and opportunities that will need to be addressed, specific tasks with adequate time to perform them can then be delegated to staff members. Most staff members will assume new responsibilities if they know they can satisfactorily integrate them into existing patterns of work.

An additional factor that influences subordinate commitment is whether they are assigned the whole task or only a part of a task. When an employee recognizes that the outcome of a project rests primarily on her own work, she will be more committed to achieving success than if she has to share responsibility with others. For example, if a hospital administrator wanted to know the possible effects of a proposed personnel policy, it would be wise to delegate that task to the personnel director rather than requesting a number of department heads to comment on it. The personnel director may choose to interview the department heads in order to obtain needed information but, because the task has been delegated to one individual, control is maximized. The personnel director will recognize that the success of the project is his responsibility. He is in a position to take credit for the project if it is done well. If it isn't, the administrator is in a position to hold one person accountable for the results.

Finally, commitment to completing an assigned task is influenced by the subordinates' perceptions as to whether they have received the necessary information to do the job. It is therefore important to level not only about what needs to be accomplished but *why* it must be completed. The subordinates need to understand the importance of the task in relation to the organization. They need to know that they can obtain background information that is relevant to the task, and, perhaps most importantly, they need to know why they were selected to do the job. When employees learn that they were selected because of their unique skills, or because of their sensitivity to a problem, or because of their record in completing projects in a timely manner, powerful motivators are tapped that contribute to the successful completion of the project.

[46] McConkey, *No-Nonsense Delegation,* p. 83.

Fourth, delegate for specific results. It is important to communicate as clearly as possible what needs to be undertaken. Such clearness of expression will help to minimize mistakes and confusion. Examples of clear statements of expectations are as follows:

"By January 1, submit a report not to exceed ten pages, outlining three models by which continuing education could be carried out in the hospital. The report should include staffings and financial projections, including proposed budgets."

"By January 1, determine the feasibility of adopting a flextime work schedule for civil service personnel. A written report should be sent to Mr. McKanna's office by January 1; an oral report should be given to the health department's executive committee on January 14."

"By January 1, list priorities for the purchase of new equipment during the next fiscal year. The maximum allowable expenditures should not exceed $335,000. Reasons justifying the purchase of each piece of equipment should be stated in writing."

Fifth, delegate authority. The delegation process often breaks down when the authority to complete a task is not stipulated. One study found that there was disagreement 50 percent of the time between first-line supervisors and their superiors over the amount of authority the subordinate had. There was either substantial overestimation or underestimation of the subordinate's authority.[47]

There are eight patterns of authority which are implicit in the following instructions:

1. Look into this problem. Give me all the facts. I will decide what to do.
2. Let met know the alternatives available with the pros and cons of each. I will decide which to select.
3. Recommend a course of action for my approval.
4. Let me know what you intend to do. Delay action until I approve.
5. Let me know what you intend to do. Do it unless I say no.
6. Take action. Let me know how it turns out.
7. Take action. Communicate with me only if your action is unsuccessful.
8. Take action. No further communication with me is necessary.[48]

An effective working relationship is facilitated when subordinates are not only given clear instructions about what is expected of them, but also understand the degree of authority they have in carrying out the assigned tasks. If such clarification is not given, subordinates will gravitate to patterns

[47] B. B. Boyd and J. M. Jensen, "Perceptions of the First Line Supervisor's Authority," *Academics of Management Journal,* 15, no. 3 (1972), 331–42.
[48] Webber, *Management,* p. 358.

1, 2, and 3 in the above list for fear that they will be criticized if they take action.[49]

Most administrators develop a basic style that reflects their willingness to delegate authority. President Dwight Eisenhower preferred delegation styles 3 and 4. He wanted his White House assistants to give him a detailed proposal that he could approve or not approve by simply giving his signature. President John Kennedy preferred patterns 1 and 2 because he wanted to be involved in early aspects of the decision-making process. President Harry Truman usually operated out of pattern 8. One high-level appointee maintained that when he once went in to report to the president, Mr. Truman cut him short by saying, "You're doing a good job. You'll hear from me when you're not. Now let's talk about the Civil War." President Nixon's style did not seem to be consistent, although many of his critics maintained that he either gave no delegation or would withdraw through patterns 7 and 8.[50] President Carter favored patterns 1 and 2, primarily because of his stated desire to be fully knowledgeable about all the background issues that might influence his decisions. President Reagan, who prefers to give wider decision-making latitude to his cabinet, favors patterns 5 and 6.

While an administrator may have a preferred pattern, it is usually better to let the nature of the work determine which pattern should be utilized. For example, a fairly routine problem that reaches the administrator's desk may be referred to a middle-level manager with the notation: "Please take action. No further communication with me is necessary unless you run into difficulty" (pattern 7). On the other hand, if a local reporter calls and asks you why there are "serious staffing problems in the pediatrics department" you may want to turn to a top assistant and state: "Look into this problem within the next twelve hours. Give me all the facts. I will decide what to do" (pattern 1).

Sixth, give feedback to the subordinate. The delegation process is not complete until the supervisor and the subordinate have an opportunity to assess what has been completed. The supervisor should give honest feedback to the subordinate concerning the quality of the work. The feedback should be specific; that is, the areas of the subordinate's strengths should be noted. If there are areas that the subordinate needs to improve, those too should be carefully delineated.

The subordinate should also have an opportunity to give feedback to the supervisor concerning the outcomes of the project. If there are instructions or patterns of authority that were not made clear, if relevant data was not provided, or if counsel from others was not given, steps should be taken to prevent those problems from recurring.

Basically, feedback between supervisor and subordinate should flow in

[49] Ibid.
[50] Ibid.

two directions. Each should try to assist the other in determining how a better job could be accomplished in the future. When that type of communication is fostered, successive work assignments will be delegated more easily and will be assumed more readily.

As you are delegating responsibilities to staff members it is important to keep a record of the tasks that have been assigned. The writing of a work-flow chart is done primarily for yourself so that you can, at a glance, determine what tasks have been delegated. Many executives also find it helpful to give a

Project	Person responsible	Interim progress report	Completion date	Evaluation of work
Submission of planning documents to the Metropolitan Health Board	R. McDonald	Mar. 15 Apr. 30 Jul. 28	Aug. 15	Aug. 28
Determination of the budget of the patient education program for next fiscal year	P. Swenson	May 1	June 1	June 15
Determination of options for salary increases for civil service personnel	F. Petersen	Feb. 15 Feb. 30	Mar. 21	Apr. 2
Determination of costs associated with proposed dental health program for employees	J. Smitheren	None	Apr. 30	May 14
Determination of continuing education programs for next fiscal year	M. Backlans	June 1	July 15	Aug. 15
Invitation to bid on repavement of parking lot submitted to four firms	F. Farnhorst	None	Aug. 1	Sept. 15
Preparation of agenda and supporting materials for board of trustees meeting, January 5-6	B. Kanter	Oct. 15	Nov. 30	Jan. 8
Determination of equipment replacement for next fiscal year	B. Caldwell	Feb. 13 Mar. 15 Apr. 18	May 15	May 21

Figure 3-5   A work-flow chart: R. McConnel, Administrator.

copy of the chart to subordinates. This not only helps to reinforce the need to complete projects by a designated date, but also keeps the subordinate informed about other work that is being carried on within the department.

A work-flow chart usually contains five types of information: (1) a brief description of the project that has been assigned; (2) the name of the individual to whom it has been assigned; (3) the date(s) of interim progress reports; (4) the date when the project is to be completed; and (5) the date of a meeting at which the work of the subordinate is to be evaluated. An example of a work-flow chart can be found in Figure 3-5.

In conclusion, the delegation process serves both the administrator and the organization when the delegator and the delegatee, working in harmony, succeed in putting into consistent practice actions in which:

1. The major objectives of the organization are broken down into manageable, challenging tasks for all levels of management.
2. All subordinates are encouraged to contribute to the maximum of their abilities and ambitions.
3. Subordinates are given the freedom to act consistent with their abilities.
4. Subordinates have a voice in determining what is expected of them.
5. A system of recognition and rewards is in place which recognizes performance.
6. The combined efforts of supervisors and subordinates culminate in a synergistic result of which the total is greater than the sum of the individual inputs.[51]

SUMMARY

A key factor that contributes to competent management is the ability to use time productively. Health administrators who are able to master this competency are aware that wasted effort, unproductive meetings, and a crisis-oriented approach to management can quickly erode their energy as well as their achievements. Time can be conserved by defining work objectives. A well-written objective is measurable, clearly stated, and perceived to be obtainable. It is equally important to delegate authority and responsibility to staff members if the work of the organization is to be carried out effectively. The prudent use of time, the achievement of important objectives, and the delegation of meaningful work are the basic building blocks in developing a productive career.

STUDY QUESTIONS

1. Identify a period in your life where you were particularly productive. What explanations can be given in accounting for that productivity? How did you manage your time during this productive period?

[51] Adapted from McConkey, *No-Nonsense Delegation,* pp. 213-14.

2. Would you rather "manage" or "operate"? What are the implications of your choice?

3. Note the following time management exercise. Under the heading of *Work Priorities* list the major tasks that you want to accomplish during the coming week. Under the heading of *Leisure Priorities* list the relationship/recreational priorities that you want to realize. Finally under the heading of *Health Priorities* write down the actions you intend to take that will protect your health. Among the items you might want to consider under this category are seven to eight hours of good sleep per night; walking, jogging, or swimming exercises; and eating three well-balanced meals per day. At the end of each day return to your list and keep a record of how well you are meeting your priorities.

A TIME-MANAGEMENT EXERCISE

Name _____   Week of _____

Work Priorities	*Leisure Priorities*	*Health Priorities*

4. Do you feel that you manage your time effectively? Can you delineate specific actions that you want to take in order to manage your time more productively?

ADDITIONAL READING RESOURCES

Douglass, Merrill E., and Donna N. Douglass, *Manage Your Time, Manage Your Work, Manage Yourself*. New York: AMACON, 1980.

Meyer, Herbert E., "The Meeting-Goer's Lament," *Fortune,* October 22, 1979, p. 95.

Pines, Ayala, and Christina Maslach, "Characteristics of Staff Burnout in Mental Health Settings," *Hospital and Community Psychiatry,* 29 (April 1978), 235.

Rohrs, Walter F., "How Time Flies," *Hospital and Health Services Administration,* 24, no. 1 (Winter 1979), 25–36.

4 Competency: Communicating Effectively

Communication is a means, not an end. It serves as the lubricant fostering the smooth operation of the management process(es).—George Terry

OVERVIEW The purpose of this chapter is to describe the ways in which interpersonal communication influences health administration. The chapter defines the nature of communication problems in organizations and suggests ways in which such problems can be minimized. Upon completion of this chapter the reader should be able to:

- Delineate three major sources of communication problems in organizations

- Describe the ways in which the self-concept influences the sending and receiving of messages

- Interpret how professionalism, status differences, and the fear of personal contact inhibit the communication process

- Define those elements in interpersonal communication that create an environment for dialogue

Everything hinges on communication. Whether the health administrator is concerned with organizational objectives, performance evaluation, fund raising, or community relations, excellence in administration is correlated with effective interpersonal communication. Administrators may be educated in the latest approach to management, yet be relatively ineffective if they are unable to adequately relate to colleagues. On the other hand, there are health administrators who have not had the advantage of formal management training but, because they are able to obtain the trust and respect of co-workers, they are able to perform credibly.

The ability to work effectively with people is a necessity if one is to be competent in an administrative position. Productivity and morale will be influenced by the quality of the supervisory communication that the staff receives. Success in obtaining funding may be contingent upon whether the administrator can persuasively communicate the needs of the organization to others. Health programs and proposals that may be excellent in their own right can be sabotaged because the decision makers do not like the personality of the designer.

Because communication and administration are closely linked, it is not surprising that managers often suggest that a major source of their frustrations is related to communication problems. In one cross-cultural study, for

Barriers to effectiveness	Percent of companies in which this is identified as one of seven key barriers		
	United States	Great Britain	Japan
1. Communication	74.24	63.63	84.84
2. Planning	62.12	63.63	65.15
3. Morale	45.45	45.45	46.96
4. Coordination	45.45	22.72	31.81
5. Critique	42.42	28.78	33.33
6. Commitment	39.39	45.45	21.21
7. Control	33.33	28.78	35.29
8. Profit consciousness	31.81	36.36	31.81
9. Creativity	25.75	45.45	48.48
10. Getting results	21.21	30.30	45.45

Managers from 198 companies, 66 each in the United States, Great Britain, and Japan representing a wide variety of businesses provided these data. Corporations from the three countries were matched with one another by nature of the business and corporate size. Managers were matched by responsibility and level in the firms. They identified corporate areas regarded as the most significant barriers to be overcome in achieving excellence in their own corporations. While barriers beyond the first two vary in importance, the first two are the same regardless of country, company, or characteristics of the managers reporting.

Figure 4-1 Foremost barriers to corporate excellence. [From Robert Blake and Jane Mouton, *Grid Organization Development* (Houston: Gulf Publishing Co., 1968). p. 4. Reproduced by permission.]

example, managers in the United States, Great Britain, and Japan stated that a significant barrier to organizational effectiveness was "communication."[1] In fact, communication problems were considered to be a greater barrier than problems relating to planning, morale, coordination, profit consciousness, and "getting results" (see Figure 4-1).

THE NATURE OF ORGANIZATIONAL COMMUNICATION PROBLEMS

What is meant by the term "communication problems"? Consider the following statements:

> "I don't think anybody in this whole organization cares about what we are doing."

> "Don't try and ask *that* department to do anything until Harry retires."

> "I swear, the only person who knows what is going on around here is the telephone operator. And she probably knows too much."

> "Those surgeons sure are prima donnas. You would think that they own this hospital."

Comments such as these are indicative that working relationships are not conducive to open communication. Stereotypes of people, incomplete information, and unmet expectations are indicators that channels of communication are not maximally effective.

There are three major sources of communication breakdowns in organizations: misunderstandings, disagreements, and misinformation.[2] *Misunderstandings* emerge when an individual does not perceive the meaning of a message as the sender intended it. The message "Next year sure is going to be austere," for example, may be interpreted in many different ways. The insecure subordinate who hears such a message may believe that employment may be terminated in the near future. In reality, the supervisor may be suggesting that there will not be financial support for new programs.

Whenever an individual sends a message, there is the possibility that it will be interpreted in different ways by different people. People read meanings in words, phrases, sentences, and nonverbal expressions. The more ambiguous the message, the greater the likelihood that it will be interpreted dif-

[1] Robert R. Blake and Jane Srygley Mouton, *Grid Organization Development* (Houston: Gulf Publishing Co., 1968), p. 4.

[2] Ernest Bormann, William Howell, Ralph Nichols, and George Shapiro, *Interpersonal Communication in the Modern Organization* (Englewood Cliffs, N.J.: Prentice-Hall, Inc., 1969), pp. 145-61.

ferently by the receiver. Unfortunately, the four words "What do you mean?" are not asked often enough in interviews and organizational meetings. The net result is that we think we know what one another means, only to discover at a later time that we misunderstood.

Disruptive *disagreements* emerge when individuals perceive that someone is attacking their "personhood." An attack on one's personhood is different from a disagreement over ideas. Most people expect that their ideas will not always receive unanimous support and approval! An attack on one's personhood, however, goes beyond disagreeing with the idea that is presented. Rather, it is a statement that implies that one is not informed, is ignorant, or is naive. People feel their personhood is being attacked when they perceive that they are being evaluated unfairly or "put down" for one reason or another. Feelings of inadequacy are also aroused if someone communicates with a tone of superiority.

Most individuals cannot tolerate an attack on their personhood. When individuals perceive that they are the objects of unfair and adverse criticism, it is necessary for them to cope with the situation and restore the image that they wish to have of themselves.

Some individuals cope by psychologically removing themselves from the conversation. If they are at a staff conference where interpersonal hostility is often verbalized, these individuals may cope by not entering into any controversial aspect of the conversation. They may choose to sit in an inconspicuous place in the room and will rarely look interested or involved in the conversation. If someone asks for an opinion on a controversial subject, they may try to double talk their way out of the situation by stating, "Well, I will need more time to think about it," or "I can see Harry's point of view, but there is something to be said about Mark's view as well. I just don't know what we should do."

The objective of this type of coping is to stay in the background in order to avoid being drawn into the conversation. Remaining aloof is perceived as a means of escaping the notice of an attacker. In more extreme instances of removal, individuals will seek to cope by becoming sick at the time of the staff meeting or by arranging schedule conflicts that preclude their being able to attend the meeting.

Another way to cope with an attack on one's personhood is to fight back. People fight back when they feel that the only way to restore their self-image is to aggressively protect their interests. Unfortunately, such fighting rarely rises above the level of the attack—if the attack is perceived as personal, the counterattack will usually be personal as well. This is generally a cyclical process in which one attack is followed by another and another.

Interpersonal warfare is not unlike military warfare. In war the combatants look for the enemy's points of vulnerability. So it is in interpersonal warfare. Immense psychological energy can be given to discerning the precise points where the other person is most vulnerable. If it is discovered that the other party was fired from the last job and that this fact has been a well-kept secret, such knowledge may be employed at a strategic moment. If it is determined that sixteen vacations days were taken last year instead of the allowable fifteen, such information will be stored until it can best be utilized. Finding chinks in the armor of individuals who pose a threat is not an idle game in most organizations.

Another way of coping with interpersonal conflict is simply to quit. Resigning from a committee that the employee finds personally disruptive, requesting a transfer to another department in the organization, or leaving the organization entirely are ways of removing the threat that the employee feels. When such action is taken, it is an indication that the individual can only cope with the situation by being removed from the perceived source of the problem.

Disruptive disagreements are self-defeating for ail concerned. Creative energy that could be focused on work-related goals and used to solve problems is given to protecting the ego. In such a situation, everyone generally loses.

A third source of communication disruption in organizations is *misinformation*. Misinformation emerges when members of the organization do not ask the critical question "How do you know?"

Many communication problems in organizations are due to the fact that employees are not dealing with facts but with incorrect inferences. When an incorrect inference is made it may be transmitted to others in the organization. They, in turn, may act as if they have factual information. For example, suppose two hospital administrators are riding in the elevator and one mentions something about a new wage scale for the coming year. On that elevator is a licensed practical nurse who thought she overheard one of the administrators state that there would be a large increase in wages. At coffee break she mentions this to several other licensed practical nurses who in turn take such information to their stations. In a very short period of time faulty information has been transmitted to people in various parts of the hospital. Whenever individuals do not ask the question "How do you know?" assumptions will be made, inferences will be drawn, and communication problems will abound.

In summary, there are three sources of communication problems in organizations: misunderstandings, disruptive disagreements, and misinformation. The extent to which an administrator is able to avoid such problems will be contingent upon whether the members of the organization can send and receive accurate messages. Effective interpersonal communication is basic to organizational effectiveness. As Lee Thayer states: "Internal communication is to an organization what the psychological/conceptual system is to the organism. It is what permits the organization to learn, to be aware of itself, to be intelligently adaptive and creatively aggressive vis-à-vis its environment."[3]

[3] Lee Thayer, *Communication and Communication Systems* (Homewood, Ill.: Richard D. Irwin, 1968), p. 20.

UNDERSTANDING YOURSELF IN THE COMMUNICATION PROCESS

*Intra*personal communication is the foundation upon which *inter*personal communication is constructed. The attitudes you hold about yourself will influence the approach you make to people, how you will interact, and what you will expect from the relationship. An administrator who enjoys challenges and feels confident that such challenges can evolve into successful outcomes will relate in one way to colleagues while the administrator who feels overwhelmed by daily problems, issues, and challenges will relate in a quite different way. An administrator who is depressed because of a family problem will probably find that such feelings will be reflected, albeit unconsciously, in his or her verbal and nonverbal communications. Likewise, an administrator who has little sense of fulfillment will probably reflect discontent. Freud suggested, and rightly so, that "No mortal can keep a secret. If his lips are silent, he chatters with his fingertips; betrayal oozes out of him at every pore."[4] Thus, a person may feel calm and self-controlled, yet be unaware that signs of tension and anxiety are leaking out in the tapping of a foot or in tense facial expressions.[5]

The importance of understanding how the self-concept shapes our behavior cannot be overemphasized.

> The most important single factor affecting behavior is the self-concept. What people do at every moment of their lives is a product of how they see themselves and the situation they are in. While situations may change from moment to moment or place to place, the beliefs that people have about themselves are always present factors in determining their behavior.[6]

Because the self-concept is critical in understanding leadership behavior it is necessary to periodically ask probing questions that will give clues as to how the self-concept might be shaping what we do at work and how we go about doing it. Questions such as the following may be helpful in unlocking the ways in which our daily routines are reflective of attitudes that we hold about ourselves:

1. What basic values do I have about myself, relationships, and work which I do not wish to change? How are these values reflected in my work?
2. Do I look forward to coming to work?

[4] Quoted in William Brooks, *Speech Communication* (Dubuque, Iowa: Wm. C. Brown, 1971), p. 112.
[5] Ibid.
[6] Arthur Combs, Donald Avila, and William Purkey, *Helping Relationships: Basic Concepts for the Helping Professions* (Boston: Allyn & Bacon, 1972), p. 39.

3. Who do I get along with best at work and who do I get along with least
   well? What factors are influencing these relationships?
4. What problems have I consciously or unconsciously been avoiding at
   work? Are the reasons for avoiding them valid?

Answers to these questions will begin to illustrate how our self-concept
alters administrative actions. If the answer to question 1 indicates that there
are no clearly delineated values to form an underpinning to administrative action, one would probably find that administrative energy is given largely to
meeting day-to-day demands rather than to activities that are designed to further those values. For example, if an administrator has a value that reflects
concern for a particular health problem in a given community, that value will
shape the direction of administrative decisions. An administrator who does
not have convictions of a similar nature will probably find that energy is given
to responding to events rather than shaping what the events will be.

Answers to the second, third, and fourth questions also give clues as to
how the self-concept is influencing daily work routines. The extent to which
an administrator feels good about her work, her relationships at work, and
the problems to be solved at work will be largely determined by the view she
has of herself.

There are two primary reasons why it is important to periodically pause
and answer questions that will demonstrate how our self-concept is influencing our work behaviors. First, a person's self-concept does, in fact, influence
the way he receives and interprets messages as well as the nature of his
response. People who have low self-esteem will tend to be sensitive to
criticism, to be overly responsive to praise, to have hypocritical attitudes, and
to feel that "nobody likes me." People with a positive self-concept will be
confident in dealing with and resolving problems, will feel equal to other persons, will accept praise without embarrassment, and will be able to admit that
they have a wide range of feelings, desires, and behaviors.[7] A positive self-
concept will also be reflected in a desire to improve. An administrator with a
negative self-concept may look upon the visionary plans of a subordinate as a
threat. An administrator with a positive self-concept might reward such
creativity. An administrator with a negative self-concept might not tolerate an
employee who is critical of administrative decisions while an administrator
with a positive self-concept will see the need and value of having someone in
the organization who raises difficult questions and asks for the rationale for
administrative policies.

A second reason why it is important to be aware of one's self-concept is
that self-concepts tend to be fulfilled. We live up to the labels that are given to
us by others or selected by and for ourselves. Students have been known to do

[7] Brooks, *Speech Communication*, p. 112.

poorly in school because of unfortunate beliefs about themselves, as seen in this example reported by Coach Darrel Mudra of Western Illinois University:

> What a boy believes about himself is really important. We had a student at Greeley who scored in the 98th percentile on the entrance test, and he thought he had a 98 IQ. And because he thought he was an average kid, he knew college would be hard for him. He almost failed in his first term. He went home and told his parents: "I don't believe I'm college caliber" and the parents took him back to school and talked with the college counselor. When he found that 98th percentile score meant that he had a 140 IQ, he was able to do "A" work before the year was over.[8]

Administrators likewise tend to live up to the labels that are self-selected or given by others. Administrators who perceive themselves as "good on the outside but poor on the inside" will probably give energy and time to outside activities. Administrators who have the label "poor on the outside" will undoubtedly expend most of their energy in the office, working out internal problems, setting internal objectives, and monitoring internal progress towards organizational goals. Administrators who label themselves as "shy and introverted" will probably behave in a manner that is unfriendly. They will avoid opportunities to talk with others and will seek seclusion. Even the outward expressions of smiling and warmth will be tempered by the label of "shy" that one might give to oneself.

Fortunately, the self-fulfilling prophecy can be a benefit to an administrator rather than a liability.

> Persons with positive self-concepts are quite likely to behave in ways that cause others to react in corroborative fashion. People who believe they *can* are more likely to succeed. The very existence of such feelings about self creates conditions likely to make them so. The nurse who feels sure of herself behaves with dignity and certainty, expecting positive response from other people. To those with whom she works, this in turn calls forth responses which tend to confirm the beliefs she already holds.[9]

A valuable source of information about how your self-concept might be influencing your administrative behavior is the people who daily see you in the work situation. John Keltner states that if we are to understand ourselves we must get information from other people about ourselves. "Indeed, it would be helpful if others could get to our center of the world we live in and see that world as we see it. Their vision of that world might help us to understand ourselves better."[10]

[8] Combs, Avila, and Purkey, *Helping Relationships,* p. 43.

[9] Ibid., p. 46.

[10] John W. Keltner, *Interpersonal Speech-Communications: Elements and Structure,* (Belmont, Calif.: Wadsworth, 1970), p. 46.

Insight from others can be valuable in confirming the view we would like to have about ourselves. On the other hand, such information can be valuable when our idealized view is not shared by others. Keltner gives an interesting illustration of an administrator whose view of himself was not shared by others:

> A department chairman discovered that the members of his department always waited until he had suggested an idea before they made any contributions to staff discussions. He perceived thereby that the staff was hesitant to initiate ideas for fear of his disapproval. This, in turn, led him to examine what his behavior said to them about him. For several months he carefully encouraged, reassured, and supported the members of his staff; finally, some of them felt sufficiently secure to express openly how they perceived him. His desire to open up his colleagues so they would not hold back ideas and impressions led him to hold back on his own suggestions and to find opportunities to support suggestions others made.[11]

An administrator who seeks feedback from others will find that his self-concept will be more consistent with reality.

In summary, your self-concept influences the way in which you communicate. It influences the way you receive, interpret, and respond to messages. Therefore, it is important to periodically pause and step outside the continual stream of occurrences and ask difficult yet essential questions related to our self-concept and our work patterns. In so doing, we will have a better understanding of the attitudes that are shaping our administrative behaviors.

BARRIERS TO EFFECTIVE COMMUNICATION

Professionalism

Rollo May has suggested that a chief barrier to establishing rapport is the professional manner that one utilizes in communicating to others.[12] Professionalism might be defined as attitudes given off in a conversation that reflect a sense of superiority. If an administrator greets an employee perfunctorily and then settles back in the chair in such a way that speaks more loudly than words that "I'm the Chief Executive Officer, and this is just another case for me," the interview is strangled before it gets off the ground.

Professionalism is rooted in an "I'm OK—You're on Trial" attitude. The feelings that are evoked by such attitudes are inadequacy and defensiveness. The coldly detached professional whose opinions are not to be questioned, whose beliefs are always "right," and who communicates with a sense

---

[11] Ibid.

[12] Rollo May, *The Art of Counseling* (New York: Abingdon Press, 1939), p. 128.

of displeasure toward those who disagree causes frustration and anger. The frustration and anger that is felt is rooted in being diminished as a human being—a feeling that one's attitudes, opinions, and beliefs somehow do not count in the professional's scheme of things.

The professional who holds an "I'm OK—You're on Trial" attitude towards others is not always the superarrogant individual we might imagine. Rather, anyone who engages in stereotyping behavior falls into this category. Repeated efforts to resolve interagency conflicts has led me to believe that one of the primary factors leading to communication breakdowns in health agencies is the way in which health workers routinely label one another. If the public health nurses believe that the environmental health sanitarians are "junior policemen," a barrier has been constructed. When the county commissioners label the development unit of county government a "bunch of ivory tower elites who plan for the sake of planning," a barrier that prevents understanding has been established. When the medical student labels the nurse practitioners as "frustrated doctors," communication between those groups will be hampered.

Stereotyping results, in part, because we do not understand one another and because we are threatened by one another. The health educator is suspicious of the social worker because of an uncertainty of what the social worker's skills might be. Worse yet, there may be a fear on the part of the community health education specialist that the social worker could organize the community power base better than the specialist can. Since community organization is supposed to be a forte of the community health education specialist, any encroachment on what is perceived to be the territory of the specialist may result in derogatory comments aimed at the social worker. The aim is to diminish the prestige of the person who poses the perceived threat and to heighten the esteem of the one who is threatened.

Stereotyping also results because we do not understand the values and the ways of working that are basic to a profession. The director of environmental services in the health department, by virtue of interests, education, and goals, may have a view of the organization, its problems, and opportunities that differs considerably from the view of the director of nutrition. The director of personnel for the hospital may approach problems in one manner while the director of nursing services approaches them in a quite different manner. These professional points of view may keep us from understanding one another, or, if we do understand one another, from agreeing with one another.

While stereotyping of a profession may be the most blatant form of professionalism, everyday communication patterns by educated health workers can also reflect a sense of superiority that intimidates other professionals and nonprofessionals. This is especially true when professionals use jargon in such a way that it keeps people from understanding what is being said. A few hours before writing this paragraph, I was in a meeting in which a systems analyst discussed the need to computerize student admission processes. His conversation was punctuated with the language of computer science as he talked about "hardware and software," "tapes," "turnaround time," "information overload," and "input." Those who understood what he was talking about (roughly a third of the group) were unabashedly enthusiastic, raised questions, and entered into the language of the moment. Those who didn't understand timidly raised a question or two but did not enter into the conversation in any significant way. After the meeting was over, I walked back to my office with a group of three individuals who had said very little. They had nothing complimentary to say about the meeting or about the systems analyst. As one member said, "When you talk to those computer types, you know less at the end of the meeting than you did at the beginning."

Why did the systems analyst talk "computerese"? It may have been that he was speaking his primary language. To put it another way, he was using words that were familiar to him much like a manager who lapses into the language of management when talking about "deficit spending," "management by objectives," or "cost accounting." A group of doctors, listening to a hospital administrator's report, could have the same reaction to the jargon of management as did the majority of the group who listened to the systems analyst.

In summary, professionalism becomes a barrier to interpersonal communication when someone communicates a sense of superiority. The autocratic administrator who is always "right" represents the most obvious example of how professionalism disrupts communication. However, whenever one stereotypes a profession so that it is diminished and whenever words are used that result in intimidating the listener, a substantial barrier to understanding has been erected.

Status Differences

An obstacle that has particular significance for administrators is related to difficulties that occur within the supervisor-subordinate relationship. Inherent within this relationship is the fact that one individual has a higher status than the other. This presents potential problems in the communication process.

When a supervisor sends a message "down" through the ranks, it is assumed that the message will be interpreted literally. People with higher status generally believe that their messages will be interpreted as they themselves would want it interpreted. Unfortunately, this often does not happen.

When messages are sent from a higher-status person, the listener will try to hear undertones of deeper meaning. Rather than taking the message at face value, the listener personalizes it. "What is the boss trying to say to me?" is a typical reponse when a subordinate receives a directive. The subordinate may try to read various meanings into the message. The subordinate may wonder whether the boss likes him, is impressed with his work, or has plans to reward or punish him.[13] The fact that administrators assume that their meanings will be taken literally, coupled with the fact that subordinates tend to personalize the messages that they hear, makes partial misunderstanding a normal result of many supervisor-subordinate conversations.

Status differences also present problems in upward communication. Administrators are generally not aware of the magnitude of the barriers related to upward communication, especially between professionals and nonprofessionals. The administrator's status, authority, and prestige set her apart from the workers. The administrator uses words differently and dresses differently. The administrator can freely call a worker to the office or walk to the worker's department, but most workers do not feel equally free to call the administrator. If the worker does not have ability to express ideas clearly, the worker may avoid communication situations with the supervisor.

When subordinates do communicate with their supervisors, the messages may not be entirely accurate or complete. Employees tend to send only those messages that will result in reward, not punishment. Therefore, it is understandable that employees will send messages that they perceive supervisors would like to hear. This can lead to disastrous results for both the administrator and the organization. The absence of negative information means that the administrator will make decisions on less than adequate information.

Because status barriers are a prime barrier to effective communication, Keith Davis suggests that it is important for administrators to carefully cultivate ways in which such barriers can be overcome.

> Management needs to "tune in" to employees in the same way a person with a radio tunes in. This requires initiative and positive action, rather than the lethargy of waiting for the signal to come in. Tuning in requires management adaptability to different channels of employee information. It requires sensitivity to the distant signals as well as those near at hand. It necessitates some selectivity to separate useless signals from the worthwhile signals. It requires first and last an awareness that signals are being sent.[14]

Fear of Personal Contact

Paul Tournier, the Swiss psychiatrist, has written:

> Each of us does his best to hide behind a shield. For one, it is a mysterious silence which constitutes an impenetrable retreat. For another, it is a facile chit-chat, so that we never seem to get near him . . . or else it is erudition, quotations, abstractions, theories, academic argument, technical jargon; or ready made

---

[13] Bormann et al., *Interpersonal Communication,* p. 150.

[14] Keith Davis, *Human Behavior at Work* (New York: McGraw-Hill, 1977), p. 410.

answers, trivialities, or sententious and patronizing advice. One hides behind his timidity so that we cannot find anything to say to him; another behind a fine self-assurance which renders him less vulnerable.[15]

The reason we "hide behind a shield" is the fear that we may be misunderstood. The fear of being misunderstood is a strong deterrent to open and honest communication. The hospital administrator who is employed by a conservative board of trustees may not share innovative and promising ideas for fear of being labeled as radical. The nursing supervisor who wishes to adopt new procedures to ensure high-quality care may share such ideas in a guarded and defensive fashion if there is a fear that the suggestions would meet with immediate resistance and misunderstandings. If the commissioner of health is perceived by department directors as not tolerating failure, the chiefs may not share negative information concerning the day-to-day operations in their departments.

If we feel that our messages will be misunderstood, we will alter them to make them more acceptable, or not communicate at all. The fear of being misunderstood can be due to a multitude of reasons. It can be due to a belief that if we share enthusiasm for an idea it will not be reciprocated. It can be due to our perception that if we share emotion-laden concerns they will not be dealt with in a rational and responsible manner. It can be due to the fact that we lack courage to address controversial subjects, especially if we feel insecure in our own position.

A basic reason why we avoid open and honest communication is that we are not comfortable with expressing emotions. Many people dislike becoming involved in situations where emotion is bound to erupt. We tend to avoid situations that are unpleasant. Therefore, when there is the possibility that hostility will erupt, we may avoid that encounter or soothe over the effects of such hostility. Positive emotions can also be avoided. One can choose not to positively reinforce a colleague for fear that the positive comments might be misunderstood. We are all wary of the backslapper who is setting us up.

Emotions, however, play an important role in the ways in which we and our colleagues function each day. People *do* become frustrated, they *do* have convictions from which they do not want to retreat, they *do* become angry when the day's events do not progress as they wish. Likewise, there is within all employees a basic desire to be affirmed—to be shown respect and appreciation for work accomplishments. In short, emotions are a basic part of our personality. Nevertheless, because of the fear that we might be misunderstood, we may choose not to make personal contact with others.

The inability to make personal contact with colleagues can have a negative effect on employees and administrators. The negative effects of not making personal contact with colleagues can mean that the individual will seldom discover a sense of belonging with the organization. Tournier has

[15] Paul Tournier, *The Meaning of Persons* (New York: Harper & Row, 1957), p. 143.

pointed out that individuals can work side by side, month after month, without ever sharing anything of significance with one another. Likewise, an individual can spend years in an organization without meeting anyone who takes the slightest interest in him as a person, in his intimate concerns, and in his difficulties or his secret aspirations. "The daily routine, together with the prevailing atmosphere of our times, makes it possible for him to associate with companions whom he really does not know, and who do not know him. He sees them only as they appear to be, and they see him as a conventional personage."[16] The net result is that the worker may put in an eight-hour day, but rarely feel a sense of strong personal identity with the organization.

Organizational communication problems can be compounded if the administrator doesn't make personal contact with colleagues. Isolation from subordinates may mean that the administrator will not learn about the true problems in a unit until it is too late to correct the effects of the situation. Likewise, if the administrator does not share with trusted colleagues the problems that need resolution, no assistance from them will be forthcoming. From an organizational perspective, if there is little personal contact with subordinates, the gulf between administration and rank-and-file workers can grow very wide.

In summary, professionalism, status barriers, and the fear of personal contact represent significant barriers to effective interpersonal communication. Before dialogue can emerge, those barriers need to be understood and, where they are prevalent, to be diminished.

THE BASIS FOR DIALOGUE

There was a knock on my office door and a colleague asked if we couldn't discuss a problem he was having with one of his classes. It seemed that the class was unresponsive to his lectures and, worse yet, was not following the carefully delineated instructions on how to write a major paper for the course. "I can't figure it out," he said. "I have told them over and over again what topics are acceptable and how to outline a major paper. But look at these papers—they didn't hear a thing I said!" His hostility to the students for not following directions could be readily seen by his additional comments that the students must be inattentive because "we went over this again and again."

If one were to go back and observe the communication that took place between the faculty member and the students, in all likelihood one would find a monological mode of communication taking place. As Ruel Howe explains, "In monological communication, the speaker is so preoccupied with himself that he loses touch with those to whom he is speaking."[17] Talking at people,

[16] Ibid., p. 42.
[17] Reul L. Howe, *The Miracle of Dialogue* (New York, The Seabury Press, 1963), p. 32.

ignoring their feelings toward the message, assuming that your message is the one that the receiver hears, making decisions without contacting the people who will be affected by the decision—such behaviors are symptoms of monologue. Monologue occurs whenever one is preoccupied with the message rather than how the receiver interprets the message.

Dialogue, on the other hand, means that there is a basic trust between individuals. It implies that both individuals have something to be gained from the relationship, and that by supporting one another it is possible to achieve mutual objectives. It implies that there is respect between the two parties and a conviction that by working together they can achieve ends that couldn't be achieved by working alone. To put it another way, dialogue means that both parties realize they have more to gain by cooperating than by competing, by being honest with one another instead of guarded and closed.

What can the health administrator do to create an environment where dialogue can emerge?

In *On Becoming a Person: A Therapist's View of Psychotherapy,* Carl Rogers shares several learnings that have particular significance to him. I would like to use Rogers' insights into his own behavior as a framework for thinking about dialogue.

Rogers' first "significant learning" is as follows:

> In my relationships with persons I have found it does not help, in the long run, to act as though I were something I am not. It does not help to act calm and pleasant when actually I am angry and critical. It does not help to act as though I know the answers when I do not. It does not help to act as though I were a loving person if actually, at the moment, I am hostile. It does not help for me to act as though I were full of assurance, if actually I am frightened and unsure. Even on a very simple level I have found that this statement seems to hold. It does not help for me to act as though I were well when I feel ill.[18]

Rogers suggests that it is not helpful or effective in his relationships with other people to maintain a facade—"to act in one way on the surface when I am experiencing something quite different underneath."[19] Our own experience undoubtedly bears this out. We generally respond most favorably to individuals whose motivations are known to us. Conversely, individuals whose motivations are obscure cause us to be uncomfortable and anxious.

The need to communicate openly has many implications for the health administrator. First, we will be most effective in our interpersonal relations when we verbalize the motivations that lead to administrative decisions. An administrator who turns down a request from a department supervisor is communicating more effectively if she gives a rationale for the turndown than if

---

[18] Carl Rogers, *On Becoming a Person: A Therapist's View of Psychotherapy* (Boston: Houghton Mifflin, 1961), p. 16.

[19] Ibid., p. 17.

she gives no explanation. Second, our greatest problems with others will occur when we project something other than what we are feeling. An administrator who feels repeated anger at an assistant creates a better environment for communication if she makes efforts to work through the problem with the assistant, rather than trying to contain her emotions until they erupt in a less-than-helpful explosion. Third, if we disclose feelings and attitudes that are germane to an issue, we can expect that honesty will be returned. Self-disclosure is essential if we are to understand one another. Keltner has observed that the more we can know about the people we are working with and the more they can know about us, the more effective will be our communication attempts.[20] According to Sidney Jourard, "You cannot collaborate with another person toward some common end unless you know him. How can you know him, and he you, unless you have engaged in enough mutual disclosures of self to be able to anticipate how he will react and what part he will play?"[21]

A second learning that Rogers shares concerns self-awareness: "I find that I am more effective when I can listen acceptantly to myself and can be myself."[22] Over the years, Rogers states, he has learned to more adequately listen to himself so that he knows more adequately than he used to what it is that he is feeling at any given moment.

> . . . to be able to realize I *am* angry, or that I *do* feel rejection toward this person; or that I feel very full of warmth and affection for this individual; or that I am bored and uninterested in what is going on; or that I am eager to understand this individual or that I am anxious and fearful in my relationship to this person. All these diverse attitudes are feelings which I think I can listen to in myself.[23]

Rogers is suggesting that there is a particular value in being aware of what it is that one is feeling and perceiving. Such awareness implies being aware of how one's psychological state is influencing the perceptions of others, the issues raised, and the decisions that need to be made. If one can be aware of how his or her psychological condition is affecting a conversation, it may be possible to alter what is said and how it is said. Most of us probably can recall a conversation (or two or three!) that we wish we could call back and handle differently. We may well say, "If I wasn't so exhausted, I wouldn't have responded that way," or "If anyone but ol' Sam would have made that request, I probably would have listened!" One of the keys to improving one's communication effectiveness is to know what is happening internally at any given moment. If we are exhausted, it may be prudent not to

[20] Keltner, *Interpersonal Speech-Communication,* p. 54.
[21] Sidney Jourard, *The Transparent Self* (Princeton, N.J.: D. Van Nostrand, 1964), p. 3.
[22] Rogers, *On Becoming a Person,* p. 17.
[23] Ibid., p. 16.

take on an emotional issue. If we know that we have a negative emotional reaction to "ol' Sam" and can monitor that reaction, it may be possible to weigh Sam's proposal without becoming defensive.

Not only is it important to be aware of how our psychological state is influencing perceptions, it is equally important to be aware of what we are communicating nonverbally. How we are perceived is greatly influenced by the nonverbal cues we give off to others. For example, if we have made a major decision and have received positive feedback from others about the decision, we undoubtedly will show the lack of tension in our facial expressions. If we are frustrated, harassed, and distraught, our internal feelings will be apparent. We may unconsciously look at our watch when a subordinate unexpectedly comes into the office. Our fingers may dance nervously on the desk or our weight will be shifted from one foot to the next.

In his book, *Sense Relaxation,* Bernard Gunther describes nonverbal communication as follows:

Shaking hands
Your posture
Facial expressions
Your appearance
Voice tone
Hair style
Your clothes
The expression in your eyes
Your smile
How close you stand to others
How you listen
Your confidence
Your breathing . . .
The way you move
The way you stand
How you touch other people

These aspects of you affect your relationship with other people, often without you and them realizing it. . . .The body talks, its message is how you really are, not how you think you are. . . . Many in our culture reach forward from the neck because they are anxious to get ahead. Others hold their necks tight; afraid to lose their head. Body language is literal. To be depressed is, in fact, to press against yourself. To be closed off is to hold your muscles rigid against the world. Being open is being soft. Hardness is being up tight, cold, separate, giving yourself and other people a hard time. Softness is synonymous with pleasure, warmth, flow, being alive.[24]

[24] Bernard Guntner, *Sense Realization: Below Your Mind* (New York: Collier Books, 1968), pp. 90–91.

The nonverbal component in interpersonal communication is very important and will greatly influence your communication effectiveness. Psychologist Albert Mehrabian has constructed a formula to explain the emotional impact of any message: Total impact = 7 percent verbal + 38 percent vocal + 55 percent facial.[25] In other words, the impact of your messages will be related to your nonverbal cues. If you give off messages that you are nonresponsive, your colleagues may not share what is really on their minds. If you give off messages that you are relaxed, they may go into depth about a situation that they would normally rush over.

As a general rule, your colleagues will trust your nonverbal messages more than your verbal messages. The reason for this is that we have learned that people can lie verbally, but it is difficult for them to lie nonverbally. The boss who shouts with a red face, "I am *not* angry with you," will not be sending a credible message. The boss who says, "I want your advice on this matter," but then looks out of the window and appears restless when the advice is being given has communicated a double and contradictory message. On the one hand, the boss has stated that advice is wanted; on the other hand, the nonverbal cues indicate that it really isn't wanted. The nonverbal cues will be the ones that are believed. As Brooks states:

> Nonverbal cues are often used to determine the authenticity of verbal messages. Thus, the blush or the frown is likely to be taken as more reliable than the accompanying verbal reassurances. When verbal cues and the nonverbal cues tell different stories, the nonverbal story tends to be believed. Words can be chosen with care, but expressive nonverbal cues cannot be chosen. The body is not so easily governed.[26]

Because colleagues will place such a high value on the nonverbal component, it is important for administrators to make certain that the verbal messages are consistent with the nonverbal messages. When we say, "Glad you stopped by the office, George; I wish you would have come to me earlier with the problem," colleagues will make a judgement *on the basis of the nonverbal component* as to whether we are sincere. Given the fact that in face-to-face communication no more than 35 percent of the social meaning is carried in the verbal message, it is critical for an administrator to send complimentary verbal and nonverbal messages.[27]

In summary, it is very important for us as administrators to understand how our feelings and emotions are shaping our perceptions. It is equally important to be aware of how those feelings and emotions are influencing the nonverbal messages we send to colleagues.

[25] Cited in Jean Civikly, ed., *Messages: A Reader in Human Communication* (New York: Random House), p. 87.

[26] Brooks, *Speech Communication,* p. 115.

[27] Ibid., p. 101.

Being able to take time to understand the person with whom he is interacting is a third significant learning that Rogers shares with his readers.

Is it necessary to permit oneself to understand another? I think it is. Our first reaction to most of the statements which we hear from other people is an immediate evaluation, or judgment, rather than an understanding of it. When someone expresses some feeling or attitude or belief, our tendency is, almost immediately, to feel "That's right"; "That's stupid"; "That's abnormal"; "That's reasonable"; "That's incorrect"; or "That's not nice." Very rarely do we permit ourselves to *understand* precisely what the meaning of his statement is to him. I believe this is because understanding is risky. If I let myself really understand another person, I might be changed by that understanding. And we all fear change. So as I say, it is not an easy thing to permit oneself to understand an individual, to enter thoroughly and completely and emphatically into his frame of reference. It is also a rare thing.[28]

In order to understand another person, it is necessary to develop a keen ability to listen. Effective listening is often an elusive quality. Tests undertaken by Ralph G. Nichols and Leonard A. Stevens demonstrate that two months after listening to a talk, the average listener will remember only about 25 percent of what was said. "In fact, after we have barely learned something we tend to forget from one-half to one-third of it within eight hours; it is startling to realize that frequently we forget more in the first short interval than we do in the next six months."[29]

If an administrator listens poorly, it means that vital information will be lost. Decisions will be based on information that is less than adequate and additional meetings will need to be called in order to "get the facts straight." Many misunderstandings in organizations can be traced directly to the fact that the participants in the conversation were not listening to one another.

There are a number of reasons why people listen poorly. Administrators can be so preoccupied with pressing issues and problems that they are not able to concentrate on the person to whom they are speaking. If those pressing issues and problems impede the listening process, they may be classified as "psychological noise." The administrator who is meeting with the head nurse on a personnel matter but who is really thinking about a forthcoming meeting with one of the members of the board of trustees is letting psychological noise interfere with the communication process. Likewise, the administrator who is very weary and can hardly wait for the day to end may have so much noise operating that the subtle, covert problems will not be observed in the final interview of the day.

The fact that most people talk at approximately 100 to 150 words per

---

[28] Rogers, *On Becoming a Person,* p. 18.
[29] Ralph Nichols and Leonard A. Stevens, "Listening to People" in *Business and Industrial Communication* (New York: Harper & Row, 1964), p. 460.

minute but have the capacity to think at approximately 450 words per minute also impedes the listening process. If the person with whom we are visiting is not animated in conversation, or if the conversation is on an issue that is not terribly important, our minds can easily wander to more interesting thoughts and concepts.

What can be done to improve one's listening capacity? L. L. Barker gives some practical advice.[30]

First, be mentally and physically prepared to listen. The ability to "center down" and to concentrate is a prerequisite for effective listening. Telephone calls that interrupt, quick glances at the clock on the wall, or looking at some papers while the other person is talking are signals that one is not tuned in to what is being said. While interruptions are often difficult to avoid, the more you can keep your private office a quiet place where people can converse with a minimum of noise and disruption, the better you will be able to establish your credibility as one who *does* listen.

Second, think about the topic in advance when possible. This suggestion is based upon research in how people learn. If you are familiar with a topic before you attempt to learn more about it, learning will take place more efficiently and is generally longer lasting. The more you can do your "homework" before an interview, the better you will be able to discuss the issues being raised. Your knowledge about the subject will also demonstrate to the other party your sincere interest in the subject.

Third, listen for main points. It is very easy to get lost in the details of a conversation. This is particularly true if you are working with someone who "rambles" and does not stick to the topic being discussed. The more you can isolate the key elements in a conversation, the more you will be able to screen out the essential material from that which is less important.

Fourth, be flexible in your views. One of the deterrents to effective interpersonal communication is the fear that the other party will not be open to a particular point of view. If some of your views are of necessity relatively inflexible, it is important to communicate the reasons why you must stick with those views. It is also important to recognize that other contradictory views may have some merit even if you cannot give total acceptance to them. If you can approach all communicative situations with an open mind, others will be more likely to share not only information they think you want to hear, but information you may not want to hear but need to hear!

A fourth self-understanding that Rogers shares is this: "I have found it enriching to open channels whereby others can communicate their feelings, their private perceptual worlds, to me."[31] What Rogers is saying, in effect, is that he has found it personally rewarding when people share what they are feeling. Most administrators know the importance of this in their work. When

[30] Cited in Civikly, *Messages,* pp. 366–71.
[31] Rogers, *On Becoming a Person,* p. 18.

we have to guess what it is that colleagues are thinking, or when we are unsure whether they are communicating their real feelings about matters that affect the organization, it makes us feel uneasy. This is particularly true for key assistants who may be closer to the working operation of a particular unit. Administrators need to know the attitudes of subordinates concerning work-related issues. When subordinates do not share such attitudes or when the sharing is closely guarded, it puts the administrator in a difficult position because the relevant information isn't being given.

In order to help evoke attitudes and feelings, it is necessary to create an environment where those attitudes and feelings can emerge. In part, this will be facilitated with the type of listening patterns that were referred to earlier. In addition, if the administrator can determine the way in which a colleague sees a situation, this will facilitate the asking of the right questions to elicit the appropriate responses.

The importance of gaining an understanding of others' perceptions is illustrated by a situation that occurred in a large metropolitan hospital where there was constant friction between pathology and the head nurse on the medical/surgical station. Each accused the other of being inefficient. The head nurse complained that the doctors criticize her when the reports from pathology are delayed. "And they are always delayed," she stated. "It takes them forever to get their reports back here." The pathology department, on the other hand, stated that they were doing the best they could in trying to serve the entire hospital and that the medical/surgical floor would just have to wait its turn.

An administrator was called in to mediate the conflict. His first task was to determine as accurately as possible how the respective parties view the situation. As Wenberg and Wilmont point out:

> A major difficulty in communication is that each of us believes his perception is the "correct" perception and that others perceive or should be able to perceive objects and events the way we do. Nearly all of us go through life firmly convinced that we see, hear, and touch what is truly there to be seen, heard, or felt. We think of ourselves as inside observers of outside reality. This is hardly the case.[32]

Because each of us do feel that what we see and hear is the "correct" perception, it is important to understand the assumptions, values, and biases which undergird the perceptions of others. This is sometimes referred to as understanding the other person's *Weltanschauung* ("world view").

In the above example, the administrator found out that pathology was, in fact, delaying their reports and this was due to the messages that they were receiving from the medical/surgical floor which they didn't like. "We don't

[32] John R. Wenberg and William W. Wilmont, *The Personal Communication Process* (New York: John Wiley, 1973), p. 113.

like the tone of their orders," stated the pathologist. "They must think we are their errand boys. One day after some secretary called down and chewed us out about something, we decided to show them who really runs this hospital. So we delayed our reports. Now they are catching h— from the doctors!"

When the administrator talked with the nurses, however, a different picture of the situation emerged. The head nurse stated that many important messages were sent to pathology by the clerk because she was "too busy" to call the lab. The clerk in turn felt put upon because she believed she had to "do all the skut work." As a net result, the clerk conveyed an abrupt, defensive, authoritarian communication style that rankled the pathology department.

The administrator who was called in to unravel the above situation was only successful when the private perceptual world of the respective parties was revealed. Only when the administrator asks questions such as the following is the internal, private perceptual world revealed:

> On what information are the statements based? Are these factual statements or inferences? If they are inferences, how good are they?

> What factors are influencing the way in which a situation is being observed? What past experiences are influencing the way in which a situation is being seen? Are the parties *expecting* to see something happen in a given way?

The careful consideration of the background out of which statements are made will be helpful in trying to understand the meaning of the message. Through careful listening and by asking questions that try to determine the types of information, feelings, and attitudes that are behind others' assertions, the administrator creates an environment where people will be more willing to share their private, perceptual world.

The fifth learning that Rogers shares relates to our ability to accept other persons. Rogers suggests that it is increasingly common in our culture for each of us to believe that "every other person must feel and think and believe the same as I do. . . ."[33] Yet on critical issues there is usually a lack of consensus of opinion as to what those issues mean or how they should be resolved. This is particularly true when people have strong personal investments in the issues.

Dialogue rests upon the conviction that we do have different ways of looking at the world and that different perspectives should be valued. Whether we can, in fact, permit the "separateness of individuals, the right of each individual to utilize his experience in his own way and to discover his own meaning in it" will largely determine whether dialogue can take place.[34]

[33] Rogers, *On Becoming a Person,* p. 21.
[34] Ibid., p. 19.

This does not imply that we must passively tolerate all attitudes that differ from our own. It does mean that different and atypical ways of looking at issues and at solutions to the problems raised by those issues need to be valued and fairly evaluated. When different perspectives are not only permitted but encouraged an environment is created in which the quality of decision making can be strengthened. To have a wide range of information on organizational problems is a critical prerequisite for arriving at the best possible solution.

SUMMARY

Because of the close link between effective administration and interpersonal communication, it is important for the health administrator to thoroughly understand those elements that foster effective communication. This means being aware of how perceptions, attitudes, and the sending of verbal and nonverbal messages are influenced by our psychological state. It means being aware of the barriers to effective communication, and realizing how professionalism, status differences, and the fear of personal contact can inhibit working relationships. Finally, it means that as health administrators, we should carefully consider whether we have an environment conducive only to monologue instead of an environment in which dialogue can thrive. If dialogue is to thrive, we must listen, we must be accepting of those whom we meet, and our messages must be clear and consistent.

STUDY QUESTIONS

1. Identify an interpersonal conflict situation. Was the conflict due to misunderstanding, disagreement, or the transmission of misinformation? What could have prevented the problem from occurring?

2. Do you believe that it is possible to "overcommunicate" (that is, to send too much information) in an organization? Why or why not?

3. If you sensed resentment in your staff due to an unpopular decision that you made, how would you deal with the problem?

4. In this chapter we noted five "significant learnings" of Carl Rogers. Which one has particular meaning for you? Why?

ADDITIONAL READING RESOURCES

DELLINGER, SUSAN, and BARBARA DEANE, *Communicating Effectively: A Complete Guide For Better Managing.* Radnor, Pa.: Chilton Book Company, 1980.

HOPPER, ROBERT, "Speech Characteristics and Employability," *Speech Monographs,* 40 (1973), 296–302.

PATTON, BOBBY R. and KIM GIFFIN, *Interpersonal Communication in Action.* New York: Harper & Row, 1981.

PETERSON, ROBIN, "Is Self-Defensiveness Keeping You from Being a Better Manager?" *Health Services Manager,* 14, no. 1. (January 1981), 6–8.

5 Competency: Selecting, Motivating, and Evaluating Personnel

"What makes a good manager?" someone asked Yogi Berra. "A good ball club," Yogi replied.

There is something that is much more scarce, rarer than ability. It is the ability to recognize ability.

—Robert Half

OVERVIEW   The purpose of this chapter is to examine three elements of human resource management. Upon completion of this chapter the reader will be able to:

- Define three phases in the recruitment process and describe the management activities that should take place in each phase

- Define six motivational principles and outline the key concepts in (a) human need theory, (b) expectancy theory, (c) content and context theory, (d) competency theory, and (e) operant conditioning theory.

- Define four prerequisites for an effective performance appraisal system

The purpose of this chapter is to discuss three concepts in human resource management: recruitment, motivation, and evaluation of employees. We will begin by focusing on the recruitment process. The effectiveness of an organization depends largely on its ability to make a good fit between the work that needs to be accomplished and the skills possessed by those who are hired to do that work. Second, we will examine six motivational principles that will assist the administrator in creating a work environment conducive to high productivity and high morale. Finally, we will discuss various performance appraisal methods through which employees can be evaluated.

THE RECRUITMENT PROCESS

The most important resource of an organization is its employees—the people who supply the organization with their work, creativity, talent, and drive. Thus, as James A. F. Stoner notes, the most critical leadership task of a manager may be the selection, training, and development of people who will best help the organization meet its goals. "Without competent people, particularly at the managerial level, organizations will either pursue inappropriate goals or find it difficult to achieve appropriate goals once they have been set."[1]

Unfortunately, despite its importance, recruitment is usually a rather haphazard process in which the most crucial decisions are made without reliable information about either the nature of the task that has to be performed or the background and skills that an applicant would bring to the job.[2] In order to avoid the errors that result from careless hiring, the recruitment process should be divided into three distinct phases: (1) searching, (2) screening, and (3) selecting (Figure 5-1).

Searching

The initial step in the recruitment process is to make a careful analysis of the position that has been vacated. You will want to become thoroughly familiar with the existing position description. If possible, you should conduct an exit interview with the person who last held the position in order to determine the accuracy of the position description. You may find it helpful to ask the employee to list the tasks that he or she did during a typical week and to estimate the amount of time spent on each. By so doing you will be able to determine if there are discrepancies between the position description and the work as carried out by the employee.

[1] James A. F. Stoner, *Management* (Englewood Cliffs, N.J.: Prentice-Hall, Inc, 1978), p. 495.
[2] Saul Gellerman, *Motivation and Productivity* (New York: AMACOM, 1963), p. 237.

Stage 1: Searching

Analyze the position.

- Conduct exit interview with previous employee.
- Discuss position with colleagues.
- Evaluate existing position description.

Decide how to recruit in order to obtain applicants.

Announce the availability of the position.

Stage 2: Screening

Examine applicants' credentials.

Examine letters of recommendation.

Develop a list of pertinent job–related questions.

Interview promising candidates.

Stage 3: Selecting

Conduct second interview with most promising applicant(s); negotiate salary; link subsequent salary increases to performance standards.

Obtain final agreement on employment responsibilities.

Send letter with the offer of employment; stipulate position requirements, salary and fringe benefit information.

Figure 5-1   The recruitment process.

Since the requirements of a position change over time, the existing position description may be outdated. In designing a new description you may want to interview others in the organization. Most employees welcome such an initiative on the part of the administration, especially if there have been problems in working with the previous employee that need to be addressed. As you listen to others and as you analyze what needs to be accomplished, write down the most important tasks that need to be undertaken. The key question that you should answer in designing a new position description is this: "During this coming year, what output from this position would I regard as representing top performance?"

After analyzing the position, you are ready to write a formal announcement indicating the availability of the position. A position announcement usually contains (1) the title and the department in which the position is administratively located, (2) the most important functions to be performed, (3) the minimum qualifications that applicants must possess, and (4) the process to be followed if an individual wishes to apply.

At the conclusion of the position announcement you should indicate that your organization is committed to the policy that all persons have equal access to its programs, facilities, and employment without regard to race, creed, color, sex, national origin, or handicap. In addition to this statement, your organization should have a formal policy that describes the commitment of management to the recruitment and retention of women and members of minority groups. This statement should be made available to prospective employees. Goals for the recruitment of women and minorities should be established. Pronouncements of salary equity should be included in the policy and, if challenged, should be verifiable by an examination of aggregate salary data. There should also be a statement indicating the procedures to be followed for resolving complaints in the event that someone believes he or she has been discriminated against.[3]

After writing the position description you will want to determine how you are going to find qualified applicants. Phillip Marvin notes that a common mistake made by inexperienced managers is that they "ride off in all directions at once" without ascertaining where the most qualified applicants may be located.[4] As a result they may find an applicant who can do the job well, but rarely will they find the person who can do the job best.

An important issue that will influence the selection process is whether you prefer an applicant with previous work experience or one who has the potential to learn the job. Some administrators prefer applicants who have a proven track record. They argue that there is no reason for searching for potential if you can have proven performance. For them the best indicator that an applicant can do the job is that he or she has done it in the past.

Others prefer to identify individuals whose academic and work background indicate that they have the potential to assume new responsibilities. There are several arguments commonly cited in favor of such an approach. First, individuals usually do not want to make lateral moves. If they are performing competently in one setting they see little personal advantage in moving to another setting where they will be performing the same tasks. Second, most individuals at mid- and top-level management positions are men from the cultural mainstream. Regrettably, if you hire strictly on past performance, women and members of minority groups will continue to be largely ex-

---

[3] Further information on hiring procedures can be found in *Health Services Manager*, 13, no. 4 (April 1980), 2.

[4] Phillip Marvin, *The Right Man for the Job* (Homewood, Ill.: Dow Jones–Irwin, Inc., 1973), p. 7.

cluded from consideration. A final advantage of hiring on the basis of potential is that you can serve as a mentor helping new employees develop their talents. Some administrators consider this one of the most rewarding aspects of their jobs.

After determining whether you would like to recruit for experience or potential you will want to determine how you are going to recruit. There are valid reasons for engaging in a nationwide search, particularly if you are recruiting for a top-level manager. A nationwide search usually yields a large pool of applicants. The applicants, because they are coming to interview from diverse occupational settings, will probably give you new insights into the tasks that need to be performed. A nationwide search also generates valuable publicity, particularly if the position description is creatively written.

In undertaking a nationwide search you will want to send the position announcement to major institutions that employ the type of people who might be attracted to your organization. You will also want to place well-written ads in major journals. In selecting the most appropriate journal you will want to inquire about the journal's circulation, including the occupational groupings of people who subscribe to it. Most editors will provide such information upon request.

Some organizations, such as IBM, General Foods, and Proctor and Gamble, have a policy of recruiting and promoting from within the organization except in very unusual circumstances. There are three major advantages of this policy. First, it is often less expensive to recruit or promote from within than to hire from outside. Second, a promotion from within policy often fosters a feeling of loyalty among employees. Finally, individuals recruited from within understand the organization's culture and may therefore perform more effectively.[5]

There are, of course, some disadvantages to recruiting from within your ranks. Unless you are a large organization such as IBM, you will probably have a small group of applicants upon which to draw. In addition, by recruiting from within you are creating a type of inbreeding that eliminates people from the outside who have the potential to bring creative insights into your operations.

Screening

The screening phase of the recruitment process is designed to winnow from the pool of applicants the very best person for the job. An announcement indicating the availability of a position will usually produce a number of applications. Those who do not meet the minimum requirements should be informed of that fact in writing so that they can look for other career oppor-

[5] Stoner, *Management*, p. 495.

tunities. The credentials of the remaining applicants should be carefully reviewed by thoroughly examining the written materials.

Most prospective employers request three types of resource materials including a letter stating why the applicant is interested in the position, a résumé containing a detailed work history, and usually two or three supporting letters of recommendation. As you begin to review the application materials you should note how the materials have been prepared. If they were written in a haphazard way you can probably deduce that the individual either isn't very interested in the position or else has only limited writing abilities.

Two criteria are commonly used in evaluating the letters of recommendation. The first is the thoroughness with which the letter has been prepared. A brief letter with little descriptive material will have little value. On the other hand, a letter that documents the applicant's work experience and the strengths and weaknesses that he or she would bring to the position is worthy of serious study. If the letter gives you insights into the person's educational background, work skills, personality traits, communication skills, and future work goals, it may prove to be a valuable resource in the evaluation process.

The second criteria to be used in evaluating letters of recommendation is the credibility of the author. If the author has been in a position to evaluate the applicant's work, you probably will want to weigh the contents carefully. Remember that, while it is helpful to learn about the applicant's character, it is equally important to know how the applicant *performed* in past jobs. Performance is your goal. Any comments that shed light on that goal should be noted.

The next step in the screening process is to invite several of the most promising candidates to your office for an initial interview. There are four commonly made errors that you will want to avoid as you interview these applicants:

1. Lack of preparation
2. Failure to probe
3. Convoluted or overdefined questions
4. Failure to translate answers into likely
   behavior in on-the-job situations

You can prepare yourself for the interview by carefully rereading the application materials. You should be thoroughly familiar with the applicant's educational background and work experience. The letters of recommendation should be carefully reread and notations made concerning information that needs elaboration. After reviewing the application materials you should make a list of specific questions that you want to ask in the interview.

The failure to probe is one of the basic problems that causes interviews to be shallow and incomplete. As we will soon see, you should ask many types of questions and give applicants ample opportunity to question you concerning the nature of the job. Your answers to questions raised will give applicants information that will help them determine whether they are interested in the position. The type of questions applicants ask also gives you some understanding of the values they would bring to the work environment.

There are certain questions that you should avoid asking. The Civil Rights Act of 1964 prohibits inquiries on marital status, credit history, homeownership, or previous arrests. It is also illegal to inquire about an applicant's religion, race, or age. The key consideration in determining what you can and cannot ask is *whether the inquiry is job related.* If it is, it probably is legally defensible. Robert Fjerstad, who has been in personnel work for twenty years, summarized the 1964 Civil Rights Act as "the best thing that ever happened to the personnel profession . . . It brought us to the premise that everything we do in personnel should be job-related and valid. It has made us back up and say, 'What is the job-related reason for asking this question?' If there is none, then you don't need to know."[6]

One problem frequently seen in interview situations is the asking of convoluted or overdefined questions. "Too many interviewers," states Ken Metzler, a well-known authority in the science of interviewing, "make bad speeches rather than ask precise questions."[7] Don't ask two questions in one sentence. Be precise. Know what kinds of information you need in evaluating the applicant.

The failure to translate answers into likely behavior in on-the-job situations is perhaps the most serious mistake that an interviewer can make. When this happens the interviewer may end up having a lot of information about the applicant but little understanding of the applicant's ability to do the job. For example, let's assume that you are hiring an assistant hospital administrator. You have two applicants that appear to hold exceptional promise. Both have an advanced degree in management. Their college records indicate a high scholastic ability. Both have distinguished themselves in extracurricular activities. The letters of recommendation for each are positive. Each seems articulate and ambitious. How, in light of the similarity, are you going to make a decision? What distinguishes one candidate from another?

The differences between two candidates who seem equally qualified may not be evident in the facts concerning their background and work experience. Rather, the differences will be seen in how and why they achieved their accomplishments. To illustrate, consider this exchange between Mary Brady, a chief executive officer at the Edina Community Hospital who is interviewing Jim Donaldson for the position of assistant hospital administrator.

---

[6] Quoted in Judith Willis, "What to Ask a Job Applicant," *The Minneapolis Star,* February 15, 1980, p. 10. Reprinted with permission. All rights reserved.

[7] Ken Metzler, *Creative Interviewing* (Englewood Cliffs, N.J.: Prentice-Hall, Inc., 1977), p. 6.

Brady: What subjects did you enjoy most in your graduate program?

Donaldson: Well, I really enjoyed my financial management course and the work I took in statistics.

The above information contributes little to an understanding of the applicant's on-the-job behavior. However, if Brady were to probe further to determine why the applicant had an interest in financial management or statistics it may give her an understanding of those work activities that would prove to be most interesting to him.

Brady: What do you think it was about the financial management and statistics courses that made them so enjoyable?

Donaldson: What I liked most about them was that there was one right answer. It wasn't like the courses in organizational behavior, where there were a lot of theories. With statistics you know that there is one answer and when you got it you were correct.

The above answer gives important clues about the applicant in terms of the job environment. It appears that he is relatively uncomfortable with ambiguity and functions best in an environment where there are clearcut expectations and answers to problems. By focused probing, Brady was able to learn something valuable about the applicant.

In order to conduct an effective job interview you may find it helpful to divide the interview into four stages.[8] In the first stage, you should tell the applicant why he or she has been asked to the interview situation. You might say, for example: "Thank you for coming here today. As you know we are looking for a director of nursing. You have come highly recommended and I thought it might be helpful to meet and explore our mutual interests." Such a statement helps the interviewee become comfortable and also conveys your interest in the applicant.

In the second stage you should outline the nature of the position: "The dirctor of nursing is responsible for all nursing services within the hospital and in our community clinic. The director is responsible for 14 head nurses who employ a staff of 210 registered nurses. The director of nursing has line responsibilities for managing the nursing budget and is a voting member of the five-person executive committee. The director reports to the chief executive officer of the hospital. The position pays $28,500 per year. We hope to find a director by September 1st."

After completing the description take a moment to see if there are ques-

[8] Modified from John D. Drake, *Interviewing for Managers* (New York: AMACOM, 1972), p. 19.

tions the applicant would like to ask. A clear understanding of the nature of the work to be performed is basic if misunderstandings are to be prevented.

In the third stage you will want to focus inquiries on technical, conceptual, and interpersonal issues. The *technical* issues relate to the applicant's background and work experience. You may want to find out about the applicant's academic background including major course pursuits. With applicants who have been out of school for a period of time you will probably want to find out how they have continued their education. You will want to inquire about their work experience including the job functions they have performed. You can find out about their interests, values, and skills by asking them what they feel they can do particularly well. They may reply that they are effective in managing people, solving conflicts, long-term planning, financial management, institutional relationships, or other areas. If you follow up by asking why they are effective in those areas you will begin to get solid technical information about their capabilities.

Conceptual issues relate to an applicant's ability to use his or her knowledge to resolve on-the-job problems. One way of examining the conceptual ability of applicants is to give them a current problem that you are facing and ask what they think could be done about it. Consider the following exchange between Mr. Britmore, an administrator who is interviewing candidates for the position of director of nursing, and Ms. Kendall, who is applying for the position:

Britmore: We are having difficulty retaining nurses. Nursing turnover in our hospital is currently over 50 percent a year. Frankly, we have not done a good job in resolving this problem. Do you have any suggestions as to how to solve this difficulty?

Kendall: That's a problem many hospitals are having. I suppose that before one should speculate about what could be done it would be important to find out from the nurses themselves why they are quitting.

Britmore: You mean that you would want to interview former employees?

Kendall: Well, probably not. But I would want each head nurse to conduct an exit interview so that we can identify the reasons for the resignations.

The above sequence would take less than a minute to complete. Yet in that minute Britmore would have learned some valuable information about the applicant. On the basis of what she said it would appear that (1) Kendall does not give snap answers to a problem; (2) she understands the concept of a line organization as reflected in the fact that she would ask the head nurses to conduct the exit interviews; (3) she is familar with a contemporary problem that would have to be addressed in her role as director of nursing; and finally,

(4) she has at least one process that could be followed in resolving the problem.

An applicant may have good technical and conceptual skills, but to be effective on the job he or she must also have skills in *interpersonal* relations. Some administrators trust their intuitive instincts in evaluating an individual's communication ability. They either like the "chemistry" or they don't. However the issue is much too important to be determined by "gut feel." The issue of interpersonal relationships within complex organizations should be discussed openly and candidly by asking questions such as the following:

If you have a difference of opinion with someone, how do you handle it?

How do you get along with your colleagues at your present job?

If you had a disagreement with your supervisor, what would you do?

How do you think your subordinates see you?

If you could speculate about your ideal supervisor, what characteristics would he or she have?

In what ways do you think committees help or hinder an organization?

In the fourth stage of the interview process you will want to gain closure about what will be done in the future concerning the position. You have an obligation to inform the applicant about the next step in the process: "We will call you by July 15th concerning your application. If at that time you would like to continue to be considered and we are in agreement to pursue employment with you, we would then like to have a second interview. At that interview you would have opportunity to meet with the members of the executive committee of the hospital. In the meantime, if you have any questions about the position or about what we discussed today, please call me."

It is appropriate for you to contact individuals who have written letters of recommendation. While you are not under a legal responsibility to do so, it is considered a courtesy to ask whether the applicant would mind if you followed up their references with a personal visit or a telephone call.

Selecting

After the initial interviews have been completed you will want to ask one or two applicants to return for a second visit. The purpose of the second visit is to discuss in greater depth the specific responsibilities of the position and to ascertain the individual's interest in moving to your organization.

Some administrators find it helpful to have other members of the management team meet with the applicant. Everyone seems to benefit from this approach. The applicant benefits by gaining insights from others about the work that needs to be done. Colleagues benefit because they feel that they have input into the hiring process. You, as the employer benefit, because colleagues will give you information about the applicant that you may not have been able to retrieve.

When involving others in the hiring process you should make clear that, while you want their input, you will make the decision as to who will be hired. This maintains your authority and clearly outlines your expectations.

Once you have determined to make an offer to someone it is customary to personally contact and inform the applicant that a letter of invitation will be arriving within a week. Such person-to-person contact will convey your interest in the person and your willingness to further discuss the position if he or she so desires.

Once having received a written offer, the applicant may wish to negotiate working conditions. This is a normal and acceptable practice and should not be perceived to mean that the applicant is being "difficult" or "disloyal." A common point of negotiation is salary. If that is a non-negotiable issue you should clearly state that in the very earliest stages of the interview process.

Setting salaries is a difficult challenge and one that is worthy of considerable thought.[9] Social scientists who have examined the concept of salary equity have arrived at two important conclusions. First, the compensation that you offer an applicant should be equitable. You should be able to document that individuals are being paid at a rate that is at least as much as their peers. Second, the salary that is offered should be *perceived* as equitable by the prospective employee. The easiest way to demonstrate equity is to give the employee aggregate salary information for their peers. For example, if you were hiring a director of nursing you might say: "You may wonder how we arrived at a salary of $28,500 for this position. Here is a study done by the State Hospital Association on professional salaries. The average salary of nursing directors within hospitals with 300–400 beds is $28,114.00."

It is important when setting a salary figure to recognize that there is a correlation between work satisfaction and the wage an individual is given. You may find it helpful in creating a good work environment to pay your employees slightly more than what their peers earn in other institutions. On the other hand, if you underpay your employees by more than 10 percent it is likely that they will be sufficiently dissatisfied that they will act to get their compensation boosted. If your underpayment is perceived to be closer to 20 percent, it is likely that you will have significant dissatisfaction and the potential for high job turnover.[10]

It is possible that the applicant will ask how future salary increases will

---

[9] Malcolm S. Salter, "What is 'Fair Pay' for the Executive?" *Harvard Business Review,* May-June 1972, p. 1.
[10] Ibid.

be determined. If that question is asked you should be prepared to outline the method that is used for arriving at cost-of-living salary increases and/or merit salary increases. Whatever method you may use, it should be based upon the fact that pay is clearly correlated with individual performance. Any policy that links pay to performance will usually be welcomed by individuals applying for management positions.[11]

THE MOTIVATIONAL PROCESS

The motivational levels of newly employed staff members are generally quite high. Most want to be perceived as competent workers who can contribute to the organization. If they are rewarded for their accomplishments, there may be little reason to be concerned about their level of motivation.

However, as Robert N. Ford has noted, many positions have inherent within them a "natural job decay."[12] Consider the comments of an assistant health commissioner working within a metropolitan health agency:

> I came to this department as soon as I received my MPH degree. I was really excited about the position. I like health planning and most of my job was going to be in that area. Everyone seemed so friendly when I arrived. Even my boss took me out for lunch the first day. But one year later everything turned sour. The politics of health planning is unbelievable. The state hospital association was mad at me for suggesting that the city had too many hospital beds. The head of health planning called me "gutless" for not stipulating how many beds were "too much." Then when the chips were down and when I really needed support my boss wouldn't back me up. There are times when I wonder whether I'm in the right job.

Job dissatisfaction is not uncommon among American workers. In fact, three national surveys conducted by the Survey Research Center at the University of Michigan have concluded that "The decline in job satisfaction has been pervasive, effecting virtually all demographic and occupational classes tested."[13] Symbolic of the dissatisfaction is the fact that 34 percent of those interviewed in the national surveys indicated that they would make a genuine effort to find a new job with another employer during the coming year.[14]

The symptoms of job dissatisfaction are identifiable. The quantity of output diminishes as does the quality. The worker's initial optimism about the

[11] Ibid.

[12] Robert N. Ford, "The Obstinate Employee," *Psychology Today,* November 1969, p. 38.

[13] Graham L. Staines and Robert P. Quinn, "American Workers Evaluate the Quality of their Jobs," *Monthly Labor Review,* January 1979, p. 4.

[14] Ibid.

organization gives way to "realism" which often reflects pessimism and cynicism. If the problems creating the work dissatisfaction are not corrected it is likely that absenteeism will increase. Finally, if workers become completely dissatisfied they may quit—often blaming their employer for their frustrations.

Many workers who assume a new position undergo a transition period in which they question their aspirations as well as their place of employment. They may recognize that their personal goals are not congruent with organizational reality. At times the obstacles that are in the way of success are more formidable than what was originally perceived.

While it may be a natural process for a worker to undergo a transition period, it is important for the worker to remain optimally productive. But how do you keep a staff member operating at high levels of performance? What can be done to keep the worker highly motivated and committed to the goals of the organization?

Few concepts in management have been studied as closely as the concept of human motivation. We will examine six motivational principles that appear to be basic in achieving high levels of worker productivity (Figure 5-2).

Principle 1: Workers are motivated by different needs.

We will begin our discussion on the motivational process by focusing on the concept of "unsatisfied need." We do so because human need theory is one of the most widely quoted and applied approaches to human motivation within organizational settings. In addition, this approach is the foundation upon which other theories are based.

While there are a number of individuals who have contributed to human need theory (including Abraham Maslow, Clayton P. Alderfer, and Edward E. Wawler III), we will focus attention on the work of David McClelland. We do so because efforts to validate his research and conclusions have met with

Principle 1:   Workers are motivated by different needs.

Principle 2:   Productive workers perceive a strong relationship between doing their job well and receiving rewards that they value.

Principle 3:   Motivation levels are influenced by the work content (intrinsic factors) and the work context (extrinsic factors).

Principle 4:   The pursuit of competence is a powerful motivator.

Principle 5:   The consequences of a worker's behavior will shape future behavior.

Principle 6:   Workers respond more positively to supervisors who are "employee oriented" than to those who are "task oriented."

Figure 5-2 Principles of human motivation.

reasonable success and also because his approach is easily transferable to organizational settings.[15]

McClelland states that there are three basic needs that all humans possess to one degree or another.

> *Achievement*—the need to excel, to achieve in relation to a set of standards, to strive, to succeed
>
> *Power*—the need to make others behave in a way they would not have behaved otherwise
>
> *Affiliation*—the desire for friendly and close relationships[16]

Achievement motivation is rooted in a desire to make a contribution to the organization. Individuals who have a high need to achieve will usually set demanding goals ("I'm going to double this budget during the next fiscal year"). They work hard as reflected in the fact that high achievers may put in sixty, seventy, or more hours of work a week. They like new challenges and often deliberately seek out situations where there may be an element of risk or even failure. While they do not like to fail, they like even less the situation where failure is not a possibility.

McClelland has noted that managers who have a high need to achieve usually share the following characteristics:

1. They eagerly take responsibility for solving problems.
2. They place high importance on receiving concrete feedback as to how well they are doing.
3. They will take calculated risks providing they see the challenge in the situation and the possibility of winning.[17]

While some individuals are motivated by the need to achieve, others are motivated by the need to obtain and exercise power. While the power motivator has not traditionally been associated with the context of motivating workers in organizations, there has been an increased awareness in recent years that it probably is one of the most important of all motivators.[18]

To illustrate its importance consider the frequent personnel changes occurring during the past ten years at the Columbia Broadcasting System (CBS). The changes in the presidency of that institution reflect the need to maintain balances of power within the corporate structure. The Watergate crisis in the 1970s was sparked by individuals whose power motivations were so strong that abuses resulted. All contemporary political revolutions, whether they be in a third-world country or in a small community in rural America, have as

---

[15] David C. McClelland, *The Achieving Society* (New York: Van Nostrand Reinhold), 1961.

[16] Ibid., p. 114.

[17] Stoner, *Management,* p. 417.

[18] David C. McClelland and David H. Burnham, "Power is the Great Motivator," *Harvard Business Review,* March–April 1976, pp. 100–110.

their foundation a struggle for power between those who have it and those who don't.

The need to obtain and exercise power is one of the wellsprings of human motivation. In fact, Clayton Reeser and Marvin Loper have found in their research on executives in large corporations that top managers must possess a high need for power, that is, a concern for influencing people. They noted, however, that the need to obtain power must be disciplined and must be directed toward the benefit of the institution as a whole and not toward the manager's personal aggrandizement.[19]

Managers with high power needs generally share the following characteristics:

1. They desire to make an impact; they want to see tangible results for their efforts.
2. They desire to be influential and, in particular, want to influence others.
3. They enjoy being "in charge."
4. They place higher priority in gaining influence over others and gaining personal prestige than they do in effective performance.[20]

The third need that McClelland identified is the need for affiliation. Of the three needs, this one has received the least attention from researchers. Yet it is generally agreed that the need for close interpersonal relationships in the work setting often serves as a motivator.

A classic example that is used to illustrate the power of affiliation needs is seen in an organization that hired a systems analyst to determine what could be done to heighten productivity. After an organizational review the analyst rearranged all the desks in the offices in such a way that productivity would greatly increase. In the process, however, he severely restricted the employees' ability to communicate with one another. Consequently productivity decreased. The analyst did not understand the affiliation needs of these workers.[21]

Managers with high affiliation needs generally share the following characteristics:

1. They search for meaningful friendships in the work setting.
2. They place high priority on working in a humane environment which they define as one where there is an absence of interpersonal conflict.
3. They are more interested in building high morale than high productivity.
4. They do not like to make decisions that go against the norms of their peer group.
5. They value being respected by subordinates.

[19] Clayton Reeser and Marvin Loper, *Management* (Glenview, Ill.: Scott, Foresman, 1978), p. 303.
[20] Robbins, *Organizational Behavior,* p. 116.
[21] Terrence R. Mitchell, *People in Organizations: Understanding Their Behavior* (New York: McGraw-Hill, 1978), p. 156.

McClelland's research into human needs has several implications for individuals in management positions. First, it is important that there be a good interface between an employee's psychological structure and the functions that need to be performed. The old adage "Select the right person for the right job" is empirically valid. The more a position enables an individual to meet his or her psychological needs, the more committed the individual will be to his or her work. If you are searching for a new staff member who will be responsible for achieving several well-defined objectives, then you probably want to employ someone with high achievement needs. High achievers respond positively to work environments in which the scope of responsibility is limited to several important functions. If you are seeking an assistant who could "clean out the dead wood in the organization" you probably want someone with high power needs. Making an impact and controlling the actions of others are high priorities for individuals with such needs. If you want to build morale, you probably want to hire an individual who has high affiliation needs providing that they also have a commitment to obtaining high levels of productivity.

The second implication of McClelland's findings is that it is important to delegate tasks that elicit enthusiasm of employees. You would not want to assign dull, simple, and uncomplicated tasks to high achievers for they would soon begin to feel that they are underutilized. Nor would you ask a manager with high affiliation needs to make decisions that would alienate peers. Rather, you would want individuals with high power needs to be assigned responsibilities that are formidable and challenging and you would want those with high affiliation needs to undertake tasks that hold promise for recognition. By constructing a good fit between the psychological needs of the worker and the tasks that need to be undertaken, you have created conditions conducive to high motivation and productivity.

You may rightly inquire as to how one should recognize such needs. How do you know whether an individual is motivated by achievement, power, or affiliation? The answer, in part, is to ask pertinent questions when individuals are interviewing for a position. Consider the following questions:

"If you could design an ideal job, how would it appear?" The answer to this question will give you information as to how much they have thought about work within the context of their values. It may also tell you about their level of aspiration: Do they see this job as a step to other positions? Do they want "big jobs"? Do they want to work independently? Do they like routine tasks? Do they want to be involved in policy issues?

"Do you like to work on many tasks or do you prefer to work on two or three major projects?" This question may tell you the degree to which they are achievement versus power motivated. High achievers usually

prefer to limit the number of tasks on which they are working ("I like to do a few things well") while power-oriented workers like to be assigned many tasks ("The more things going on the better I like it").

"Do you prefer working alone or with others?" Individuals high in affiliation will report that they enjoy working with others ("I'm a team player"); individuals who have high achievement needs will enjoy working with others if it helps them meet their own goals ("Committees work well when members give you information you don't already have"); individuals with high power needs usually prefer to work alone due to the fact they they don't believe in shared authority ("When I finish a task I like to know that it is something that I have accomplished").

"Do you like to take on projects where there is high visibility and a risk of failure, but also a chance for recognition if you succeed?" Individuals with high achievement needs would likely ask for clarification of how much risk is involved; individuals with high needs for power would enthusiastically respond in the affirmative while individuals who have high affiliation needs might reply: "Well, if something like that was assigned to me I would do it, but I would want to know that I had the support of the administration if I ran into problems."

Once an individual has been hired you should periodically examine the fit between the worker and the job. Perhaps the best indicator of whether the interface between psychological needs and work is a good one is reflected in the quality of work that is produced. If the subordinate's work is of high quality you can reasonably assume that the fit is satisfactory. If the caliber of work consistently declines, the subordinate is sending you a message that the work is not meeting his or her needs for power, achievement and/or affiliation.

Principle 2: Productive workers perceive a strong relationship between doing their job well and receiving rewards that they value.

Expectancy theory suggests that the strength of a tendency to act in a certain way is dependent on the strength of an expectation that the act will be followed by a given outcome that the individual perceives to be attractive. Three variables form the basis of this approach to human motivation: attractiveness, performance-reward linkage, and effort-performing linkage.[22]

Victor Vroom defines expectancy as an action-outcomes-association.[23] It is a belief on the part of the worker that a certain action will result in a par-

---

[22] Stephen P. Robbins, *The Administrative Process* (Englewood Cliffs, N.J.: Prentice-Hall, Inc., 1980), p. 301.

[23] Victor H. Vroom, *Work and Motivation* (New York: John Wiley, 1964), p. 483.

ticular outcome. *Attractiveness* has to do with something that one does not now have but would like to have in the future. It may be a promotion, a merit salary increase, the chairmanship of a committee, a lateral transfer to another department, or even a change in jobs or career.

Performance-reward linkage might be defined as the individual's perception that if he or she takes certain actions it will lead to a desired reward. The outcome can take on a mathmatical value from zero, which is an absolute belief that no outcome will result from an action, to +1, which represents complete certainty that an outcome will follow a particular event.[24] An x-ray technician who believes that longevity in the organization automatically results in a promotion would have a +1 expectancy. On the other hand, if she believes that those technicians who are better educated than herself will receive promotions, she might have a zero expectancy.

Effort-performing linkage might be defined as the worker's perception that a desired reward is worth the effort necessary to achieve it. If a custodian knows that it is possible to obtain a $500 bonus he might first examine the attractiveness of that sum of money ("I sure could use it right now to fix up the house.") Subsequently, he would determine what kinds of work he would have to do to ensure that he received that bonus ("I'd probably have to work the dog shift, keep my coffee breaks brief, and quit talking back to my boss"). Finally he would make a decision about what action he would take by making an assessment of whether the goal is worth the effort[25] ("Five hundred bucks isn't worth working any dog shifts").

There are several important implications for management that arise out of expectancy theory. First, the degree of commitment that workers bring to their jobs will be determined by their perceptions as to whether they can accomplish what has been assigned. If a subordinate has twelve major tasks it is unlikely that he can complete all twelve at the same level of quality. Confronted with twelve tasks the worker will tend to undertake those which he knows can be accomplished.

Second, expectancy theory suggests that workers will expend energy on those tasks that they perceive will result in some personal benefit. This implies that if you are unhappy with how subordinates are spending their time you may want to focus on what they perceive to be the rewards for what they are undertaking. For example, if a financial controller believes that he will receive recognition from the hospital administrator for controlling costs it is likely that he will fight hard to trim expenses even at the risk of alienating various hospital constituencies. On the other hand, if the comptroller believes that hospital administrators come and go but that chiefs of staff stay around

[24] Richard M. Steers and Lyman W. Porter, *Motivation and Work* (New York: McGraw-Hill, 1975), p. 221.
[25] Adapted from Robbins, *Organizational Behavior,* pp. 130–31.

forever, it is likely that he will perceive that his rewards will come from the hospital physicians. If that this is the case, whatever cost-saving trimming that might be done will carefully circumvent the interests of the physicians.

William Howell's observation that "People do things for their reasons, not yours,"[26] aptly sums up the third implication of expectancy theory. Everyone is motivated differently. What motivates one person will not necessarily incite others to action. Expectancy theory reminds us as managers that workers will not necessarily respond to *our* motivations, lofty and important as they may seem. Rather, they will respond to their own motivations.

Over fifty studies have confirmed the validity of the expectancy-theory approach to motivation.[27] As the theory predicts, the workers who perform best in an organization have clear performance goals that they know can be performed. They also see a strong relationship between doing their job well and receiving rewards that they value.

Principle 3: Motivation levels are influenced by the work content (intrinsic factors) and the work context (extrinsic factors).

One of the most intriguing theories of motivation has been proposed by Frederick Herzberg.[28] The focal point of Herzberg's research was to answer the question "What do people want from their jobs?" He requested workers to describe situations when they felt particularly good or bad about their jobs. Their responses were carefully recorded and are summarized in Figure 5–3.

According to Herzberg, organizational rewards can be listed under two broad categories which are called the "hygienes" and the "motivators."

HYGIENES (EXTRINSIC FACTORS)	MOTIVATORS (INTRINSIC FACTORS)
1. Company policy and administration	1. Achievement
2. Supervision	2. Recognition
3. Relationship with supervisor	3. Work itself
4. Work conditions	4. Responsibility
5. Salary	5. Advancement
6. Relationship with peers	6. Growth
7. Personal life	
8. Relationship with subordinates	
9. Status	
10. Security	

[26] E. Bormann, W. Howell, R. Nichols, and G. Shapiro, *Interpersonal Communication in the Modern Organization* (New York: Holt, Rinehart & Winston, 1969), p. 224.

[27] Steers and Porter, *Motivation and Work*, p. 220.

[28] F. Herzberg, B. Mausner, and B. Synderman, *The Motivation to Work* (New York: John Wiley, 1959).

Herzberg's research led him to conclude that the hygienes (extrinsic factors) are primarily related to job dissatisfaction while the motivators (intrinsic factors) are primarily related to job satisfaction. Herzberg stated that if an employee had all the hygiene factors present at an acceptable level it would produce a *neutral* feeling about the job. That is, the employee would neither feel particularly satisfied or particularly dissatisfied. If the hygienes were at an unacceptable level, job dissatisfaction would likely result. If managers wanted to develop a highly motivated work staff, said Herzberg, they should focus not only on the hygienes but on the motivators, which are the true initiators to action. If there is adequate recognition, responsibility, advancement, and room for achievement the typical worker will be highly motivated and productive.

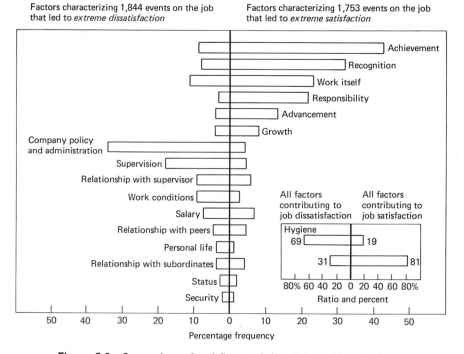

Figure 5-3 Comparison of satisfiers and dissatisfiers. [Reprinted by permission of the Harvard Business Review. An exhibit from "One More Time: How Do You Motivate Employees?" by Frederick Herzberg (*Harvard Business Review*, January-February, 1968), p. 57. Copyright © 1968 by the President and Fellows of Harvard College; all rights reserved.]

This model of motivation has become popular with managers because it has sharpened the focus on what motivates employees. Historically organizations have spent huge sums of money in training and development efforts that sought to strengthen the hygienes. Herzberg's research put up a warning flag which said in effect: All the energy you put into making the hygiene factors more conducive to meeting employee needs will, at best, only result in a neutral reaction by the employees. Therefore, if you seek to eliminate those factors that create job dissatisfaction you may bring about peace, but you will not necessarily bring about motivation.[29] The net result of this insight is that training programs are now emphasizing those management activities that will strengthen the motivators. The contemporary willingness of management to have workers involved in planning and controlling their work can be largely attributed to Herzberg's findings and recommendations.[30]

While Herzberg's research has thrown new light on what motivates employees it should be noted that the "motivation-maintenance theory," as it is often referred to, is not without its detractors. There are some who have questioned Herzberg's methodology. For example, when employees like what they do they credit themselves (motivators) but when the job does not go well they blame the environment (hygienes). The reliability of the research has also been questioned. The raters who examined the data had to make interpretations and the findings may have been contaminated by such interpretations. Nevertheless, Herzberg's theory has been widely utilized and his findings appear to be consistent with general surveys of worker opinions about what they want from their work in nationwide polls conducted in the 1970s by the National Opinion Research Center.[31]

What practical use does the motivator-maintenance model have for health administrators? First, if you want to have a highly motivated staff, effort must be made to have a reasonably satisfactory work environment (hygiene factors). You will have difficulty convincing an employee that the work should be a reward in and of itself if the wages are perceived to be considerably below what other individuals with equal training and work experience are receiving. The current issue about nursing salaries is a case in point. Consider the comments made by a nurse:

> A highly trained nurse in a neonatal unit may make $12,584 a year. Think about that salary in terms of what other people in society are making. And then think about her responsibilities. If she makes even the slightest error in a medication

[29] Robbins, *Organizational Behavior,* p. 124.

[30] Ibid., p. 125.

[31] Ibid., pp. 124–25.

schedule, the baby could be a vegetable for the rest of his life. And the state could end up paying a million dollars for the care that person would need over a lifetime. [32]

The principle that the hygiene factors must be reasonably satisfied if employees are to be optimally productive cuts across occupational lines. You can give a great deal of recognition to the hospital dietitians, yet if they have little status or security within the hospital it is unlikely that they will be highly motivated. What good is it to give a pat on the back if the basic desire for a decent work environment is not being met?

The second implication of Herzberg's research is that if you can provide opportunities for growth, additional responsibility, and advancement, it is likely that the employees will be highly motivated. To provide such opportunities is to "enrich" those positions where employees have the potential to assume additional responsibility.

Job enrichment is the "deliberate upgrading of responsibility, scope, and challenge in work." [33] It is based upon a philosophical premise that most workers' talents and abilities are not adequately utilized in contemporary organizations. It is also based on a belief that most workers want to have new responsibilities and opportunities for growth.

An example of job enrichment is illustrated in the experience of a plant supervisor. Upon taking his job he found that fifteen janitors reported to him directly. There was no foreman to supervise these individuals. One day the new supervisor was looking at the files of each of these janitors and discovered that the former plant supervisor had made negative notations about each of them on their performance review form. The janitors were characterized as being lazy, unreliable, and generally unmotivated.

The new supervisor was determined to do something about the situation and called a meeting of the fifteen men. He started the meeting by saying that he realized that there were a number of housekeeping problems that had existed for years but that he didn't know how to solve them. Since the janitors were the experts in the housekeeping area he asked if they could work together and try to resolve the difficulties. A deadly silence resulted. Seeing that there was no response he sat down and said nothing for almost twenty minutes. Finally one of the janitors told about a problem he was having in his area of responsibility and made a suggestion. Soon the others told about the way they would solve the problem and eventually there was a lively discussion while the superintendent wrote down all the ideas.

Judging from the way the janitors responded the superintendent realized that they had the ability to resolve many of the difficulties his department was

[32] Robert L. Veninga and James P. Spradley, *The Work/Stress Connection: How to Cope with Job Burnout* (Boston: Little, Brown and Co., 1981), p. 248.
[33] Paul Hersey and Kenneth Blanchard, *Management of Organizational Behavior* (Englewood Cliffs, N.J.: Prentice-Hall, Inc., 1977), p. 70.

having. As a routine procedure he then began sending any housekeeping problem to the janitors for their review. For example, when the salesmen for the various cleaning and supply companies came to the organization the superintendent did not visit with them but asked the janitors to do so. In fact, the janitors were given an office so that they could meet with the salesmen. Regular meetings were also set up so that the entire group of fifteen individuals could meet and resolve the problems they were experiencing.

All of this activity on the part of the superintendent had a tremendous influence on the behavior of the janitors. They became a cohesive, work-oriented team that took pride in its work. Their appearances also changed. Prior to the job enrichment activities they appeared a grubby lot. Now they came to work clean and well kept and looked like they were anticipating the work that had to be done. Interestingly the superintendent was continually stopped by other administrators and asked, "What have you done to those lazy, good-for-nothing janitors, given them pep pills?" Even the superintendent was amazed at what was happening. It was not uncommon to see the janitors running floor tests to see which agent was cleaner or which one did the best job. If they were going to make the decisions about which supplies to purchase they had to make certain that they knew which one was the best.

It is important to note that none of these activities detracted from their work. It is true that the janitors took on additional responsibilities but they worked harder and more efficiently than ever before.[34]

The third implication of Herzberg's research is the understanding that objectives that *make sense to the worker* will be the ones that will motivate the individuals to high levels of productivity. When you delegate tasks to others you should explain both the importance of the task and the reasons why these particular workers were selected for undertaking the project.

To illustrate this process, consider the task of hospital incident reporting. The tabulation of incidents that are harmful to patients is usually a tedious, time-consuming, and thankless job. However, it is an important task since litigation usually centers on one or more "critical incidents." When a hospital administrator assigns responsibility to a staff member for coordinating the incident reporting system, that staff member may only grudgingly accept the responsibility. This is especially true if the task is portrayed as "something that has to be done by someone." However, if the hospital administrator genuinely believes that incident reporting is a way to prevent harmful problems from occurring and that the task is so important that the person responsible should be given the authority to resolve damaging problems, then the probability increases that the task will be competently and enthusiastically undertaken.

---

[34] Illustration modified from ibid.

Principle 4: The pursuit of competence is a powerful motivator.

One of the newest theories of motivation has been proposed by Edward L. Deci.[35] Deci's theory expands our knowledge in that it highlights the concept of "competence" as a principal motivator.

Deci has built on Herzberg's work which differentiates extrinsic and intrinsic factors. Deci states that intrinsic motives are those activities for which there is not apparent reward other than the activity itself. Deci suggests that children and adults seek out novel experience in which the only reward for doing an acitivity is the act itself. The infant will crawl towards a television set because of the blinking lights. The crawling might involve a considerable struggle for the infant but there is something inherently enjoyable in moving towards the strange patterns in a lighted box. A child will climb a tree for the simple joy that comes from scaling new heights. Likewise an adult who has never water-skied might attempt it even though there may be doubt that the effort will result in success.

Deci stated that most people will actively look for stimulation in their environment. In fact, the central nervous system, if it is to develop normally, must be stimulated. Prisoners of war living in small cells will make up games, develop coverts patterns of communication with other prisoners, and fantasize about how to regain their freedom. All this is undertaken to keep their minds active.

It is also true that individuals can become overly stimulated. When this happens the results may be unhealthy. The child may look down from the tree and panic when it is apparent how high she has climbed. The adult who takes a hard plunge in an initial attempt at water-skiing may decide that golf is a better sport. When there is overstimulation the individual will pull back, regroup, and reaffirm competence in another area.

From a management point of view, workers are optimally motivated when the stimulation is in some type of balance. Because workers are stimulated by opportunities for growth they will search for puzzles, problems, and novel experiences and attempt to master them. Once mastered, however, such opportunities cease to motivate because they are no longer puzzling, problematic, or novel. The search will then begin anew. To stay optimally productive a worker must find an emerging challenge.[36]

While workers desire acceptable levels of stimulation it is equally true that they can become overstimulated. When the in-box becomes too full, when requests for information can no longer be answered, when reports cannot be written in a timely fashion, and when there simply isn't enough time to do the job, the workers' motivational levels decrease. And, in all probability, so will their commitment to their jobs.

[35] Edward L. Deci, *Intrinsic Motivation* (New York: Plenum Press, 1975).
[36] Robert Ullrich and George Wieland, *Organizational Theory and Design* (Homewood, Ill.: Richard D. Irwin, 1980), p. 241.

A major implication of Deci's theory is that administrators should seek to provide a work environment that has a healthy balance between overstimulation and understimulation. In pursuit of such balance, training opportunities should be provided. The staff member who is assigned responsibility for coordinating incident reports needs to be trained in how to evaluate incident reports, how to investigate alleged errors, and how to prevent the problems from recurring. Even the janitors whom we discussed need an opportunity for continuing education. If they are going to make decisions on what types of cleaning supplies to buy they ought to know how to evaluate the effectiveness of their purchase.

Principle 5: The consequences of a worker's behavior will shape future behavior.

The theory of operant conditioning has its roots in the research of B. F. Skinner. Skinner stated that behavior that is followed by a rewarding experience will tend to be repeated while behavior that is followed by negative consequences will tend to be extinguished.

The operant conditioning process can be portrayed as follows:

$$\text{Stimulus} \longrightarrow \text{Response} \longrightarrow \text{Consequences} \longrightarrow \begin{array}{l} \text{Future response} \\ \text{to stimulation} \end{array}$$

In the work environment, the stimulus may be a delegated task, a work objective, or a service to be performed. The individual's response (or lack of response) to that stimulus will lead to certain consequences (praise or punishment). Such consequences will determine the future response of the individual when confronted with the same stimulus.[37]

The focus of Skinner's theory is represented in four variables: positive reinforcement, extinction, punishment, and avoidance learning. *Positive reinforcement* is by definition a consequence that makes it more likely that a given behavior will recur. *Extinction* is designed to eliminate undesirable behaviors rather than to help shape desired actions. To encourage extinction, the supervisor withholds reward. Oftentimes extinction is carried out by ignoring an individual rather than by direct application of sanctions. Therefore, if a worker is disruptive in staff meetings the supervisor may choose to ignore the behavior rather than communicate directly with the employee. *Punishment* is a negative reinforcer designed to inflict enough pain so that the behavior will cease. Giving harsh criticism, reducing an individual's rank, denying privileges, and taking away freedom are frequently used methods of meting out punishment in a work setting.[38] *Avoidance learning* takes place when individuals have learned to behave in ways that will help them avoid or escape unpleasant consequences.

[37] Stoner, *Management*, pp. 422–24.
[38] Ibid., pp. 422–24.

Skinner's "Law of Effect" has strong appeal to administrators because of its practicality. As has often been noted, there is nothing as practical as a good theory and, in this case, the theory has numerous applications to organizational settings. W. Clay Hammer has identified six rules by which operant conditioning can be used effectively in management.[39]

First, administrators should not reward all individuals uniformly. Reinforcers should be based upon performance. When they are not, it diminishes the ability of the reward to motivate high levels of productivity. To reward high, middle, and low achievers in the same way has the effect of reinforcing poor or average performance and ignoring high performance.[40]

Second, it is important to be aware that failure to respond also modifies behavior. The absence of feedback does not result in a neutral reaction. Generally the absence of communication from a supervisor is interpreted as a negative reinforcer. Administrators influence subordinates by what they do and also by what they do not do. An administrator who does not give positive reinforcement to a high-performing worker may find that the employee's performance levels will decline over time.

Third, it is important to inform individuals what they must do if they are to be rewarded.[41] Subordinates need to know the criteria by which they are being evaluated and that a desired consequence will follow if a task is performed competently.

Fourth, subordinates need to be informed when they are doing something wrong. Informing workers *while the task is being accomplished* that their performance is substandard is more effective in reducing error than waiting until the task is finished. Likewise, if rewards are withheld but the subordinate does not know why they are being withheld, it is unlikely that performance will improve.

The fifth implication of Skinner's theory has become almost a cardinal rule: Never punish a subordinate in front of others. When workers are punished in public they are humiliated. Workers dislike public reprimands and usually seethe with resentment at a boss who does not understand that fact. It is interesting that workers will often come to the defense of a peer who has been publicly humiliated. This often compounds the severity of the problems between supervisor and subordinate.

Finally, be fair. It is important that the consequences of a behavior be appropriate to performance standards. Workers should be given the rewards or punishments that are deserved. No more, no less. Overrewarding undeserving subordinates, or severely punishing those who are only marginally

[39] W. Clay Hammer, "Reinforcement Theory and Contingency Management in Organizational Settings," in *Organizational Behavior and Management: A Contingency Approach,* ed., Henry L. Tosis and W. Clay Hammer (Chicago: St. Clair Press, 1974), pp. 221–224.
[40] Stoner, *Management*, p. 425.
[41] Ibid.

substandard will usually result in bitterness, recriminations, and low productivity.[42]

These principles of reinforcement theory can be utilized in modifying the behavior of individuals.[43] To illustrate how this can be done consider a six-step process that Judy Kindall, a hospital administrator used in modifying the behavior of her assistant Fred Maridam (Figure 5-4).

The basic problem that Judy had with Fred was that he simply could not complete projects on time. Often he would ask for extensions, claiming "I just haven't had time to get at it." Other times Fred would defend his tardiness by saying that he had "too much to do." In other instances he would say that a report is "just about finished"—yet it would not appear for another week or two.

In reviewing the situation, Judy defined the problem as follows (Step 1): "My assistant, Fred Maridam, is not able to complete delegated tasks punctually." Having defined the problem, Judy began to chart the frequency of the targeted behavior (Step 2). A review of the projects that had been delegated to Fred indicated that 50 percent of them were completed from two weeks to two months late. Requests to delay the completion day of projects and reports were made on 60 percent of the delegated assignments. In three instances a task was never completed.

Judy Kindall listed the possible explanations for Fred's conduct (step 3):

1. He is overworked.
2. He can't prioritize responsibilities.
3. He loses perspective on the dates by which tasks are to be completed.
4. He is lazy.
5. He feels that I won't crack down on him.
6. My instructions aren't clear.

After reviewing the list, Judy met with Fred (Step 4) in order to (a) develop an intervention strategy, and (b) implement the strategy. She also began charting the changes in Fred's behavior. The strategy that Judy decided to implement was to meet with her subordinate for one hour every Friday

Step 1: Define the behavioral problem as precisely as possible.

Step 2: Measure the extent of the problem; summarize the findings.

Step 3: List possible explanations for the behavior.

Step 4: a. Develop possible intervention strategies.
          b. Implement the intervention strategy.

Step 5: Provide appropriate reinforcement.

Step 6: Evaluate and determine whether the intervention was successful.

Figure 5-4 A behavior modification process.

[42] Ibid.
[43] Ibid.

morning. At that meeting the expectations for the next week were delineated and an agreement was arrived at as to the dates by which delegated tasks were to be completed. At the following week's meeting a written progress report was to be given by Fred to Judy outlining the progress that had been made.

Judy carefully kept a record of the tasks that were assigned and whether they were being completed punctually. Happily 80 percent of the tasks were now being completed on time. The progress that Fred was making in his patterns of punctuality was rewarded (Step 5). Only in one instance did a negative reinforcer have to be used and that had to do with a particularly important report whose deadline Fred missed. After considerable efforts to encourage him to finish the report (positive reinforcement) and finding that Fred continued to put if off, she informed him that if it was not completed by the end of the following week the task would be delegated to someone else (negative reinforcement). Not wanting to fail and not wanting someone else to be given an area of his responsibility were sufficient stimuli to goad Fred into action. The report was completed over a weekend.

Six months later Judy reviewed the progress that had been made and determined that the problem had been effectively resolved (Step 6). Meeting on a weekly basis did seem to improve performance. In an effort to help Fred become more independent she began meeting with him on a biweekly basis and subsequently on a once-a-month basis. The subordinate's performance did not drop because of this strategy. As Skinner has suggested, once an individual has learned a new behavior only intermittent (periodic) reinforcement needs to be carried out. If the intermittent reinforcement is effective, newly acquired behaviors will not be extinguished.

There have been many encouraging results when Skinner's approach to motivation has been applied in organizational settings. Luthans and Lyman discovered that supervisors trained in the operant conditioning procedure that we have just described were able to improve the performance of their departments.[44] One survey of major and complex organizations such as Standard Oil, Michigan Bell, Emery Air Freight, and General Electric found that positive reinforcement strategies resulted in major gains in efficiency, cost saving, attendance, and productivity.[45]

Principle 6: Workers respond more positively to supervisors who are "employee oriented" than to those who are "task oriented."

An employee-oriented supervisor is one who is interested in the well-being of subordinates. They indicate their confidence in workers by giving them ample freedom to define the process by which tasks are to be undertaken. They permit workers to have a say in the decisions that will affect

[44] Cited in ibid., p. 427.
[45] Cited in ibid.

them. They solicit suggestions about strategies that will make the work environment more conducive to high performance. They provide timely feedback so that workers know how they are doing. If a problem arises, the employee-oriented supervisor will give the necessary assistance. Finally, an employee-oriented supervisor is more likely to reinforce behavior with rewards than with punishment.

Task-oriented supervisors tend to see employees as secondary to the product or service being rendered. Workers who are supervised by task-oriented individuals report that communication is essentially one way, that is, from the top down. When errors are made, task-oriented supervisors assume that the fault rests with the worker rather than in a misunderstanding or a breakdown within the system. Task-oriented supervisors seldom give feedback, assuming that workers only need to be told what to do and informed if they are not performing to the desired level.[46]

There is considerable data available that seems to confirm that employee-oriented supervisors are more effective in developing a highly motivated staff than those who are task oriented. A pioneering study was undertaken over a three-year period of time in the offices of the Prudential Insurance Company in Newark, New Jersey.[47] Matched pairs of work groups with twelve in each sample were carefully studied. Each pair of work groups was statistically matched with regard to sex, marital status, average age, education, years of experience, salary, grade average, distance from job to home, and average scores on a battery of psychological tests.

The researchers noted statistically significant differences in the productivity levels of the groups. Some groups were producing at a high level and others were not. Prior to the study it was hypothesized that the demographic characteristics of the supervisors such as age, education, experience, and salary would explain the differences in the group productivity. The study at Prudential, however, demonstrated that none of these factors made a difference.

According to the research, the key difference between the high-productivity groups and the low-productivity groups was whether or not the supervisors were employee oriented.[48] The high-productivity groups had supervisors who talked with their workers and seemed genuinely interested in what they were accomplishing. They supervised in a more general manner that permitted workers to apply their own unique competencies to their jobs. Interestingly, however, they were more critical of sloppy work and did not hesitate to reprimand if it were appropriate. The supervisor in the low-producing groups tended to overinstruct their subordinates about what they

---

[46] Robert Blake and Jane Mouton, *The New Managerial Grid* (Houston: Gulf Publishing Co., 1978).

[47] W. Earl Sasser, Jr., and Frank S. Leonard, "Let First Level Supervisors Do Their Job," *Harvard Business Review*, March-April 1974, p. 117.

[48] Ibid., p. 118.

were to do and how they were to do it. They watched their workers closely, which subordinates often took as an indicator of low trust. It is interesting to note that the high-productivity supervisors talked about their people; the low-productivity supervisors talked about their jobs.

Rensis Likert followed the Prudential study with a number of similar studies in a variety of occupational settings. His work confirmed, in part, the earlier Prudential studies. He found that the better supervisors spent more time in meetings with their employees and did a better job of keeping subordinates informed. They solicited the opinions of workers and took a general interest in them.[49]

Saul W. Gellerman, in a later study, analyzed the jobs of twelve supervisors by following each through an entire work shift.[50] He noted every move and questioned them on each course of action that they took. He found three patterns of supervision particularly interesting. In the "excellent" pattern of supervision, the supervisor would give reassurance when employees were discouraged but leave them alone if they did not need supervisory help. In the "good" pattern of supervision, the supervisor would frequently check to make certain that the employees were following the correct procedures. In the poor or "mediocre" form of supervision the supervisor would check to make certain the subordinates were in the proper location, would energetically rush around, and would seldom sit behind the desk. Clearly the best form of supervision was that in which the supervisor took an interest in subordinates, yet gave them enough freedom so that the job could be completed in an appropriate manner.

The significance of these studies is that the perceptions of workers about their supervisors appears to be an important variable in the motivation process. Their commitment to the organization is influenced by the extent to which they perceive that their boss is interested in their well-being. This does not imply that supervisors have to be on a friendly first-name basis with every employee. Nor does it imply that punishment cannot be given when appropriate. (In the Prudential study, it was found that the more effective supervisors were more critical of subordinates' work than the supervisors in the low-producing groups.) What it does mean is that higher levels of motivation are generally achieved by supervisors who are perceived to be open to suggestions, fair in evaluating subordinates' work, and consistent in giving rewards.

In summary, we have examined six motivational principles that should be thought of as guidelines rather than rigid rules. Remember, all employees are not alike. Nor are all situations alike. Nor is there one best way of motivating employees. The competent manager is one who recognizes that there are various insights into motivation that are set forth in over 3,350 ar-

---

[49] Rensis Likert, *The Human Organization* (New York: McGraw-Hill, 1967), pp. 1–42.
[50] Cited in Sasser and Leonard, "Let First Level Supervisors Do Their Job," p. 118.

ticles, books, and dissertations published to date on job satisfaction. If we were to sumamrize the key concepts, the list would be as follows:

1. The need for achievement, power, and affiliation will influence individuals to act in ways that will fulfill such needs (McClelland).
2. Workers will exert energy on tasks dependent upon whether they see the completion of the task as leading to a desired reward (Vroom).
3. The context and content of work are motivators. Of the two, the content (intrinsic) appears to be the more powerful in motivating human behavior (Herzberg).
4. The desire to be competent is a motivator providing that workers believe that the outcomes will be intrinsically or extrinsically rewarded (Deci).
5. Behavior in organizations can be shaped through positive and negative reinforcement. In general, it is more effective to reward desired behavior than to punish undesired behavior (Skinner).
6. If workers perceive that their supervisors are interested in their well-being, it is likely that they will perform at higher levels than if such an interest is not shown (Likert).

THE EVALUATION PROCESS

In our discussion of motivation we learned some important facts about organizational behavior. We learned that behavior is largely a function of its consequences. That is, what people do in organizations is shaped by their perception of how they will be rewarded. We also learned that most individuals want to be competent and to master their work environment. We now want to expand these concepts by applying them to one of the toughest tasks that management faces—performance appraisal.

Managers are often reluctant to systematically review the performance of subordinates. Some resist because they do not have knowledge of performance appraisal methods. Others resist because they dislike the task of informing individuals that their work is unsatisfactory. Some managers philosophically feel that performance evaluation comes dangerously close to a violation of the integrity of others. "Managers are uncomfortable," said Douglas McGregor, "when they are put in the position of playing God. The respect we hold for the inherent value of the individual leaves us distressed when we must take responsibility for judging the personal worth of a fellow man."[51]

Nevertheless there are three compelling reasons why performance appraisal must be one of the primary functions of management. First it is the responsibility of management to ensure that the organization succeeds as a

[51] Douglas McGregor, "An Uneasy Look at Performance Appraisal," *Harvard Business Review,* May-June 1957, p. 90.

total system. To do that it is necessary to coordinate and evaluate the work of employees. If an employee's output is satisfactory, it is management's unique prerogative to reward such a behavior to ensure that it will be continued in the future. But if an employee's output is unsatisfactory, it is also management's prerogative to offer inducements or punishments that will help the employee become more productive.

Second, performance appraisal does, in fact, improve performance. We will soon see that the effectiveness of an evaluation system has much to do with the method that is used and the skills of the evaluator. However, when employee evaluations are carried out in an objective manner and when the intent of the evaluation is to assist employees in becoming competent, the net result is that evaluation improves rather than detracts from productivity.[52]

Third, most employees want and need to know how well they are performing. They want to know that they are perceived as competent and that the quality of their output is meeting acceptable standards. They also want to know if their performance is substandard. Learning that one's performance is not meeting acceptable standards is apparently less threatening than not knowing how one is being evaluated.

Historical Background

Performance appraisal has been associated with work for centuries. The emperors of the Wei Dynasty in A.D. 221–65 designated an "Imperial Rater" whose task it was to determine the effectiveness of the royal family. Centuries later, Ignatius Loyola defined a system for rating the members of the Jesuit Society.[53]

In the 1800s, European companies designed formal methods to evaluate employee performance. One of the most interesting concepts was developed by Robert Owens in Scotland. When employees arrived at their jobs they found a colored block indicating how they had performed the previous day. Different colors indicated various levels of performance.

The first formal appraisal system in the United States was initiated by the federal government and city administrators in the late 1800s. In 1916, Walter D. Scott developed a "man-to-man" rating chart that was used to evaluate the military leadership during World War I. After the war, Frederick Taylor began to apply statistical measures to business settings in an attempt to make work more efficient. Because of his success many business firms initiated time management studies that sought to evaluate the speed by which employees were accomplishing their tasks.

---

[52] D. Yoder, *Personnel Management and Industrial Relations* (Englewood Cliffs, N.J.: Prentice-Hall, Inc., 1970), p. 229–31.

[53] This section has been adapted from Linda Pohlman Haar and Judith Rohan Hicks, "Performance Appraisal: Derivation of Effective Assessment Tools," *Journal of Nursing Administration,* September 1976, p. 37.

Graphic scales were introduced in the 1920s that required supervisors to evaluate subordinates on a continuum from "poor" to "excellent." The human relations school of management theory, in seeking to counteract what seemed to be impersonal time-management studies, emphasized the need to evaluate personality variables. Many current evaluation forms that measure an individual's friendliness and cooperative spirit can be historically traced to human relations theorists.

But by mid 1950s management by objectives (MBO) was beginning to have an impact on the performance evaluation system of many organizations. General Electric was one of the first organizations to establish MBO when they undertook an extensive planning and reorganization program in 1952.

In the 1970s judicial court decisions and interpretations of those decisions by the U.S. government further defined what should take place in performance evaluations. In *Griggs* v. *Duke* Power Company (1970) the U. S. Supreme Court mandated that any type of testing procedure through which a person is hired or promoted must relate directly to the job duties that are to be performed. It is illegal, said the Court, to use any test of mental ability for purposes of selection or promotion if no correlation can be established between the test and job performance.[54] The Equal Employment Opportunities Commission further stated that any criterion used in hiring or promoting individuals must be directly related to the job. Employers must be able to substantiate that any test that has been used is reliably predictive and significantly correlated with important elements of work that must be performed.[55]

Prerequisites for Effective Performance Appraisal

Several important conclusions emerge from the historical efforts to evaluate the work of employees. We will discuss four that appear to be the basic building blocks in constructing a formal performance review system:

1. Performance evaluation should involve the total organization.
2. Employees need to know the criteria that will be used in the evaluation, when the evaluation will take place, and who will conduct the evaluation.
3. Performance appraisal is most productive when the evaluator and the evaluatee trust one another.
4. Rewards must follow satisfactory performance.

The first prerequisite is to have an explicit policy indicating that *all employees are subject to periodic performance appraisals.* This implies that

[54] Ibid.
[55] R. McCormick, "Can We Use Compensation Data to Measure Job Performance Behaviors?" *Personnel Journal,* December 1972, pp. 918–22.

evaluation of performance will be occurring at all levels of the organization, including the highest-paid employee as well as part-time hourly reimbursed workers.

If an organization has never had a formal performance appraisal system, any step in developing such a mechanism will probably be met with resistance. Employees will be suspicious, wondering what management has up their corporate sleeves that will make life more difficult.

To diminish resistance it is helpful to make explicit the rationale of performance appraisal and why management is initiating such a system at this point in time. It should be emphasized that everyone will take part. It is also important to state that the results of the evaluations will be confidential.

To reinforce the importance of performance appraisal some governing boards now insist that chief executive officers and other top executives be evaluated by the board of directors after a designated period of time. Such a policy makes explicit the importance that the board places on performance evaluation. It also gives feedback to executives about their performance and helps them determine what changes should be made if board expectations are to be realized.

A second prerequisite for effective performance appraisal is that *employees should understand the criteria on which they will be evaluated, when the evaluation will take place, and who will be responsible for carrying it out.*

It is particularly important for employees to know the criteria on which they will be evaluated. There are a number of evaluation methods available to managers; each has its own strengths and limitations.

One method is an *essay technique* in which the evaluator writes a description of the worker's strengths and weaknesses. The recorded information is usually impressionistic. Some essay evaluations will be general while highlighting the critical points the evaluator wishes to make. Others essays are grouped under headings such as performance, cooperativeness, and job knowledge. The primary advantage of an essay is that it can provide an in-depth analysis of performance as well as descriptive information that is not found on checklist evaluation forms. Essays are, however, time consuming to write and vary greatly in length and content depending upon the evaluator. Their success in changing employee behavior is often contingent upon the writing skills of the supervisor.

Rating scales require an evaluator to make a judgment ranging from superior to unsatisfactory on a number of performance-based criteria. Most evaluators using this method commonly examine the quality and quantity of an employee's work, cooperation, initiative, and dependability. A typical graphic rating form used for nonsupervisory personnel is seen in Figure 5-5.

A *checklist* is an efficient method of evaluation. The basic difference between a checklist and a rating scale is the type of judgment that is required. Rating scales permit evaluators to express degrees of satisfaction; checklists usually require only a "yes–no" response on performance-related criteria. The primary advantage of checklists is that performance expectations are clearly delineated in behavioral language. Because checklists are efficient they can be used with large groupings of employees. They are, however, difficult to construct and do not have the benefit of providing the descriptive information given in essay methods.[56]

Figure 5-6 illustrates one particularly effective checklist method of evaluation. Note how thoroughly the measuring instrument has been constructed. Each criterion is stated in behavioral terms easily identifiable by the reader. Upon receiving this evaluation the professional staff nurse will have considerable information concerning her planning, decision-making, assessment, teaching, and supervisory skills.[57] In addition, she will receive valuable information as to how she is perceived as a nurse clinician.

A *field review method* is undertaken when several supervisors rate one employee. The ratings of the supervisors are aggregated and an average score is then assigned to the employee. The major advantage of this method is that group judgments tend to be more valid than individual ratings.[58] In addition, the evaluators are able to identify areas of interrater agreement and disagreement. The major disadvantage is the amount of time it takes to review the performance of many employees.

With the *comparison method* employees are ranked on the basis of their overall job performance with others in their peer group. Typically the evaluator will list from top to bottom the best to worst employee. This method has the advantage of letting employees know exactly how they are valued in comparison with other employees. The primary disadvantage is that it is difficult to compare individuals. To overcome this weakness some managers prefer to rank subordinates as being in the top third, middle third, and lowest third.

Some managers find *face-to-face* interviews to be the most effective way of informing employees about the quality of their work. Those who prefer informal interviews note that the time to evaluate employees is not necessarily June 30 or December 31. They also point out that the best time to reinforce behavior is when it is occurring. It you wait until some future date to discuss what is happening, it is likely that the passing of time will color your perception of the event. "Thus if a subordinate's performance is less than it might be or the employee is failing to a degree in interpersonal relations, it is not only unnatural but unwise to wait three months—or six or twelve—to talk about the situation."[59]

[56] Haar and Hicks, "Performance Appraisal," p. 37.

[57] Ibid., pp. 44–45.

[58] W. Oberg, "Make Performance Appraisal Relevant," *Harvard Business Review,* January-February 1972, pp. 61–67.

[59] Aaron Q. Sartain and Alton W. Baker, *The Supervisor and the Job* (New York: McGraw-Hill, 1978), p. 254.

Non-Supervisory Employee Appraisal

Employee's Name: _____ Division: _____

Title: _____ District: _____

Date Current Title Obtained: _____ Present wage rate: _____

Review carefully and check one block as appropriate

	(A)	(B)	(C)	(D)	(E)	Consider employee's efforts since the last review dated _____ and show by a check (X) any changes in each of the categories		
						HAS IMPROVED	LITTLE OR NO CHANGE	HAS GONE BACK
1. Safety Performance — Consider all facets of safety in connection with his or her present job title, in carrying out company safety policies. During past 2 years No. disabling work injuries ___ No. medical treatment injuries ___ No. motor vehicle accidents ___	☐ Careless of safety of self and others.	☐ Occasionally causes mishaps.	☐ Accepts safety as part of job.	☐ Practices good safety habits and is considerate of others.	☐ Exercises great care and foresees hazards to self and fellow employees.	☐	☐	☐
2. Attendance and Punctuality — Consider attendance on the job and reporting on time. During past year No. days incidental absence ___ No. days benefit absence ___ No. times tardy ___	☐ Undependable, absent or late without proper notice.	☐ Frequently absent or late.	☐ Some absence with good cause.	☐ Occasionally absent or late. Notifies in advance.	☐ Record is perfect.	☐	☐	☐
3. Quality of Work — Considers the completeness, neatness, and acceptability of work done.	☐ Considerably below job requirements.	☐ Has not reached expected level.	☐ Acceptable.	☐ Definitely better than the expected level.	☐ Exceptionally high quality.	☐	☐	☐
4. Quantity of Work — Considers amount of work done within a given time compared to expected results.	☐ Considerably below job standards.	☐ Has not reached expected level.	☐ Acceptable	☐ Definitely better than the expected level	☐ Exceptional productivity	☐	☐	☐

	(A)	(B)	(C)	(D)	(E)			
5. Job Knowledge Consider the completeness of knowledge of job duties.	Has very little knowledge of job duties. (A)	Has fair knowledge of job duties. (B)	Average job knowledge. (C)	Knows most all job knowledge well. (D)	Unusually detailed knowledge of job. (E)	☐	☐	☐
6. Cooperation Consider attitude toward work, associates, and supervision Willingness to work with and for others.	Poor team worker. (A)	Fair team worker. (B)	Generally cooperative. Works reasonably well with others. (C)	Good team worker—works and cooperates well. (D)	Excellent team worker—goes out of way to cooperate. (E)	☐	☐	☐
7. Initiative and Application Consider to what extent the employee is a "self starter," also the attention and effort applied to his work.	Wastes time, never looks for work, needs abnormal amount of supervision (A)	Inclined to take things easy. Requires occasional prodding (B)	Steady and willing worker. (C)	Energetic, demonstrates initiative. (D)	Exceptionally industrious, resourceful, and attentive to all of his or her duties. (E)	☐	☐	☐
8. Dependability Consider the manner in which the employee applies himself or herself to work, and consider other items regarding dependability.	Cannot be relied upon. Has to be closely checked. (A)	Good worker but needs more checking than others on same type of work. (B)	Can be entrusted to do a job with a minimum follow-up. (C)	Applies himself or herself well. Requires only an occasional check. (D)	Justifies utmost confidence. Carries out his or her work in all details. (E)	☐	☐	☐
9. Physical Fitness Consider energy, endurance, physique, and general health in relation to the employee's ability to do work.	Poor health. Handicapped. (A)	Health below normal. Flexibility limited. (B)	Good health. Only occasional illness. (C)	Good health and energy. Rarely ill. (D)	Excellent health. Very active, lots of energy and endurance. Never ill. (E)	☐	☐	☐

Date of Evaluation _____

Evaluator _____

Figure 5-5 Rating scale evaluation form. [From John M. Ivancevich, Andrew D. Szilagyi, Jr., and Marc J. Wallace, Jr., *Organizational Behavior and Performance* (Santa Monica, Calif.: Goodyear Publishing Co., Inc., 1977), pp. 432–433.]

Professional Staff Nurse—Performance Appraisal

Directions—Please respond to the following checklist by completing separate checklists for each staff nurse in your area. Put a checkmark (√) in the "Yes" column if a nurse demonstrates a given behavior most of the time. Put a checkmark in the "No" column if the nurse either does not demonstrate the behavior at all, or demonstrates it infrequently. If the behavior is not relevant to your situation, put a checkmark in the "N/A (Not Applicable)" column. Any additional comments may be added in the areas designated, following the checklist.

1. General behavior to be evaluated:
Assessment

Does the staff nurse . . .

	YES	NO	N/A
a. identify in writing as well as verbally the present physical and emotional condition of the patient, the history of the disability, and the patient's expectations of rehabilitation?			
b. utilize physical assessment skills in initial contacts with patients to determine appropriate nursing intervention as evidenced by written and verbal communication regarding patient?			
c. identify and evaluate patient and family needs, abilities, and readiness to learn, as evidenced by both written and verbal communication and contact with patients?			
d. demonstrate ability to assess appropriate nursing intervention for the various types of patients in the rehabilitation setting?			
e. assign appropriate available personnel to the patient reflective of the degree of skilled nursing care required?			

Comments:

2. General behavior to be evaluated:
Planning

Does the staff nurse . . .

	YES	NO	N/A
a. indicate in the patient chart and in the nursing care plan, both long- and short-term goals for patients following assessment of nursing care needs?			
b. formulate a written nursing care plan for each of the patients assigned, based on collection of information from patients?			
c. anticipate the work flow and delegate appropriate tasks, as evidenced by completion of own work within allotted time?			
d. demonstrate flexibility by response to: emergencies, scheduling changes, or adverse conditions?			

Comments:

Figure 5-6 Checklist evaluation form. [Reprinted with permission from "Performance Appraisal: Derivation of Effective Assessment Tools," by Linda Pohlman Haar and Judith Rohan Hicks, *Journal of Nursing Administration*, September 1976, p. 37.]

3. General behavior to be evaluated:
Delivery of Patient Care

Does the staff nurse . . .

	YES	NO	N/A
a. provide skillful, safe nursing care to own patient caseload as indicated in written report found in patient chart and nursing care plan; outlining the plan, treatment, and patient response to nursing intervention?			
b. evaluate and intervene when necessary in nursing care delivered by other non-RN personnel to patients on his/her team?			
c. administer prescribed treatments and medications and alter the same within limits of professional judgments based on patients' physical and emotional needs?			
d. report observed physical and emotional reactions to treatment and medications and indicate in writing in the nursing care plan and in the patient chart implications of such reactions?			
e. identify and appropriately utilize nursing resource persons to facilitate delivery of quality nursing care?			

Comments:

4. General behavior to be evaluated:
Decision making

Does the staff nurse . . .

	YES	NO	N/A
a. utilize sound judgment on the basis of critical thinking and problem-solving criterion, as evidenced by ability to provide rationale for decisions, in both written and verbal communication?			
b. suggest constructive changes in the delivery and monitoring of patient care, as evidenced by updated written care plans, and consultation from appropriate sources?			
c. request and accept constructive criticism regarding nursing judgments from appropriate resource persons?			
d. inform head nurse and/or clinical nurse specialist of unusual or difficult nursing care problems?			

Comments:

5. General behavior to be evaluated:
Patient and Family Teaching

Does the staff nurse . . .

	YES	NO	N/A
a. teach the patient and his family to relearn former skills of daily living or mastering patterns of adaptation to compensate for lost abilities, as evidenced by evaluation of patient and family's understanding prior to discharge?			
b. provide the family with information necessary to support the patient in the relearning process?			
c. plan activities for the patient designed to integrate new learning into daily life?			
d. reinforce with the patient and his family information and skills taught by physical therapy, speech therapy, occupational therapy, etc.?			
e. communicate prepared plan of care to other members of the nursing team, giving rationale for decision?			
f. present in behavioral terms, directions for care of patients, testing to see if directions are interpreted appropriately?			

Comments:

6. General behavior to be evaluated:
Supervision of Co-Workers

Does the staff nurse . . .

	YES	NO	N/A
a. demonstrate leadership ability in team conference situation, as evidenced by use of problem-solving techniques, use of probing questions, and organizing personnel for action?			
b. demonstrate the ability to constructively plan and use time . . . daily, weekly . . . by rotation of shift?			
c. guide and supervise non-professional nursing staff in accomplishment of established goals of care?			
d. accurately evaluate skills of personnel and make assignments in accord with assessed capabilities?			
e. demonstrate the ability to confront team members with issues concerning patient care?			
f. give and accept feedback from staff members regarding appropriate or inappropriate behavior for purposes of improved patient care?			
g. demonstrate sensitivity to fellow worker's needs as they relate to the job, by providing support, giving advice, or referring to appropriate sources of help when necessary?			
h. seek help from appropriate resource person when unusual or difficult problems of a supervisory nature occur?			

Comments:

7. General behavior to be evaluated:
Utilizing Interdisciplinary Approach

Does the staff nurse . . .

	YES	NO	N/A
a. communicate observations of nursing staff to appropriate members of interdisciplinary rehabilitation team?			
b. implement and reinforce plan of speech therapist?			
c. incorporate and reinforce new skills being learned in physical therapy when patient returns to the nursing unit?			
d. engage patient in appropriate occupational therapy as designated in interdisciplinary conference?			
e. contribute constructive changes and observations to members of rehabilitation team, giving rationale for suggested changes?			

Comments:

Comments by Employee:

Employee's Signature _____

Head Nurse's Signature _____

Department Head's Signature _____

Date _____

Advocates of formal systems of evaluation emphasize the importance of having established time periods that are specifically set aside for performance appraisal. Advocates note the employees prefer structured interviews as compared with informal conversation. They also note that the formal system usually produces a written statement concerning each employee's performance that can later be used for promotion or disciplinary action.

Managers who have been surveyed on the issue of informal versus formal evaluations generally prefer the more structured approach. They frequently characterize the informal plan as not having any plan at all and insist that a "systematic, logical approach is obviously better than its opposite."[60]

One way of initiating a formal interview is to prepare yourself by writing an essay evaluation based on four categories of information:

1. Quality of employee performance
2. Utilization of resources
3. Demonstrated competencies
4. Problems to be resolved

The first task is to evaluate the quality and quantity of the employee's work. This means reviewing the employee's work objectives and noting whether they have been completed in a timely manner. Most managers will want to note whether the employee has been spending time on tasks that are extraneous to the work objectives. As you write a paragraph or two, focus on outputs by asking yourself whether desired objectives have been satisfactorily met.

Under the second category, evaluate the financial and human resources that have been used in meeting the work objectives. Are the financial expenditures consistent with earlier projections? Are they reasonable? Does the employee have adequate financial resources to do the job? You will also want to examine how the subordinate employs the talents and expertise of others. Does the subordinate utilize the theoretical and technical information of other employees? Does the employee give assistance to others on work-related problems? Does the employee delegate work when it is appropriate to do so?

Under the third category you should list, point by point, the employee's strengths. If the employee has done a good job it should be stated with ample documentation.

Finally, under the fourth category, list problems associated with the performance of the subordinate. Succinctly write the problem. Elaboration can be done at the time of the interview.

You will note that we have not included a fifth category called "interpersonal relations" although many formal rating systems contain such a reference. We have excluded this category because we want the evaluation to be strictly job related. This is not meant to imply that you should avoid discussing interpersonal issues. However the interview should not focus on

[60] Ibid.

whether the employee is extroverted or introverted, friendly or shy. *The issue is whether or not the job is being done.* If interpersonal factors have a bearing on performance it would be appropriate to focus on such concerns but only if they have relevance to the employee's productivity. An example of an essay evaluation can be found in Figure 5-7.

The written confidential essay evaluation should be sent to the subordinate's office several days prior to the interview. It is helpful to include a note with the evaluation indicating your willingness to discuss the issues and, if there are errors of judgment, a willingness to rewrite the evaluation.

The formal interview should begin with a clear statement of the purpose of the evaluation—that it is to assist the employee in doing the best possible job. After such a statement has been made you will want to review the strengths of the employee in an effort to reinforce high-quality work. Next, you will focus on the quality and quantity of output as well as how well the subordinate has utilized resources. Out of this discussion should come agreement on the shortcomings and the problems associated with the employee's work. The last phase of the oral interview should result in agreement about approaches to be taken in solving identified problems. The date by which the problems are to be solved should be jointly determined. Some managers find it helpful to have subordinates sign the essay evaluation form to signify their agreement with the evaluation; others ask subordinates to sign only to indicate that the document has been read and understood.

As you conduct the interview it is important to remember that subordinates need ample opportunity to discuss the problems and frustrations that have been occurring. It is also wise to find out the nature of the employee's goals and work aspirations. If you have given adequate encouragement, the subordinate should leave feeling that it is possible to be more effective. As Claude George states, "Given the proper encouragement most employees will emerge from an evaluation interview with renewed vigor and determination to do a better job."[61]

A third prerequisite for effective performance appraisal is related to *the degree of trust between the evaluator and the evaluatee.* Trust develops when there is a desire to use objective data in evaluating performance. Trust also develops when there is agreement that the primary purpose of an evaluation is to help one another be more effective.

There are four errors committed by evaluators that erode trust.[62] The first is *leniency error* which comes about when an evaluator consistently grades an employee in a highly positive or highly negative way. While some employees may merit consistently high or low ratings, most will succeed or fail to various degrees. When an evaluator consistently downgrades an employee's

[61] Claude S. George, *Supervision in Action* (Reston, Va.: Reston Publishing Company, 1979), p. 197.
[62] Adapted from *Organizational Behavior*, pp. 355-60.

Essay Evaluation

Name ___ __ Marilyn Braested __ __ __ __ __
Title _____ Director, Comm. Health Educ.
Date _____ July 25, 1981 __ __ __ __ __
Evaluator __ Judy Shannon __ __ __ __ __

I. *Quality of Employee Performance*

At the time of the last evaluation it was determined that Marilyn Braested would plan and carry out educational programs in (a) smoking cessation, (b) stress management, and (c) diabetes education.

The results of the smoking cessation program were, according to evaluations by participants, positive. Six weeks after the program began, 65% of the participants quit smoking, which is considerably better results than what is obtained in most smoking cessation programs. The educational program was well planned and administered.

The stress management program did not have uniformly positive evaluations by participants. Only 25% who participated felt it was "worth their time." Written objectives for this program were apparently not prepared. Only 16 adults participated. The target enrollment was 45 individuals.

The diabetes program is scheduled for next week. Objectives written in behavioral terms have been prepared. Enrollment seems to be higher than what was projected. Competent workshop leaders have agreed to participate.

Summary: The smoking cessation program was a success demonstrating high quality work by Marilyn and the health education programs. The stress management program had a number of weaknesses which should not reoccur. The diabetes program holds promise to be highly successful.

II. *Utilization of Resources*

A. Financial Resources: The financial projections for these three programs is consistent with earlier projections. If the enrollment in the diabetes program is as high as it now appears, the department will be making money on its educational efforts.

B. Human Resources: The participants in the smoking cessation program indicated that the instructors were of unusually high quality which is a tribute to the selection of workshop leaders by Marilyn. The Public Health Nursing program was not consulted on the diabetes education program which seems to be contributing to the irritations between the health education and nursing programs.

III. *Demonstrated Competencies*

Among the competencies which Marilyn Braested has demonstrated are the following:

1. Good organizational skills as evidenced by the success of the smoking cessation program.

2. Good faculty selection skills as evidenced by the quality of the faculty who were recruited in the smoking cessation program.

3. Able to competently administer a budget.

IV. *Problems to Be Resolved*

1. Should the Public Health Nursing department be consulted on educational programs in which they have expertise?

2. Should workshops be cancelled if there are fewer than 20 registrants who have pre-enrolled?

3. Why did participants in the stress management program rate the educational effort as "ineffective?"

Figure 5-7 Essay evaluation form.

contribution it is referred to as negative leniency error; when high scores are consistently given it is called positive leniency error.

Subordinates generally distrust any evaluator who consistently errs in either of the two directions. The back-slapping boss who always tells subordinates what a great job they are doing is distrusted because objective feedback is not being given. Negative bosses who only tell employees how bad they are doing are distrusted because they have an inability to recognize accomplishments.

The *halo error* is a tendency to let our assessment of an individual on one trait influence our evaluation of that person on other traits. For example, a supervisor who rates a worker high on conscientiousness and dependability may also tend to rate him high on many other attributes. On the other hand, if the worker has an abrasive personality the supervisor may tend to minimize the employee's accomplishments because of a preoccupation with his communication behavior.

Similarity errors take place when an evaluator rates other people according to those qualities that he perceives in himself. Evaluators who perceive themselves as assertive may look for that quality in others. Subordinates who demonstrate that quality will benefit while those who don't will be penalized. Most employees distrust such an evaluator for they recognize that they are not being judged on performance but rather whether they copy their supervisor's attributes.

The error of *low differentiation* means that everyone in a work group is given the same rating by the supervisor. Evaluators who are low differentiators tend to ignore or suppress differences because they perceive their work universe as more uniform than what it really is. High differentiators will utilize all available information in searching out the differences between employees and rewarding those whose work output is of greater quality. For objective evaluation to take place and for trust to develop evaluators must be high differentiators.

The best way to prevent these errors is to be aware of each and to reaffirm that your objective is to evaluate in a fair and honest manner. Your willingness to rewrite parts of the essay evaluation if new data emerge will help to build a trusting relationship. In addition, if you indicate an interest in obtaining feedback on your performance you will improve the climate in which evaluation takes place.

The final prerequisite for effective performance appraisal is to give adequate rewards for high performance. As indicated in our discussion on motivation, people do things for their reasons—not yours. What they do is largely a function of perceived rewards. Therefore, if you are seeking to change behavior in a performance review appraisal you must link potential rewards to a desired outcome.

The types of rewards that an organization can offer are more complex than many realize. There is direct compensation, but there also is indirect compensation and nonfinancial rewards. In Figure 5-8 we see a modification

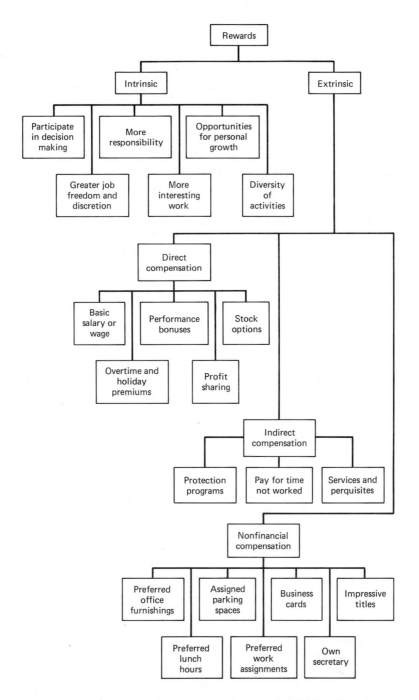

Figure 5-8 Types of rewards. [From Stephen P. Robbins, *Organizational Behavior: Concepts and Controversies* (Englewood Cliffs, N.J.: Prentice-Hall, Inc., 1979), p. 365. Copyright © 1979. Reprinted by permission of the publisher.]

of Hertzberg's motivational system in which intrinsic and extrinsic rewards are listed. Intrinsic rewards are perceived differently by employees. Some might prefer more responsibility while others would choose greater job freedom. Some might prefer to be transferred to a department where they could do more interesting work; others might like to be more involved in decision making. Each of these intrinsic rewards should be made available to employees depending upon the quality of work that is achieved and the opportunities that exist within the organization.

If you have the authority to do so, you may want to consider giving expanded extrinsic rewards to employees. Unfortunately, in most health organizations there has been little use made of performance bonuses, additional vacation days, and expanded fringe benefits. The private sector has long recognized the power implicit in such rewards and carefully utilizes them to reward performance and to keep talented employees committed to their organization.

SUMMARY

We have examined three concepts basic to effective human resource management: recruitment, motivation, and evaluation of personnel. We learned that the recruitment process has three phases: searching, screening, and selecting. In each phase there are specific responsibilities that the health administrator should carry out if the best possible person is to be selected for the position.

We also examined six motivational principles based on theories of human need, expectancy, content and context, competency, and behavior modification. Although these theories differ from one another, each has relevance to the health administrator in building a climate where employees are highly motivated.

Finally we reviewed the advantages and disadvantages of various evaluation methods. We noted that performance is the key variable to examine when conducting a performance appraisal.

STUDY QUESTIONS

1. Identify an individual who has had experience in hiring personnel. Interview this person and ask questions that will give you insight into the recruitment/hiring process. Among the questions you might want to ask are the following: (a) What process does your organization follow in hiring new employees? (b) What interviewing techniques have you found to

be helpful in learning about the applicant's background and suitability for the job? and (c) What can applicants do to increase the likelihood of obtaining employment in your organization?

2. Identify a work situation in which you have been particularly productive (or unproductive). Analyze the *nature of the work* that you were undertaking, the *supervision* you received, and the *rewards* that you obtained. Can you identify reasons for your level of productivity?

3. What motivates you in the work you are now doing?

4. You are supervising a staff member who has been one of your most effective employees. However, during the past twelve months the employee's productivity has gradually declined. The employee's optimism has given way to periodic cynical remarks. You note that the employee occasionally comes to work late and is frequently tardy at staff meetings. How would you go about correcting this situation?

ADDITIONAL READING RESOURCES

Recruitment

HUGHES, DAVID G. "Can Marketing Help Recruit and Retain Nurses?" *Health Care Management Review*, 4, no. 4 (Summer 1979), 61–66.

METZLER, KEN, *Creative Interviewing*. Englewood Cliffs, N.J.: Prentice-Hall, Inc., 1977.

WALSH, DIANA CHAPAN, and RICHARD H. EGDAHL, eds., *Women, Work and Health: Challenges to Corporate Policy*. New York: Springer-Verlag, 1980.

Motivation

ALDAG, RAY, and ARTHUR BRIEF, *Task Design and Employee Motivation*. Glenview, Ill.: Scott, Foresman, 1978.

BABNEW, DAVID, "What Motivates People to Work Effectively?" *Hospital and Health Services Administration,* 25, Special II (1980), 43–53.

HURKA, SLAVEK J., "Need Satisfaction among Health Care Managers," *Hospital and Health Services Administration,* 25, no. 3 (Summer 1980), 43–54.

SLAVITT, DINAH, PAULA STAMPS, and EUGENE PIEDMONT, "Measuring Nurses' Job Satisfaction," *Hospital and Health Services Administration,* 23, no. 3 (Summer 1979), 62–76.

Evaluation

BLAKE, ROBERT, and JANE SRYGLEY MOUTON, *Productivity: The Human Side* (New York, AMACOM, 1981).

BRIEF, ARTHUR, "Developing a Usable Performance Appraisal System," *Journal of Nursing Administration,* 9, no. 10 (October 1979), 7–10.

COUNCIL, JON D., and ROGER J. PLACHY, "Performance Appraisal Is Not Enough," *Journal of Nursing Administration,* 10, no. 10, (February 1980), 2, 20–27.

HOLLEY, W. H., and H. S. FIELD, "Performance Appraisal and the Law," *Labor Law Journal,* 26 (1976), 38–65.

O'REILLY, CHARLES A., III, and BARTON A. WEITZ, "Managing Marginal Employees: The Use of Warnings and Dismissals," *Administrative Science Quarterly,* 25, no. 3 (September 1980), 467–84.

6

Competency:
Developing Productive
Committees

*Search all your parks in all your cities . . . you'll find
no statues to committees.—Anonymous*

OVERVIEW The purpose of this chapter is to describe concepts that can
assist in developing an effective committee structure. Upon
completion of this chapter the reader should be able to:

- State the advantages and disadvantages of groups in
  problem-solving situations

- Define six theoretical propositions relating to small-
  group behavior and state the significance of each

- Describe how procedural, critical thinking, and social
  norms are established within a group

- Define the critical components in the PERT process

- Define strategies through which group cohesiveness can
  be strengthened

- Define the functions of a governing board

Administrators spend a great deal of their work life in meetings. A study undertaken by Henry Mintzberg of McGill University found that executives spend an average of 69 percent of their work life in meetings with two or more people.[1] A Kriesberg survey among seventy-five organizations found that executives averaged ten hours per week in formal meetings and that the more responsibility the executives had, the more likely it was that they would spend time in committee deliberations.[2]

Given the large investment in time that executives devote to meetings, one might rightfully inquire as to whether the time is well spent. The purpose of this chapter is to give you the conceptual tools with which you can evaluate the effectiveness of committees within your organization. We will examine six propositions which, if understood and implemented, can create the necessary environment for a productive committee structure. We will learn about the importance of selecting task-oriented group members and what can be done to create conditions where the membership will be highly motivated to accomplish specific objectives. We will examine how people communicate within groups and note various ways that groups go about making decisions. But most importantly, we will examine the crucial role that you as a leader enact in the life of the group. Indeed the key variable influencing the success of committees appears to be the nature of the leadership. Let's begin our discussion with an analysis of the benefits and costs of committee work within contemporary health organizations.

BENEFITS AND COSTS OF GROUP MEETINGS

George Homans, one of the pioneers in the construction of group theory, suggests that it is important to see meetings as consisting of activities that are valued but achieved at a cost.[3] Therefore any committee meeting can be ascribed a value, cost, and profit. For example, a health commissioner might meet with department heads on a weekly basis. At times these meetings are productive because unfamiliar information is processed and conflicts are mediated. At other times the discussion wanders and little is accomplished. Occasionally disputes are not resolved and department heads return to their offices with increased anxiety and concern.

If Homans were to critique such a meeting he would examine the "exchange" that takes place. He would ask what rewards the members receive

[1] Herbert E. Meyer, "The Meeting-Goer's Lament," *Fortune,* October 22, 1979, p. 96.
[2] Alan C. Filley, Robert J. House, and Steven Kerr, *Managerial Processes and Organizational Behavior* (Glenview, Ill.: Scott, Foresman, 1976), p. 143.
[3] George G. Homans, *Social Behavior: Its Elementary Forms* (New York: Harcourt, Brace, Jovanovich, 1961), p. 81.

and whether members perceive that the meeting is worth their time. He would examine the product/outcome(s) of the deliberations and determine whether the costs (the psychological energy expended and the salary monies consumed) are acceptable to the person leading the group. In brief, Homans would want to know *whether the results are worth the expenditures.*

In assessing benefits and costs it is important to recognize that there are various pressures impinging upon health administrators to spend more and more time in meetings. Perhaps the most fundamental force is the trend of movement since World War II from rigid, authoritarian management structures to more participative and democratic forms. As Herbert E. Meyer notes, the American family has changed dramatically during the past thirty years and has become less and less authoritarian.[4] As the family has changed so have other institutions. The next result is that "there is a definite trend these days toward fewer and fewer followers . . . everyone wants to be a part of the action."[5]

Because professionals want to participate in the decision-making process, most health administrators carefully weave a committee structure that enables such participation. Some do so reluctantly and reflect what Harold J. Leavitt and Jan Lipman-Blumen term a *direct management style.*[6] "Direct types of people do it themselves, organize and compete to win it—no matter what the 'it' happens to be."[7] Such administrators view committees as a necessary evil. You have to have them to keep people content, but they are burdensome, cumbersome and notoriously unproductive. Administrators who have direct management styles insist that most of the work done by committees could be undertaken more efficiently by top management, providing that the organizational norms would permit it. Since the norms often support shared decision making, committees are established only with great reluctance.

Other administrators value committees because they believe that they can achieve ends through shared decision making that they would not likely achieve if they acted in a direct, authoritative manner. Leavitt and Lipman-Blumen refer to this as a *relational management style.* Such administrators "help, support, and back up other people—often getting kicks from contributing to the success of others, or from a true sense of belonging."[8] Such managers see committee work to be a valuable end in itself as individuals learn to work with one another, come to understand the challenges and problems of

[4] Meyer, "Meeting-Goer's Lament," p. 96.
[5] Ibid.
[6] Harold J. Leavitt and Jean Lipman-Blumen, "A Case for the Rational Manager," *Organizational Dynamics,* AMACOM (Summer 1980), p. 28.
[7] Ibid., p. 28.
[8] Ibid., p. 28.

the organization, and tap one another's creativity in making the enterprise as effective as possible.

Leavitt and Lipman-Blumen suggest that the direct style of management is the predominant mode being practiced in contemporary organizations. They forcefully argue, however, that important changes are taking place in organizations and that researchers will "discover some years from now that successful managers are more relational than they had believed and less competitive or power oriented."[9] Recent research tends to substantiate this prediction as evidenced in works of Victor Vroom, Phillip Yetton, and Fried Fiedler who have noted that a key skill of contemporary administrators/supervisors is the ability to manage the people side of the enterprise.[10]

A second pressure producing more meetings has been the explosion of federal regulations that necessitate group deliberations to assure compliance. Most health administrators now serve on audit, affirmative action, and health planning committees that simply did not exist a few years ago. We can probably expect additional institutional committees as long as legislative actions mandate consultation among various groups.

Finally, committees are frequently established because one person does not have the information necessary to make *quality* policy decisions. The array of services in the typical hospital and health department is truly impressive in terms of quality and quantity as compared with only a decade ago. Few administrators are likely to have in-depth knowledge about each service, the technology necessary to support each service, and the personnel qualifications needed to carry them out. Therefore, when a question is raised about a service, the administrator will usually consult with others who have the most accurate information about the issue at hand. For example, at the time of this writing, there is concern about the quality of drinking water in the upper-midwest region. To resolve the problems associated with waste contaminates, the expertise of many individuals—including health administrators and practitioners, legislators, corporate administrators, and research scientists—will have to be tapped. Undoubtedly this will necessitate the formation of more than one committee to examine the problem.

As we view the pressures that result from having more and more meetings we could lament the passing of an era where efficient authoritarian decisions could be made by a single individual. That lament would probably be a mistake, not only because the modern era often demands the credibility that comes from concensus decisions, but also because group participation has a number of positive attributes that strengthen the decision-making process.[11]

[9] Ibid., p. 29.

[10] Cited ibid., p. 35.

[11] The section on the advantages and disadvantages of group problem solving has been adapted from James A. F. Stoner, *Management* (Englewood Cliffs, N.J.: Prentice-Hall, Inc., 1974), pp. 299–302. Reprints by permission.

Advantages of Committees

Group problem solving has five major advantages over individual problem solving. Let us examine each of these advantages in detail.

Greater knowledge and information   In general the total information possessed by all members within a group is bound to be greater than the knowledge of an individual. Think, for example, of the challenge of changing the behavior of lake property owners who, through their indiscriminate use of lawn fertilizers, are slowly changing the character of a lake. An environmental health sanitarian might have the best technical information as to why toxic chemicals are killing the fish population; a health educator might have the best information about what communication channel should be used (door-to-door interviews, leaflets inserted in mailboxes, "town" meetings) in informing the property owners about the consequences of their actions in destroying the quality of the water; and a public health nurse might have the best demographic information concerning the residents. By working as a multidisciplinary team these three persons are able to pool their information and determine the most effective strategy for resolving the water pollution problem. It is likely that they will arrive at a higher-quality solution by working together than they would if each worked separately.

It is prudent to form a group when a problem is of such a magnitude that no single individual has adequate information by which to resolve the situation. If one individual has the information necessary to make a quality decision it is usually unnecessary to call a committee meeting.

More approaches to a problem   Most individuals have a process by which they approach problems and make decisions. David Kolb, Irwin Rubin, and James McIntyre have identified four approaches to learning.[12] The first approach is through *concrete experience.* Some individuals enjoy here-and-now learning. They generally do not think abstractly but are present oriented. One of their chief attributes is that they help a group stick to its task and point out when the discussion is rambling without purpose or direction. They are particularly valuable in helping a group focus on the known facts in a situation. Others learn through *reflective observation.* They enjoy analytical thought and the synthesis of facts, opinions, and perceptions. Often reflective observers will prevent a group from "shooting from the hip"—taking actions based on too little thought. Other people learn best through *active experimentation.* Like those who approach learning through concrete experiences, these individuals are pragmatic. They enjoy learning by doing. An environmentalist who learns through active experimentation would not simply want a group to "think" about the toxic substances seeping into a lake; he would want the

[12] David A. Kolb, Irwin M. Rubin, and James M. McIntyre, *Organizational Psychology, an Experiencial Approach* (Englewood Cliffs, N.J.: Prentice-Hall, Inc., 1974), pp. 21–40.

group to go out to the lake, test the water, and see for themselves what is happening. Active experimenters are often risk takers and for that reason alone they are a benefit to a group. Finally, some individuals approach problems through *abstract conceptualization.* Like the reflective observers they are analytical. However, they often take actions that help the group see the entire problem rather than simply one part of it. When the group becomes bogged down on one aspect of a problem the abstract conceptualizer will force the group to see how that issue relates to a larger problem. Abstract conceptualizers also like to follow a process for carrying out discussion. Such a process-oriented emphasis to problem solving is usually beneficial to the entire group.

One of the chief benefits of multidisciplinary work is that an individual's approach to learning and problem solving is complemented by other styles. The more complex the issue, the more the different modes of learning will be needed if a thorough examination is to be made. While it is true that the presence of four different learning styles can create conflict within a group, it is equally true that when the four styles are blended together problems can be efficiently and effectively addressed.

Increased acceptance of solutions   There are many instances where staff members are responsible for implementing key policy decisions. In such situations it can be helpful to have them involved in the defining of the policy and in determining the ways that it could best be instituted within the organization. When staff have input into the decision-making process they are generally more committed to implementing the decision than if they were not involved.

Lower economic costs   A final advantage of group decision making is that groups can be cost effective. For example, when a supervisor and four subordinates meet together for one hour, they collectively spend five working hours in the meeting. If the supervisor had to meet with each of the four subordinates individually a collective total of eight working hours would be needed. Moreover the extra three hours would all be at the expense of the supervisor's own schedule. This difference between the two modes—group versus individual meetings—can be further highlighted when cost figures are attached to each alternative. If you assume that the supervisor earns $20,000 per year and the subordinates earn $15,000 the total cost of the individual meetings would be $84.10; the group meeting would cost $45.66 or 54.3 percent of the cost of the individual meetings.[13] Note that the group meeting could last almost twice as long as the individual meetings and still cost less. Likewise it should be noted that as the size of the committee increases, the

[13] Filley, House, and Kerr, *Managerial Processes,* p. 143.

cost advantage increases; and as the mean earning of the committee members increase, the cost advantage also increases.[14]

Disadvantages of Committees

While there are advantages to committees, there are also disadvantages that should be weighed prior to initiating group deliberations. The three disadvantages commonly cited are premature decisions, individual domination, and disruptive conflicts.[15]

Premature decisions   Earlier we noted that a decision made by a group is generally superior to a decision made by an individual. That statement is true providing the group has done its homework and carefully examines potential solutions to a carefully defined problem.

Unfortunately, groups often do not spend the time necessary for rational problem solving. In addition, groups may decide on solutions that are popular but that are not necessarily effective. In other instances groups may think of more effective solutions after a consensus has already been reached but will not give full consideration. Their attitude is "Well, we made our decision. We better stick with it."

Individual domination   The quality of discussion can be undermined by the domination of one or two individuals. Dominators seek to exploit their power in order to arrive at decisions that they feel are in their best interest. The power may be legitimate, as evidenced by a hospital comptroller who is determined to see a given financial policy come out of the meeting, or it may be assumed, as evidenced by a house physician who has little formal authority but much technical expertise.

The domination of one or two individuals within a group dampens the enthusiasm of others. Some withdraw and become quiet. They may cease to attend the committee meetings citing the fact that "it's all wired; they (the dominators) will get their way." Still others respond to the domination by fighting back. Allegedly the fights are over an issue but in reality they are over the use of power within the group.

The success of group decision making is contingent upon a perception that everyone in the room has a chance to speak, to be heard, and to be taken seriously. When that perception is present, group members will share their ideas and, once a decision has evolved, will tend to support it.

[14] Ibid.
[15] Adapted with permission of the publisher from James A. F. Stoner, *Management,* pp. 299–302.

Disruptive conflicts   Seldom are there visible conflicts in the early stages of a group. Conflicts usually emerge when a position is defined that is perceived to have an adverse impact on one or more of the group members. When people feel threatened in a group they often stake out a counterposition. As they argue for their position they become psychologically invested in it. When other group members disagree, a competitive atmosphere emerges. Soon the issue is not finding a policy or a procedure or a decision that will best help the organization; rather, the issue is who will win the argument.

When a group is weighted down in win-or-lose issues, the energy of the membership is no longer focused on task-oriented outcomes. The *raison d'être* for the group is usually lost. Consequently, high-quality solutions that have high acceptance are rarely found.

Factors That Can Be Assets or Liabilites

There are several variables that can be considered strengths or weaknesses depending upon how they are managed by the leader and by the group membership.

Risk taking   A common myth about groups is that they are more conservative in decision making than individuals. Researchers have found that groups often make what they term "risky shifts," which are solutions to problems that are more innovative and daring than individuals would consider prudent if they were to make a decision on their own.[16] For example, in dealing with a hypothetical situation in which a worker must decide whether to stay in a secure job or go to one that is less secure but that offers a higher salary, groups have been more likely than individuals to recommend the riskier option.[17]

Disagreements   As we have seen, win-or-lose disagreements can erode the productivity and the morale of a group. However, disagreements are also a strength, providing that individuals are willing to learn from one another. It is through disagreements that new ideas are born and old ideas are examined. If a group does not have any task-oriented disagreements it probably has low cohesion which usually results in low productivity.

Vested interests   It is a rare situation where group members don't have a vested interest in a particular solution to an organizational problem. A vested interest is a weakness if the investment is so great that individuals can-

---

[16] There have been hundreds of studies published on the "risky shifts" phenomenon. Those who would like to study this intriguing concept are encouraged to read Russell D. Clark, "Group-Induced Shift Toward Risk: A Critical Appraisal," *Psychological Bulletin,* 76 (1971), 251–70.

[17] Stoner, *Management,* pp. 300–301.

not be objective about a situation. However, it can also be a strength. Usually those with vested interests are strongly committed to being in attendance and will argue forcefully for their position. Often they will have considerable technical information that can be used in group problem solving.

There are two basic principles that should be followed in working with individuals representing vested positions. First, if possible, the vested interest should be made public. Sometimes this can be most adeptly handled by asking all group members at the initial meeting to state what they hope to accomplish in the group. The more you can help members discuss their privately held positions, the less chance there is that they will later sabotage the decision-making process. Second, the basic norm that should be reinforced is objectivity. The group leader should repeatedly ask the group to examine all the facts in a situation rather that to consider only how a decision will alter one person's (or one department's) political position.

In summary, task-oriented groups and committees are an integral part of every formal organization. It is likely that there will be increased pressure to form additional committees and ad hoc groups as technology expands and regulations increase. Committees are not inherently "good" or "bad" although there are specific advantages and disadvantages that should be considered when establishing a committee structure within an organization.

BASIC CONCEPTS: THE DYNAMICS OF TASK-CENTERED GROUPS

We began our discussion of small-group communication by examining the assets and limitations of committees. As an administrator, your objective should be to maximize the strengths that committees bring to problem solving and to minimize their limitations. To do this it is important to understand the dynamics of task-centered groups. Each of the following propositions will give you insight into why some groups are productive, cohesive, and efficient while others fail to capture the imagination and interest of its members.

Proposition 1: Groups function most productively when there is a sharply focused goal.

The key words in the above proposition are *sharply focused goal*. The starting point in developing a successful committee structure is to write a charge. The word "charge" is an old military expression in which troops were assigned a target to be conquered. The success of the operation was contingent upon a clear understanding of what was to be achieved, how it was to be carried out, and the ramifications of what would take place if the unit was not successful in achieving their objective.

If a committee is to succeed, it also must have a defined task. Therefore, every committee should be given a charge that includes (1) a precise statement of the task, (2) the rationale as to why the task should be undertaken, and (3) a time frame that stipulates a terminal date for the completion of the assignment.

The *task* should be a straightforward description of what needs to be accomplished and can usually be written and confined to one or two sentences. The wording should be clear, concise, and understandable. Consider the following tasks, each of which is sharply focused:

Group	Task
Executive Committee, Salem Community Hospital	To produce by May 15 a certificate of need outlining a justification for the expansion of the hospital's department of obstetrics
Nursing Executive Committee, Parkview Nursing Home	To specify by June 30 administrative policies that can be used to *recruit* and *retain* staff nurses
Programming Committee, Public Health Nursing Department, State Health Department, State of Michigan	To determine by November 15 a minimum of ten educational programs that will be offered within the city of Benton Harbor during the next calendar year
Budget Accounts Committee, Health Services Division, State of Texas	To produce by May 30 three budgets—one that is 5% lower than the current budget, one that reflects current year's expenditures, and one that is 5% higher than this year's allocations

The second part of the charge contains the *rationale* as to why the assigned tasks must be accomplished. It is important for the membership to know the history of the issues they will be discussing and why they have been asked to participate. It is also helpful to list the qualifications of the person who is chairing the committee and to explain why he or she has been appointed to lead the group.

Finally, it is important to stipulate a *time frame* in which tasks should be accomplished. Sometimes the terminal date will be written into the tasks, as can be seen in the above examples. At other times administrators will write a separate section within the charge that specifies both the time frame and the nature of the product that is to be produced. It is not uncommon for administrators to ask for interim reports to ensure that the committee is making adequate progress in realizing its goals.

An effective method of communicating a charge to a committee is through a written memorandum as seen in Figure 6-1.

To: The Council of Department Heads
State Health Department

From: Bob Wexler, M.D., Health Commissioner

Subject: Evaluation of the Lead-Screening Programs

Task defined

During this coming year I am requesting the Council of Department Heads to review and make recommendations concerning the Lead-Screening programs which have been offered during the past five years. Specifically, I am asking you to *determine the effectiveness of these programs and to recommend by May 30th whether they should be continued, modified, or expanded.*

Rationale

This is a critical issue for our community and for our Health Department. We have had two deaths during this past year due to lead poisoning and thirteen youngsters were hospitalized for toxic reactions from digesting lead base paint.

I am asking the Council of Department Heads to address this issue, because most of your departments are involved in the current lead-screening and educational programs. Each of you brings your expertise to this community problem; each of you has resources within your departments which can be used in assessing the magnitude of the problem and possible remedies.

I have asked Ms. Francis Moore, R.N., M.P.H., the Director of the Public Health Nursing program, to chair your meetings. Ms. Moore has had considerable experience with community based educational programming. She also has perhaps the best data concerning the incidence of lead poisoning in this community and across the nation. I know of her interest in this topic and I am pleased that she has accepted this responsibility.

Time frame

I would like a final report from you by May 30, including specific recommendations as to what the Health Department's response should be to the lead-poisoning problem. I also would like an interim report concerning your programs by February 15th. If I can be of any assistance, please let me know.

Figure 6-1   Example of a charge to a committee.

Proposition 2: Productive committees are composed of productive individuals.

As one might anticipate, there is a positive correlation between the effectiveness of a group and the effectiveness of individual members. Yet this fundamental fact is often lost when committee members are haphazardly selected without forethought as to who should be on the committee, what they can contribute, and whether or not they will be effective.

While membership selection is often based on hunches as to who might do a good job, behavioral scientists have in recent years been able to define guidelines that can help you select the most appropriate people.[18] Let us look at five of the most important of these guidelines in more detail.

1. Before selecting the membership, determine how many people are actually needed to carry out the task. There is a tendency in many human service organizations to have committees consisting of a large number of individuals.

[18] For further information on group membership see Kenneth Wexley and Gary Yukl, *Organizational Behavior and Personnel Psychology* (Homewood Ill.: Richard D. Irwin, 1977), pp. 123–43.

The rationale for this is that anyone who has a stake in the issue should be included. While that rationale is understandable it often results in unwieldy and unproductive groups.

Think a moment of the groups that you have belonged to. Most of us have experienced membership in groups that ranged in size from three to twenty individuals. When you met with the larger-sized groups, how did you feel? Were you more inclined or less inclined to speak in the larger group? Did you feel your contribution carried as much weight in the larger as in the smaller groups? How satisfied were you with the decisions made in these respective groups?

If your experience is typical, you probably found that you spoke fewer times in larger groups and that a small number of individuals actually made the decisions. You may recall that the large groups were boring and slow moving. If so, you probably left the large groups with lower levels of satisfaction than you gained from the smaller groups where you actively participated.

Group size affects performance as well as satisfaction. We know that larger groups tend to take more time reaching decisions, particularly if consensus or near-consensus decisions are required. We also know that subgrouping takes place in large groups. Unless there is strong leadership that prevents the large group from splintering into subgroups there is often a split between conservative and liberals, those who are for something and those who are against, and those who want change and those who resist.

You can understand how easily subgroups form when you consider the communication relationships within groups of various size. In two-member groups, only two relationships are possible. But in a triad there are nine possiblilities (Figure 6–2). To demonstrate how rapidly the complexity of a group increases R. Bostrom[19] calculated all the communication relationships possible within groups from three to eight members:

Number in group	Interactions possible
2	2
3	9
4	28
5	75
6	186
7	441
8	1,056

For problem solving purposes *a group from five to seven members is ideal.* The reasons for this are threefold.

First, a group of five to seven members permits sufficient heterogeneity of ideas. Usually there will be three or four perspectives on a given issue;

[19] R. Bostrom, "Patterns of Communication Interaction in Small Groups," *Speech Monographs,* 37 (1970), 257–58.

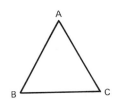

1. A to B	4. B to C	7. A to B and C
2. A to C	5. C to B	8. B to A and C
3. B to A	6. C to A	9. C to A and B

Figure 6-2 Possible relationships within a three-member group.

seldom will there be more than seven. A group with five to seven members is usually able to represent the various bodies of opinion on a given subject.

Second, a group of five to seven members permits everyone an opportunity to speak. No one has to fight to be heard. No one needs to feel inhibited by the sheer number of people in the group. The possibility for subgrouping is diminished because most members know the points of view of one another.

Finally, a group of five to seven members tends to be efficient. If consensus decision making is needed it will more likely be obtained by a committee of this size than by those that become increasingly larger. Therefore, when establishing a committee, keep the size of the group membership manageable. While five to seven members is not an ironclad rule, it does represent the optimal size when undertaking problem solving.

2. Select members on the basis of their technical abilities. The quality of decisions made within groups can usually be correlated with the quality of information that the committee has at hand. The key question you should ask when selecting committee members is "Who has the best information concerning this issue?" Interestingly the individual who has the best information may not be the person with an administrative title. While top-level executives and mid-level managers frequently serve on institutional committees, we are learning the importance of having staff members involved in deliberations on policy issues. They not only bring certain types of technical information to the discussion but often bring a perspective on the issue that administrators may not have.

3. Select members on the basis of their ability to implement decisions. One of the reasons that committees have poor reputations in many organizations is that decisions arrived at in committee meetings are often not implemented. At times this is because the decisions are impractical. At other times the decisions are made by individuals who do not have the formal authority to initiate action. In still other instances decisions are not implemented because they are not consistent with organizational policies or practices.

When committees deliberate for long periods of time and then find that their recommendations are not put into effect, the result is highly negative. Committee members resent the time they have wasted and will usually become critical of the administrator who they believe is not taking their work seriously. If the recommendations of committees are repeatedly shelved, managers and staff members will be reluctant to serve on subsequent committees.

To solve this problem it is important that individuals appointed to committees have enough administrative authority to implement their decisions. But if the recommendations cannot be implemented in whole or in part, it is equally important that the committee receive specific feedback as to why it cannot be done. Usually this implies that the chief administrator will meet with the group and inform them of the disposition of their report. While the group may disagree with the disposition they will respect the administrator who forthrightly communicates with them about their work.

4. Select members who have an interest in the topics to be discussed. If an issue does not have personal meaning to participants, it is likely that their interest in the group will be reflected in tardiness, missed meetings, and a general lack of interest.[20]

5. Finally, it is important to select individuals who have appropriate interpersonal skills. While it is hoped that those who serve on committees will be able to ask pertinent questions, process large amounts of data, mediate conflicting opinions, and logically think through the implications of the discussion, there is one interpersonal skill that is basic to effective group participation. The *ability to listen* should be the chief communication attribute you look for when selecting members for a committee. All other productive communication behaviors within groups are based on that key skill.

Proposition 3: Effective and efficient formal group operations require a leader who is directive and task oriented, yet concerned about the social structure of the group.

Most studies on committee effectiveness have found that productive groups usually have strong, task-oriented leadership. L. Berkowitz, for example, found in a study of seventy-two management conferences that a high degree of "leadership sharing" was *inversely* related to participant satisfaction and group output.[21] While it is generally recognized that there is a close correlation between group effectiveness and leader effectiveness often it is not clear what characterizes strong, task-oriented leaders. Is it the leader's personality? Is it the leader's knowledge of the topic or the ability to persuade others? At just what point does "strong, directive" leadership become overbearing and counterproductive?

[20] Wexley and Yukl, *Organizational Behavior,* pp. 123–30.
[21] Cited in Filley, House, and Kerr, *Managerial Processes,* p. 148.

To answer such questions we must turn to the body of theory and research associated with small-group communication. Much of this research, initiated after World War II, focuses on the issue that we are now exploring: What makes a person effective in a leadership role?

Much of the early research hypothesized that personality traits distinguished leaders from followers. The notion that leaders are born, not made, had evolved through centuries of religious and political thought. Conventional political wisdom has suggested that individuals such as Roosevelt, Lenin, Hitler, and Churchill had certain traits through which they could evoke the trust of their followers. It is interesting to note that during the 1980 presidential campaign there was a lamenting that the candidates didn't seem "presidential"—that is, they didn't have the necessary traits of vision and magnetism.

In testing the assumption that leaders were somehow different from followers, researchers began measuring all sorts of characteristics including the weight and height of leaders and contrasted such statistics with those of nonleaders. They gave intelligence, vocabulary, and personality tests with the hope that the resulting data would delineate specific traits endemic to those who occupy leadership positions. But it was to no avail. In 1948 R. M. Stogdill reviewed the studies and declared that it was impossible to delineate any inherent personality traits that differentiate leaders from nonleaders.[22] The long-held belief that leaders are born and possessed inherent leadership qualities simply did not stand up under scientific study.

After Stogdill's research was published, a second assumption was tested: the assumption that effective leaders had desirable *communication styles*. The researchers compared autocratic and democratic styles of leading groups and compared leaders who were group oriented (that is, concerned about the social dimension of groups) with those who were production oriented (that is, concerned with the task dimension of groups). The initial studies demonstrated a superiority for democratic styles of leadership as measured in terms of production, group participation, and morale. It appeared that individuals who shared authority with group members were more successful in achieving high productivity and morale than were authoritarian leaders. However, the notion that one particular leadership style is inherently more effective than other styles was soon discredited. Researchers were able to demonstrate that, while one particular style might be effective on a particular situation, it did not follow that such a style would be effective in all situations. An autocratic military leader might be effective in war; however, those same autocratic approaches might fail if tried in a civilian work setting.

The realization that the situation partly determines what leadership

[22] R.M. Stogdill, "Personal Factors Associated with Leadership: A Survey of the Literature," *Journal of Psychology,* 25 (1948), 35–71. Note as well, R.M. Stogdill, *Handbook of Leadership: A Survey of Theory and Research* (New York: Free Press, 1974).

behavior is more effective led small-group theorists to advocate a *contextual* approach to the study of leadership. Today the contextual approach is by far the most popular and most common perspective in studying group leadership.

From a contextual perspective, an effective group leader is one who can master the environment in which the group exists. To do that, a group leader must look upon every group as unique for every group has its own norms, talents, potentials, and modes of communication. Therefore a leader grounded in contextual theory would not necessarily utilize skills and behaviors that had been successfully used in the past and transpose them on a new group. Rather the leader would examine the group's context and determine what leadership behaviors are appropriate in this new situation.

One of the most important concepts to emerge out of contextual theory is that of group norms. A norm is a "shared expectation of right action that binds members of a group and results in guiding and regulating their behavior."[23] There are several norms that are particularly important in influencing the group's productivity: procedural norms, norms of critical thinking, and norms of social support. Anyone who wishes to successfully lead a group must understand how norms are established, how they can be modified, and how they correlate with effective task-oriented discussion. Let's begin by examining some of the most basic norms that are established in the very early stages of a group's deliberations.

Establishing procedural norms   When a group comes together for the first time there usually is a high degree of primary tension.[24] Primary tension is represented in the social unease and stiffness that often accompanies the first group meeting. This is particularly true if group members do not know one another. Each will want to make a good impression on others. Each will be concerned with whom they can trust and who might pose a threat. Each will make an assessment as to whether the group will be worth their time. Often the primary tension will be seen in extreme politeness, apparent boredom, or tiredness accompanied with considerable sighing or yawning.[25]

Figure 6–3 is a hypothetical construct that helps explain the effect of social tensions within a group. The horizontal line on the figure indicates the amount of social tension a given group can tolerate and still be productive. However, when tensions rise above this level the group cannot function effectively. The group may go through the motions of talking about an issue and even try to solve problems. However, unless the primary tensions are diminished the possibility that the group will make sound decisions is very low.

Contextual theory suggests that skilled leaders should recognize that one

[23] Ernest G. Bormann, *Discussion and Group Methods: Theory and Practice* (New York: Harper & Row, 1969), p. 260.

[24] Ibid., p. 107.

[25] Ibid., p. 172.

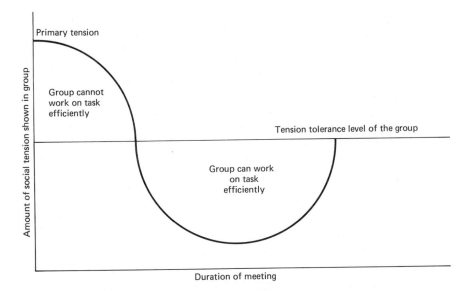

Figure 6-3   Primary tension curve. [From *Discussion and Group Methods: Theory* and *Practice*. Copyright © 1969 by Ernest G. Bormann. Reprinted by permission of Harper and Row Publishers, Inc.]

of their immediate goals ought to be the reduction of primary tension within the group. To reduce such tension procedural norms will need to be established. These norms are rooted in some of the most elementary, yet important questions that group participants have on their minds.

"What is the purpose of this meeting?" A skillfull leader needs to set forth the context of the meeting. One way to accomplish this is to stipulate the underlying purpose of the deliberations. Generally meetings fall into one of four categories. The *briefing meeting* provides members with information necessary to carry through on plans that have been previously determined. In such meetings the objective is clear and the group members only need to find out who is to do what, when, and where. *Instructional meetings* are designed primarily to give group members information that will help them become more proficient in their task or give them background information that will assist in making decisions in subsequent meetings. For example, if a health agency is asked to respond to a legislative mandate, the chief executive officer might invite legislators to describe the new legislation with the heads of the various departments. If this were an instructional meeting no effort would be made to evaluate the legislation or even to determine how the health agency should respond. Rather, the purpose would be to obtain the best possible information about all facets of the legislation. A *consultative meeting* is one where an individual responsible for a decision asks for advice from members of the group. The group is seen as a reservoir of information that should be

tapped if a quality decision is to be made. In such a setting the group is not responsible for making the decison but only for providing information. Finally there are *decision-making meetings.* Most group members prefer such meetings because they have an opportunity to formulate courses of action. If the decision is important, the discussion will be spirited as individuals shape the final product of the group.

Primary tension increases when there is confusion within the group concerning the fundamental purpose of the meeting. If members come expecting to make decisions but it turns out that they are only to receive a briefing, they may resent that their time is not being used in a more valuable way. Conversely if they come expecting to only listen to someone present an issue and suddenly find that they are in the middle of a heated decision-making process they may wish that they had arrived better prepared.

To reduce the primary tension a group leader should carefully delineate the specific purpose of each meeting. A well-written agenda can assist if it contains a brief paragraph outlining what is to be accomplished and the topics that will be discussed. As you examine the agenda in Figure 6-4, determine how the leader is seeking to reduce the primary tension within the group.

"Will this committee take up much of my time?" One of the concerns that heightens primary tension is the degree to which a committee might con-

---

AGENDA

Executive Council

Date of next meeting: March 29th

Meeting time: 3:00–5:00 P.M.

Place of meeting: A-306

Several physicians have raised questions concerning the scope of the hospital's liability insurance program. Mr. Frank Brenner, Assistant Vice-President of the Prudential Insurance Company will be with us to describe the key points of our coverage and to compare our policy with that of other hospitals.

The purpose of this meeting is to provide information necessary to evaluate our insurance program. In subsequent meetings we will determine whether a recommendation should be made to the Board of Trustees concerning the modification and/or expansion of our insurance coverage.

In order to make this meeting as productive as possible, specific questions which you would like Mr. Brenner to address should be forwarded to Dr. Gerald Anderson prior to March 24th.

    3:00   Coffee
    3:15–4:00   Overview of the hospital's Insurance Program—Mr. Brenner
    4:00–4:45   Discussion of questions/issues identified by members of the Executive Council
    4:45–5:00   Identification of agenda items for future meetings of the Executive Council
    5:00   Adjournment

If you cannot attend but would like a briefing on this meeting please contact Ms. Shirley McDonald at 373-8106.

Figure 6-4 An example of an agenda.

sume valuable work time. Most group members are eager to have the amount of work that will be required sharply defined.

There are a number of ways to address the time issue. You may choose to be direct and indicate that you have scheduled a series of meetings in order to complete the task. Or you may prefer asking the group to determine when they would like to meet and for how long. Committee members usually prefer this approach and will quickly begin to identify what needs to be done and how many meetings should be scheduled in order to achieve the task. By asking the group to resolve this issue you are implicitly stating an important norm about your leadership behavior: You expect the group to determine solutions to problems that will emerge during the life of the group. An additional advantage of having the group determine meeting times is that it gives members an opportunity to determine when they can be most productive. Breakfast meetings may be difficult for parents who want to see their children off to school. Likewise there will be times during the workday that are more desirable than others, given each person's work priorities.

"What happens if we miss a meeting?" An important question that is seldom overtly discussed concerns the consequences of not attending meetings. This is an important issue and probably should be addressed by the group leader in one of the early meetings.

Some leaders find it helpful to reinforce the necessity of attending meetings, yet give members the freedom to miss if other work priorities arise. Consider the following comment of a group leader:

> I would hope that we would have high attendance at these meetings. Given the tasks that are before us we will probably be able to arrive at decisions more efficiently if we are in regular attendance. However, in a busy hospital such as ours I do know that, on occasion, you may need to miss a meeting. When that happens I would appreciate it if you would let me know beforehand. Minutes of the meeting will be circulated to you within one week of the committee meeting. As you read the minutes of a meeting that you missed please feel free to call me or another member of our group to obtain additional information about what took place. At any rate, I hope that you will find this group to be so stimulating that it will be a rare event when you can't attend!

Comments such as these reinforce important expectations. On the one hand the leader is indicating that he or she recognizes that emergencies do arise and that some meetings may be missed. On the other hand, the leader is indicating that this should not take place frequently. And, when members can't attend, they have certain obligations—not the least of which is to become knowledgeable about what took place in the meeting.

"How will we handle conflict when it comes up in this group?" Most groups can release their primary tensions by determining the nature of the task, how it should be approached, and how they can best work together. However, as discussion ensues, misunderstandings, disagreements, and per-

sonality conflicts may emerge. Ernest Bormann describes the symptoms of the *secondary tension* as follows:

> Secondary tension causes a different group climate than does primary tension. It is loud, noisier and more dynamic. Voices are louder and more strained. Long pauses may appear but often two or three people speak at a time. Everyone is highly interested in the proceedings. No one seems bored or tired. Members may fidget in their chairs, half rise, pound the table, get up and pace the room, run their hands through their hair, gesture excitedly and exhibit a much higher level of excitement and involvement.[26]

It is common for members to cope with secondary tension in one of two ways. Those who do not enjoy conflict situations will withdraw. They may sit through an entire meeting and not offer a single comment. Others whose anxiety has been heightened to such a degree that it must be dissipated will fight. They are the ones who become loud, noisy, and more dynamic.

It is important to help the group work through the secondary tension that may be causing anxiety and conflict. At times this can best be accomplished by asking questions that invite individuals to diagnose the dynamics within the group: "Do you think we are making adequate progress?" "What is keeping us from being able to make decisions?" "If we could change one thing within our group, what would it be?" "How can we restructure next week's discussion so that it is more profitable?" Such forthright questions will establish a norm of conduct that indicates that "in this group, our problems will be confronted."

Establishing norms of critical thinking   Effective problem solving is contingent upon analytical thought. An effective leader will prod the group to think, use logic, test ideas, demand evidence, and refute that which does not appear to be valid.

Group members frequently emulate the leader in determining how analytical and critical they should be within the discussion. If the group leader is amiable, doesn't want to offend anyone, and isn't eager to test the ideas of others, it is likely that the group will follow such norms. On the other hand if the group leader values reasoning, asks for clarification, and critically examines statements made by group members, it is likely that others will also approach issues analytically.

Analytical thought is based on these three questions:

1. What do you mean?
2. How do you know?
3. What does this mean for us—right now?

[26] Ibid., p. 171.

These three questions can keep a group from becoming intellectually lazy. Consider a conversation among three nurses concerned about the working conditions within their hospital. Note how skillfully Joan Hastings is able to move the conversation from opinion to an analysis of facts.

Mary Fraser: Working around here sure is dreadful.

Judy Kizer: Yeah, they are always shorthanded. I'm not sure I can take another year.

Joan Hastings: What do you mean? A year ago, before I came to work here
(1)   you told me that this was the greatest place in the world to work!

Judy Kizer: I did? Ha, ha. That's what you get for accepting my advice.

   [*Long pause*]

Joan Hastings: I take it from things you have mentioned last week that you
(2)   really don't like this hospital.

Mary Fraser: Oh, I don't mean to imply that everything is bad. But it just doesn't seem that they care about the nurses.

Joan Hastings: Well, last year the raises were better than what we received in
(3)   a long, long time. And we did get an additional paid holiday this year.

Joan Hastings: What is it specifically that bothers you?
(4)

Mary Fraser: I can't put my finger on it. I sometimes think it is that rigid scheduling office. Other times I think I've just been doing oncology nursing for too long. And still other times I wonder whether my feelings about nursing aren't more a reflection of problems I've been having at home.

Joan Hastings: If you were to make one change around here that would make
(5)   you feel better, what might it be?

   [*Long pause*]

Mary Fraser: I probably would like to do a different kind of nursing—like work with kids in pediatrics.

Judy Kizer: That's possible for you to do isn't it?

[*From here the discussion centered on positive actions that they could take to increase work satisfaction.*]

As you reread the above conversation note how Joan, through the use of thought-provoking questions, is able to help Mary rethink her situation. Joan first asked for clarification (1) of what Judy meant when she stated that she couldn't "take another year." Second, Joan summarized the feelings implicit in Mary's opening comment (2) and challenged the belief that their particular hospital was a poor place in which to work (3). She asked Mary to define what she didn't like in her position (4) and finally challenged her to determine constructive action (5).

An effective group leader should make an assessment of the intellectual climate at each meeting for it will change over time. If group members are unwilling to undertake critical thought, the group leader will need to ask questions, test assumptions, and—by example—compel the group to deal with the issues. This can be accomplished through two types of inquiries.

First, ask for a definition of concepts and words being expressed within the group. Terms are frequently defined arbitrarily, particularly when they have emotive meanings. In a context of a bitter strike between hospital administration and employee unions words such as "solidarity" "picket lines" and "lockout" will be given an almost idiosyncratic definition by the one using such expressions. The terms "capping of costs" or "health services competition" will be perceived in one way by a hospital administrator who is seeking to balance a budget and in another way by a government official who is seeking to restrain hospital expenditures.

Second, test the premises upon which statements are made. When a group member advances an argument the first step in testing the conclusion is to be certain that the premises are true. If it turns out that one or more premises are false, the conclusion will be unacceptable. For example, someone might state that the basic reason for having a nursing union is "to increase our wages." That may be correct—but it may not be. It may be that the real reason for a nursing union is to upgrade the status of nursing and that one method by which that status will be improved is through the increase of wages.

To repeat, *the quality of a group's product/outcomes will reflect the amount of analytical thought that takes place within the meetings.* The group's leadership has the primary responsibility to ensure that deliberative thinking takes place.

Establishing norms of social support   An effective leader will establish procedural norms and, through role modeling, help establish norms of critical thinking. But it is equally important for the leader, if morale is to be high, to ensure that members receive social support.

Traditionally the literature in small-group communication has contained much prescriptive advice on how to develop positive social norms. Group leaders were told of the importance of helping group members learn about one another prior to working on the task. It was suggested that leaders should be friendly to participants, give everyone the right to speak, disagree without becoming disagreeable, protect the rights of group members representing minority positions, and, when a group member fails to attend a meeting, let the member know that he or she was missed.

Contemporary small-group theorists do not minimize the significance of these basic communication behaviors; however, they suggest that *meaningful norms of social support evolve out of meaningful tasks.* You can help the group become acquainted with one another, you may model superb communication skills as evidence in giving everyone a chance to speak, but unless the tasks that the group are addressing are *perceived to be meaningful,* the norms of social support will usually not emerge.

When groups address significant issues the norms of social support become established in an almost incognito fashion. Consider a governing board of a health systems agency that is designing a health systems plan. The board's task will be to identify the most significant health problems in their region and determine an annual implementation plan.

At the initial meeting there may be a great deal of primary tension. Members may not know one another and will probably have little knowledge about what it is they are to accomplish. Usually the board will consist of representatives from nursing, medicine, hospital administration, and public health. In addition, half of the board members will usually be consumers, some of whom may have little knowledge of the complex issues that will be addressed. As the discussion begins it is likely that each member will reflect on how his or her comments are being interpreted; it is probable that each will speculate about the motivations of others for serving on the board.

After several meetings, group members will begin to feel more comfortable with one another. They now have a better understanding of the tasks that are to be addressed and they will have a better idea of what contributions each can make. If board members are being positively reinforced for their contributions, most will go away from the meetings feeling that their presence is valued and respected.

After the third or fourth meeting, the group environment will be such that members will feel free to disagree with one another. This usually represents the first test as to whether the social norms are strong enough to withstand the tension. If the disputing parties seek to understand one another's perspective it is likely that the cohesion within the group is of sufficient durability that it will be able to withstand the secondary tensions that arise.

If, after seven or eight meetings, you were to analyze the board's deliberations, you would find that social norms have been firmly established. If the group is productive you may be able to identify positive social norms as reflected in comments made by participants:

"I really look forward to these meetings. This is one of the hardest working groups that I have ever been in."

"I don't always agree with what's going on, but I don't hesitate to speak up. And I don't hang back if I've got a disagreement with someone else."

"What we are doing is important. We might not always agree with one another, but you know that you always have a chance to say what is on your mind."

"This committee is worth my time. I'm glad I'm here."

In helping a group develop positive social norms the group leader should ask, *What can I do to help the group members see the significance of this task?* If a group understands the importance of their deliberations they will be less likely to show up late or miss meetings. They also will be more inclined to do their homework and dig for facts that will be useful in the discussion. When disagreements occur, group members will try to understand what is being said so that a quality product can be produced that will withstand the critical scrutiny of outsiders. But if the membership does not see the significance of the meeting and if they come to believe that the group is "treading water," "spinning its wheels," or a "waste of time," undesirable social norms will be formed. In all likelihood the existence of these negative social norms will be reflected in low group productivity, low morale, and a desire to get off the committee as soon as possible. In summary, directive leadership occurs when the person who is chairing the committee establishes positive procedural, critical thinking, and social norms. If the leader can resolve the procedural issues quickly, the group will soon be able to move into a discussion of substantive issues. If the norms of critical inquiry are present the group will be able to synthesize large quantities of information and outline issues in an efficient manner. If the group understands the significance of the task and if each member believes that his or her contribution is important, strong social norms will develop and will be particularly useful in resolving conflicts and tensions that may emerge.

Proposition 4: Effective group decison making is facilitated through the use of decision-making models.

The traditional method of teaching students how to make decisions is based on John Dewey's "Five Phases of Reflected Thought." Virtually all authorities in small-group communication have elaborated on these phases and usually advocate the following major steps as agendas for the discussion process:

1. Making a precise statement of the nature and scope of the problem
2. Finding information about the problem

3. Determining causes of the problem
4. Specifying the goal to be achieved in the solution
5. Stipulating limitations on the group's problem-solving and implementation ability
6. Proposing a variety of possible solutions
7. Testing these solutions against goals and limitations
8. Defining a final solution
9. Implementing the solution into operation

While a knowledge of the above process is important, it does not specify what actually should be done in each step to help a group arrive at a high-quality decision. This weakness in decision-making technology has been rectified by the advent of information systems. In recent years quantification has been playing an ever more important role in the theory and practice of decision making. In fact, the term, *decision sciences* is becoming more commonplace in the vocabulary of practicing administrators as they become more aware of various quantitative and quasi-quantitative decison-making models.

There are a number of decision-making models available to health administrators who wish to improve the decision-making capabilities of their institution.[27] Each has its strengths, limitations, and potential uses in human services organizations. We will focus on one model called the Program Evaluation Review Technique (PERT) because it is a method that has been successfully used in human service organizations and is adaptable to committee deliberations.

The U.S. Navy introduced PERT in 1958 as a response to some of the problems arising in designing the Polaris missile program. Later it was adopted by the Air Force and numerous other government units and private industrial enterprises because it is well suited to program planning and management control.

PERT procedure consists in a group working together to plot a network of the activities that must be undertaken to achieve a specific outcome or goal.

---

[27] Among the most widely known quantitative techniques are the following: *Game Theory*—used to determine the optimum strategy in a competitive situation; *Linear Programming*—used to allocate scarce resources in an optimum manner in problems of scheduling, service mix, etc.; *Simulation*—used to imitate an operation or process prior to actual performance; *Waiting-Line Theory*—used to analyze the feasibility of adding facilitites and to assess the amount and cost of waiting time; and *Sampling*—used for market research and internal audits of employee productivity. A concise summary of quantitative methods of analysis can be found in Joseph L. Massie, *Essentials of Management* (Englewood Cliffs, New Jersey: Prentice-Hall, Inc., 1979), pp. 155-71. Further information on quantitative approaches to decision making can be found in Harold Bierman, Jr., Charles P. Bonini, and Warren H. Hausman, *Quantitative Analysis for Business Decisions* (Homewood, Ill.: Richard D. Irwin, 1977).

The completed network serves to define and coordinate what must be accomplished as well as revealing weaknesses in the implementation plan.

The steps involved in PERT decison making are summarized by Gerald M. Phillips:[28]

1. Define a *final* "event" or occurrence that will mark the completion of a problem-solving effort or program. The final event might also be thought of as the goal that is to be achieved. The term "event," which is used in several of the PERT steps, is defined as an incident that takes no time but that marks the beginning or completion of a process.

2. List the major events that must take place before the final event can happen. You do not need to list events in order but care should be taken to evaluate each item listed to ensure that it conforms to the definition of an event and does not name a process. The group utilizing PERT should make certain that no major element of implementation is left out in listing of the events.

3. The events are now ordered in sequence of occurrence, if it is possible to do so (Figure 6-5). By listing these events you may find that some can occur simultaneously; that is, they are not dependent on each other. Sometimes events are discovered that depend on the completion of more than one precedent event. It should be emphasized that the ordering of events is based upon what *must* occur immediately before each named event. "This is not a matter of preference", states Phillips, "but of logic. If you find that it makes no difference whether one event precedes another it cannot be listed as a precedent."[29]

4. Fill the event chart together into a diagram as represented in Figure 6-6. This diagram is a skeleton description of the entire program. Its chief benefit is that it can be examined visually for logic. "If two lines happened to cross, for example, it would likely mean that two activities would interfere with each other. If the lines looped it would reveal an endless activity probably carried on for no reason. If a visual examination indicates that some of the lines do not connect, it would indicate either an error in planning or scheduling an unnecessary activity."[30]

5. If the logic of the PERT diagram is satisfactory to the group, the planning of the activities that must take place should be undertaken. Usually in this phase the group will estimate the time that each of the activities require and this is recorded on the "track" *between* each event (t_e). In calculating estimated time, group members are asked to make three calculations: an optimistic estimate indicating the least amount of time

---

[28] The section on the PERT Technique has been adapted from Gerald Phillips, "PERT as a Logical Adjunct to the Discussion Process," *The Journal of Communication,* Vol. XV, Number 2, (June 1965), pp. 89–99.

[29] Ibid., p. 95.

[30] Ibid., pp. 95–96.

Agency: City Health Department

Goal: Community Education Drive on Air Pollution

Program: Television Documentary

Event no.	Event	Necessarily preceded by:
1.	Campaign planning meeting adjourns	0
2.	Campaign proposal presented to supervisor	1
3.	Approval letter from supervisor received	2
4.	Film selected	3
5.	Film ordered	4
6.	Film received	5
7.	Meet with TV station manager	4
8.	TV schedule confirmed	7
9.	Publicity items written	8, 13
10.	Publicity items mailed to newspaper	9
11.	Film discussants selected	4
12.	Film discussants invited	11
13.	Film discussants accept invitation	12
14.	Spot announcements drafts completed	4, 13
15.	Spot announcements played	14
16.	Film delivered to TV studio	6
17.	Film discussants arrive at studio	13
18.	*Final Event:* Televised documentary film off air	17, 10

Figure 6-5   Sequencing of events. [From Gerald Phillips, "PERT as a Logical Adjunct to the Discussion Technique," *Journal of Communication,* 15, no. 2 (June 1965), 95.]

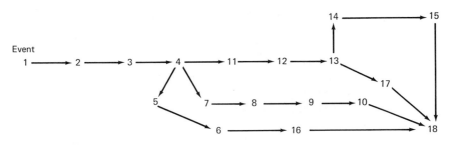

Figure 6-6   PERT diagram for TV show. [From Gerald Phillips, "PERT as a Logical Adjunct to the Discussion Technique," *Journal of Communication,* 15, no. 2 (June 1965), 96.]

that it will take to undertake the activity (a), a pessimistic estimate (b), and an estimate of the most likely time (m). Estimated time is determined from a weighted average as follows:

$$t_e = \frac{a + 4m + b}{6}$$

After calculating the estimated time, it is helpful for the group to calculate a variance (δ^2) for each combination of events:

$$\delta^2 = \frac{b - a}{6}$$

6. The basic task in step 6 is to determine how long it will take to accomplish each event (T_e). The very latest date by which each event will be completed (T_l) is calculated by working backward from the starting date for the project (T_s). By using these figures the group can now fill in the blanks on their network and determine what is called a "critical path," which is the path to the final outcome that has the least slack time. The slack time is computed by subtracting T_l from T_e.

The path with the least slack time becomes the critical path in the program. The estimates of how long the program will take to complete will depend on the critical path. The estimate is made by calculating Z from:[31]

$$Z = \frac{(T_s - T_l)}{\sqrt{\Sigma \delta^2 T_e}}$$

Z will be subsequently checked on a table of the normal curve for an estimate of the probability that the entire program will be completed on time. Figure 6–7 is an example of a completed activity chart.

The PERT process is orderly, deliberative, and logic oriented. But does it actually work in an orderly way when used by groups whose membership has varying opinions, vested interests, and perceptions? Does PERT actually rule out differences of perception, interpersonal conflicts, and outright disputes between group members?

PERT theoreticians do not deny that orderly process can be disrupted by psychological and conceptual differences between members of a group. However, they suggest that the nonrational elements can be controlled by using a very deliberate problem-solving methodology from start to finish that incorporates the essential elements of the PERT process is as follows:[32]

[31] Ibid., p. 96.

[32] Adapted from Gerald M. Phillips, "PERT as A Logical Adjunct to the Discussion Process," *The Journal of Communication,* Vol. XV, No. 2 (June 1965), pp. 91–92.

Between events	Activities	Time in days				
		a	m	b	t_e	σ^2
1 & 2	Committee appointed to write report Report draft written Report approval obtained Report delivered to supervisor	7	14	28	15.2	11.25
2 & 3	Supervisor reads report Approval granted					
3 & 4	Committee appointed and meets Screening and acceptance of films Previewing films Approval letter received Film selected	7 21	10 42	14 56	10.2 40.8	1.44 33.99
4 & 5	Letter written Check obtained Order mailed and received	7	10	14	10.2	1.44
4 & 7	Meetings held with TV director	7	10	14	10.2	1.44
4 & 14	Copywriter hired Drafts written and approved	21	28	35	28.0	5.29
5 & 6	Film shipped and received	21	28	35	28.0	5.29
6 & 16	Film inspected, packaged, delivered	0.25	1	2	1.0	0.08
16 & 18	Film played	0.25	0.27	0.50	0.3	0.004
7 & 8	Schedule prepared and approved	7	14	21	14.0	1.37
8 & 9	Drafts written and approved	21	28	35	28.0	5.29
9 & 10	Releases mimeographed and mailed	1	2	3	2.0	0.11
10 & 18	Releases received and run 5 times	5	6	8	6.2	0.25
4 & 11	List of possible discussants made Discussants and alternates selected	14	21	28	21.0	5.44
11 & 12	Phone calls made	1	2	3	2.0	0.11
12 & 13	Details given discussants Alternates contacted if necessary Final confirmation of discussants	7	14	21	14.0	1.37
13 & 14	Notification sent	0.1	0.1	0.1	0.1	0
14 & 15	Announcements delivered Run for one week	8	12	15	11.8	1.35
15 & 18	Interval to program	0.25	0.25	0.25	0.25	0
13 & 17	Instructions given discussants Discussants preview film Discussion rehearsal	14	21	28	21.0	5.44
17 & 18	Warm–up discussion	0.12	0.20	0.25	0.2	0.04
13 & 9	Biographies and background obtained	7	10	12	9.9	0.69

Figure 6-7 PERT activity chart. [From Gerald Phillips, "PERT as a Logical Adjunct to the Discussion Technique," *Journal of Communication,* 15, no. 2 (June 1965), 97.]

1. The *source* of the problem under discussion is defined.
   a. Statement of group feeling concerning the source of the problem.
   b. Subgroup assigned to investigate the source of the problem and report back to the group.

2. Leader states problem.
   a. Terms and phrases are defined.
   b. Background information is analyzed.

3. Factual statements offered, classified, and tested.
   a. Statement should not be opinion or evaluation.
   b. Statement must be a "fact"; if in doubt the criteria for a "fact" is examined.
   c. Statement must be pertinent to the problem.

4. Leader restates problem in the light of the facts; terms and phrases are redefined until group agrees they understand problem.

5. Causal statement offered.
   a. Cause must relate to observable phenomena.
   b. Cause must relate to controllable elements.
   c. Cause must be pertinent to problem.

6. Group authority and limitations defined.
   a. Group determines power, scope of authority, time, money, and personnel available.
   b. Group establishes legal, moral, and practical limits on activity.

7. Goal statement offered.
   a. Goal must be pertinent to redefined problem.
   b. Goal must fit within authority and limitations.
   c. Group agrees list of goals are complete.

8. Group determines extent to which goals are realized or in process of realization through ongoing problems.

9. Solution proposed.
   a. Solution must be goal directed.
   b. Solution must be feasible.
   c. Solution must fit within authority and limitations.

10. PERT plan developed for program.
    a. Event list established.
    b. Event list ordered.
    c. Activities listed.
    d. Time (T_e) estimates calculated.
    e. Variances calculated.
    f. Expected times calculated.
    g. Scheduled completion time set.

h. Latest completion times calculated.

i. Probability of completion calculated.

11. Program activated and completed.

12. Program evaluated against goals.

a. If goals not satisfied, group attempts new solution.

b. If goals satisfactorily met, group may receive new problem.

In summary, one of the principle advantages of the PERT procedure is reliance on logic and rational step-by-step problem solving. Its success in both public and private sectors has been noteworthy. While it cannot guarantee that the best solution to the given problem will always be found, it can give a reasonable estimate of the time it will take to finish a task and a probability that the solution will achieve specific objectives agreed to at the outset of the process.

Proposition 5: Group cohesiveness, or solidarity, is an important indicator of how much influence the group as a whole has over individual members.

Human beings have been aware of the importance of cohesion since they began to record their history. Military commanders, athletic coaches, political leaders, and employers have long discovered the importance of teamwork, group loyalty, and high morale if certain goals were to be accomplished. The troop, team, or business staff that functions as a well-integrated unit can often accomplish tasks that would be impossible to achieve if members were only concerned with themselves. Members of cohesive groups are loyal to one another, look forward to the group meetings, and often speak with pride about the group's accomplishments. Students of small-group behavior refer to this feeling of loyalty and *esprit de corps* as group cohesiveness.

During the past two decades researchers have sought to document the importance of cohesion in contemporary work groups. They have found a positive relationship between group cohesiveness, performance norms, and performance itself, indicating that cohesion is a valuable asset. You will note in Figure 6-8 that high performance is contingent upon high performance norms and high cohesiveness. High performance norms signify that the group has demanding yet achievable goals and is committed to realizing those goals during a predetermined time period. High cohesiveness implies that the group members respect one another, value one another's contributions, and will support one another even in task-oriented conflict situations.

Figure 6-8 also demonstrates that a group may have high performance norms but, if cohesion is low, will be able to obtain only medium performance. You can probably verify this from your own experience if you have been a member of a group where the performance goals were acheivable but the group's cohesion was low because of disruptive misunderstandings.

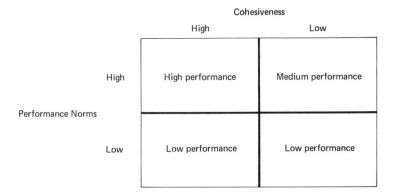

Figure 6-8 The relationship between cohesion and performance. [From John M. Ivancevich, Andrew D. Szilagyi, and Marc J. Wallace, Jr., *Organizational Behavior and Performance* (Santa Monica, Calif.: Goodyear Publishing Co., Inc., 1977), p. 219.]

One may ask whether performance is *always* contingent upon high cohesion. The answer is a qualified no. It is possible to have high performance without high cohesion for short periods of time. In their pennant-winning years the Oakland Athletics baseball team had many interpersonal disputes. There was constant complaining and bickering and players demanded to be traded. Yet they won baseball games. Likewise, an autocratic boss may be able to achieve high productivity for a short period of time but it is unlikely that high performance will be maintained *over time* without an element of cohesion among the staff. It is interesting to note that shortly after winning their division titles, the Oakland Athletics became a losing, mediocre baseball club.

Whether a group is cohesive can be detected by listening to how its members talk to one another and the character of their conversation. In highly cohesive groups you will see a lot of social interplay. Group members will greet one another by their first names. They will quickly get down to the task at hand. There will be little strategizing as to what to say or how to say it; rather members will state what they are feeling at the present moment. The conversation will be lively and task oriented. After the meeting has adjourned you will hear comments such as "We sure got a lot accomplished today," or "That hour really went by fast," which are indicative of a highly cohesive group.

Interestingly, researchers have found that there often is more conflict rather than less in cohesive groups. In highly cohesive groups, members feel free to disagree with one another and to challenge one another's perspectives. Robert F. Bales and his associates at Harvard studied a number of different groups and found that the most disagreements occurred when husbands and wives were in the same group.[33] The reason for this is that families tend to be highly cohesive units where people speak their minds. It's a safe environment for disagreement. Therefore when husbands and wives come to the same group meeting they may be the first to disagree with one another.

The signs of low cohesion are equally easy to identify. If you sense that everyone is overly polite to one another, the chances are good that there is low cohesion. If group members are bored, disinterested, yawning, or looking out the window you can be assured that the group is communicating a not-too-subtle message: "Let's get this meeting over with as quickly as possible."

There are a number of actions that a group leader can take to strengthen the cohesion with the group. Among the most important are the following:

Keep the size of the group manageable   It was earlier recommended that the membership of task-oriented groups be limited to five to seven members. In a well-known study of group cohesion, Stanley Seashore collected data on almost 6,000 people in industry and found that cohesion *declined* as group size *increased* up to about twenty members.[34] Beyond twenty members the cohesiveness diminished dramatically. Seashore noted that group size has more of an influence on group cohesiveness than such variables as the education and age of the participants. The basic reason for this is that interaction between group members is a basic prerequisite for high cohesion.

Build a group identity   Cohesion begins to evolve when the leadership thinks and talks in terms of the unit as a group. Frequent use of such terms as "we," "our group," "our division," and "what we hope to accomplish" appears to be a necessary prerequisite to building cohesive groups.

Stress teamwork   The leader can set the tone of teamwork by accepting the basic principle that athletic coaches have operated on for years: "I don't care who gets the credit as long as we win." During the 1980 baseball season George Brett of the Kansas City Royals baseball team threatened to be the first player in many decades to bat .400. As the Royals went from city to city Brett was besieged with the same questions: "Will you break the record?" "How many hits do you think you will get this year?" Brett was well versed in the principle of teamwork. His answer was predictable as he stated that he didn't care how many hits he made as long as his team won. As any baseball coach knows, a winning team cannot be built on any other basis.[35]

---

[33] Cited in Bormann, *Discussion and Group Methods,* p. 63.

[34] Stanley F. Seashore, *Group Cohesiveness in the Industrial Work Group* (Ann Arbor, Mich.: Survey Research Center, University of Michigan, 1954), pp. 90–95.

[35] Ernest Bormann, William Howell, Ralph Nichols, and George Shapiro, *Interpersonal Communication in the Modern Organization* (Englewood Cliffs, N.J.: Prentice-Hall, Inc., 1969), p. 103.

A group leader concerned about building cohesiveness must be committed to the team principle which is: Do not worry about credit but do worry about whether the team will achieve its goals. If a group leader is unduly interested in taking credit, other members will follow and a star system with every man for himself will result. It is important to remember that *a group will never work as hard for a leader, as they will for the good of all.*[36]

Give group rewards   Reaching a group goal is rewarding in and of itself. However, a leader who wants to help build a group tradition will give additional rewards. For example, you may ask the group to select several individuals to give a report to other groups within the organization. By so doing you are indicating your confidence in the group's membership to accurately represent what it has accomplished. In the case of important committees you may even wish to have their report bound in book form to serve as a tribute to their work. You may also want to give the group additional responsibilities and challenges as a reward for their achievements. Or you may simply want to invite the group members out to dinner or have them into your home for a social occasion. Regardless of which method you employ, the message that they did an effective job should be given unambiguously.

In summary the cohesive group fulfills the need for each of its members to believe that what they are doing for the organization amounts to something worthwhile. A cohesive group is not "just putting in time" but, rather, working on activities that will make a positive difference in the performance of the organization.

Proposition 6: There is a positive correlation between group output and the quality of participation of individual members.

Up to this point we have examined group structure primarily from the point of view of the leader. We have noted how important it is to establish a purpose for the group and to select competent group members. We have seen that the context of a group changes from meeting to meeting and that a skillful leader needs to be aware of how procedural, task-oriented, and social norms are established. Finally we have seen the important role of cohesion within groups and have noted several actions that you can take to facilitate the emergence of solidarity.

However, you will not always be the formal leader. And, because you are not in the chairperson's role, it may appear to be more difficult to exert leadership. Nevertheless you can, as a group member, influence the direction of the group to ensure that it is productive, cohesive, and worth your time. Four actions can be taken to increase your effectiveness:

[36] Ibid.

Do your homework   Understanding the *history* of a problem is indispensable if you are to comprehend its significance. Requesting background materials that are pertinent to an issue will enable you to make perceptive and to-the-point comments within the group meeting. Pluralistic ignorance is a common occurrence in many groups. The best antidote to ignorance is to gain a historical perspective on that which is being discussed.

Keep the end point clearly in focus   You will recall from our discussion of PERT that an effective group is one that clearly identifies its desired end result. One of the contributions that you can make to a group is to periodically ask what the current discussion has to with that end goal. If it has nothing to do with it, you would help the group by asking for clarification as exemplified in the following comment: "Our goal was to determine a *process* for the allocation of salary merit increases. I am not certain why it is that we are now evaluating every department in the hospital." Such a comment can help the group determine whether the discussion is, in fact, furthering the group towards the completion of its objective.

When you examine group discussions you will find that there are many *fantasy chains* that group members pursue. A fantasy might be thought of as an idea that is suddenly put forth in the group. The idea often does not relate to the agenda of the meeting. For example, consider five individuals who begin their work and soon discover that they have disagreements over how they should proceed. One member wants to adjourn the meeting because he doesn't believe that anything else can be accomplished at this time. Another advocates spending time in the library in order to "get all the background information." Still another group member wants to use a problem-solving process such as PERT. Unfortunately there is no agreement as to the direction the group should take. The conversation begins to wander. Somebody mentions a forthcoming social event. There is a pause and the individual who wanted to do problem solving tries to bring the group to the task at hand. The individual who wants the meeting to adjourn responds, "Oh, you're just like my boss." Another member quickly picks up the comment. "My boss is always telling us to solve things logically and rationally by using problem solving. The problem with all that stuff is that you just can't relax and sit and talk." Another member says, "Ya, that's just like my supervisor. He's all work and no play." The group continues this fantasy chain conversation as they discuss their experiences with authority figures. Somebody may bring the group back to reality and again focus on the purpose of the meeting. But if the group doesn't wish to interact on the task, some other fantasy will emerge and the group will be off talking about something else that is extraneous to the discussion.[37]

[37] Modified from Ernest G. Bormann and Nancy C. Bormann, *Effective Small Group Communication* (Minneapolis, Minn.: Burgess Publishing Co., 1975), pp. 58–59.

The leader of a group has the primary responsibility to ensure that the group is working on productive tasks. However the leader often needs a strong ally to keep the discussion task oriented. A valuable and indispensible role of a group member is to assist the group leader in keeping the discussion focused on specific objectives. If you can't figure out how the conversation relates to the objective, the chances are good that the group's conversation is not relevant to the task at hand. By asking for clarification and by restating the objective that is to be achieved, a member of the group can help focus the discussion on what is truly important.

Speak to the point   Just as it is important to help the group see the relationship of its communication to the end goal it is also imperative that you periodically evaluate your own comments. Many individuals are more interested in making speeches than being understood. If you want your thoughts to have an impact on a group's deliberations you should, when speaking, confine yourself to *one basic point*. Make that point slowly and deliberately—but confine yourself to conveying one idea at a time.

Build on the comments of others   If you were to talk to a building contractor about how to construct a new home, the contractor would tell you that everything moves sequentially. First, the financing is secured by the owner. Contracts are signed. The bulldozer clears the ground. The foundation is laid. Strong supporting beams are put into place. The electrical work begins. The home is roughed in. The finishing takes place and, finally, the keys are turned over to the new owner.

Group discussion is seldom so systematic. Yet if you were to examine the conversation within effective task-oriented groups you would find a fairly systematic construction taking place. The group members would initially determine the process for reaching their goal. The agenda would be agreed to and the discussion of the issues would commence. Group members would listen to the contributions of others and would build on them. There would be few "off the wall" comments that didn't relate to the previous discussion. If the group began to move into fantasy chain conversations, someone would call it to their attention. Quickly they would return to their immediate work.

As you participate in groups you should listen for what is being said. If you don't understand the communication you should ask for clarification. Undoubtedly others in the group share your confusion. Building does not necessarily imply agreement. But building does mean that your comments are relating directly to what is being said.

In summary, when you agree to be a member of a group you should seek to understand the background issues that have led to the meeting. When you speak, keep to the point while building on the comments of others. And most of all, keep the end goal of the group's deliberations clearly in focus.

WORKING WITH GOVERNING BOARDS

It is the rare institution that does not have a board of directors, sometimes referred to as the board of trustees or simply the governing board. It is interesting to note that such boards exist in every industrial country and are even formalized in Soviet law.[38] Legally, governing boards are considered the representatives of the owners. In public institutions the owners are the state; in private institutions the owners are usually individuals. To the law, the governing board is the principle legal organ of the enterprise and, in the event of litigation, is largely responsible for what transpires within its jurisdiction.

As one reviews the history of governing boards, it becomes apparent that we have passed through an era in which boards were little more than what Peter Drucker terms "shadow kings."[39] As assertive administrators "took charge" and left the governing board with little to do, oftentimes it became a "mere showcase, a place to inject distinguished names, without . . . influence or desire for power."[40]

However, rapid change has taken place as reflected in a new relationship between health executives and governing boards. To comprehend this change it is necessary to understand how the field of health care and public health has been shaped by economic, legal, and political considerations during the past three decades.

In the 1950s and 1960s the economic pie seemed to be almost unlimited. The federally mandated Hill-Burton legislation provided considerable resources for new hospitals and for the training of health workers. Technology was being refined at a rapid rate which meant new and better services. The escalating costs of the new technology was perceived to be manageable as health insurance programs became the center piece in fringe benefit programs. National Health Insurance, which was trumpeted as being "around the corner," was expected to provide still more resources.

The 1950s was a decade of growth for public health institutions as well. Public health agencies were able to add personnel and to provide new services. There was a deep sense of pride in being in public health. The major communicable diseases had been conquered; the dreaded disease of polio had been eradicated.

During this period of growth, private and public institutions often saw little need to utilize the expertise of members who sat on governing boards. Most health organizations were moving forward, offering increased services with increased resources. There seemed to be few major policy problems that demanded extensive board member involvement. Likewise board members

[38] Peter Drucker, *The Practice of Management* (New York: Harper & Row, 1954), p. 178.
[39] Ibid.
[40] Ibid.

felt relatively little need to intervene in the administrative affairs of the institution—especially when the balance sheet produced black ink.

In the late 1960s and 1970s, however, dramatic changes in the political, economic, and legal environments altered the relationship between governing boards and chief executive officers. In the public domain, administrators became the target of complaints of inner-city residents who felt that public programs were not responsive to their health and housing needs. The smoke hovering over the Watts district in Los Angeles and the inner city of Detroit were poignant symbols of frustration. Unfortunately public health administrators were caught between the high expectations of consumers and limited state and federal resources.

In the private sphere there was a growing recognition that the economic pie was not unlimited. Shareholders in nonhealth industries became critical when they saw that long, sustained periods of economic growth could not always be projected. The cost of staying in a hospital continued to rise, giving way to political criticisms that health expenditures were out of control.

In light of these developments governing boards became the focal point of criticism by consumers, shareholders, and legislators. The media often rebuked board members who did not take their jobs seriously as evidenced in the Penn Central bankruptcy case where the inability of board members to exercise adequate control over policy decisions was stated as an important cause of Penn Central's economic collapse.

The legal environment was also changing during the 1960s and 1970s. Lawsuits against institutions were being filed more frequently, often implicating the governing board. As these suits were adjudicated it became apparent that just one case brought successfully against an organization could significantly damage its reputation and possibly its financial structure for years to come.

In view of these changes, governing boards have begun to take their role much more seriously. In many instances they have reorganized themselves in order to be more productive. One of the best-known changes occurred at General Electric when the board of directors formed five new committees, each chaired by an outside director. The committees were charged to deal with such critical policy areas as audit issues, management development and compensation issues, public issues, science and technology issues, and operations.[41]

While one may lament the passing of an era in which administrators largely controlled what took place in the institution, it should be noted that this increased activism on the part of governing boards has a number of advantages. Perhaps the prime advantage is that individuals serving on governing boards often have wisdom, experience, and skills that can be useful in

---

[41] "GE's New Strategy for Faster Growth," *Business Week* No. 2236, July 8, 1972, p. 53.

finding creative solutions to complex organizational problems. In order to maximize the relationship between chief executive officers and the governing board it is important to understand some of the most basic functions that governing boards commonly perform.

Board Functions

Perhaps the most important function of a governing board is *the selection of the administrative officers who are responsible for the day-to-day operation of the enterprise.* Some have even gone so far as to suggest that the board might be ornamental with respect to other functions and still be a useful and constructive board if it performed this function thoughtfully and constructively.

It is a common procedure for governing boards to form a search committee which, in turn, will recommend to the entire board the names of one or more individuals who could serve as the chief executive officer. Usually the search committee will have on it several members of the board as well as individuals representing professional and consumer groups.

A second function of a governing board is to *review major policies.* In practice, governing boards approve or disapprove major policies that are initiated by the chief executive officer. It is not uncommon, however, for board members to propose major policies for the institution. Usually this is undertaken with the concurrence of the chief executive officer. If such concurrence doesn't exist, it may be a sign that trust between top executives and board members has been eroded.

A third function of a governing board is to *review the performance of the chief executive officer.* This function can make chief executives apprehensive. It need not, however, if the evaluation process is objective and fair.

Many chief executive officers recognize the value of being reviewed on a three or five-year evaluation cycle. Two advantages of such review are commonly cited. First, problems between the board and top mangement become known. All too often board members will complain in private, not sharing their concerns with the chief executive. There have been instances where chief executives learned only after being dismissed of the depth of the feelings that board members had about their administrative performance. An evaluation of top management identifies problems and gives administrators an opportunity for rebuttal. If the criticisms are justified it gives the administrator an opportunity to straighten out the difficulties.

The second advantage of formal reviews is that positive evaluations give new, implicit authority to top management in carrying out its tasks. A public vote of confidence implies that the actions of top management will be backed by the board. Such public confidence will enable the chief executive officer to make difficult decisions and to make them stick.

The above functions represent three of the most important tasks for which governing boards are responsible. There are however other functions that can be equally important:

1. Giving final approval to the *objectives* of the organization and the *measurements* that will be taken to judge the progress in achieving these objectives.
2. Examining the *economics* of the institution including its capital investment program and its managed expenditures budget.
3. Serving as the *final judicial judge* when serious disputes arise within the organization. The board can serve as a "Supreme Court" in mediating serious differences of opinion over major policy issues.
4. Providing *advice and council* to top management in exercising its authority.[42]

Guidelines for Working with Governing Boards

There are a number of actions that the chief executive officer can take to foster a productive working relationship with the governing board. First, *their relationship should be defined.* Some suggest that the chief executive officer should be an official board member. The primary advantage of the formalized relationship is that it tends to dissipate the antagonism that can emerge between the administration of an organization and the members of the governing board. When the chief executive officer is a member of the board, there is an opportunity to listen to discussions, provide relevant information, help formulate policy issues, vote on them, and subsequently implement them. When the chief executive officer is actually working "shoulder to shoulder" with the board, a feeling of "we are all in this together" arises and an opportunity for productive collaboration often ensues.

The constitution of some organizations precludes the chief executive officer from holding an official position on the board. Nevertheless the role of the chief executive officer should still be delineated. Among the issues are: Should the chief executive officer be in attendance at all meetings of the board? To what extent should the chief executive officer initiate issues for discussion, prepare agendas, and undertake the staff work necessary to make the board meetings productive?

Most chief executive officers will work closely with the chairperson of the governing board, even when they are not officially on the board. Generally it is the responsibility of the chief executive officer to identify issues requiring discussion or action at board meetings. Most chief executive officers prepare bimonthly reports to the governing board which usually include (1) *major developments* affecting the institution, (2) *major policy* questions that need to be addressed by the board, (3) a statement indicating how *past*

[42] Modified from Peter Drucker, *Practice of Management,* p. 178.

decisions of the board are now being implemented and (4) a *financial statement*.

Second, a good working relationship between the chief executive officer and the governing board evolves out of trust. *Trust is always built when individuals respect the honesty of one another.* It is admittedly difficult for chief executive officers to describe to board members situations that may adversely reflect on their administration. Nevertheless, if the chief executive officer is perceived to be conscientious and honest, most board members will have enough confidence to know that the problems will be resolved. It is important to remember that when truth is fudged and when board members begin to feel that they are receiving incomplete or inaccurate information the seeds of distrust are sown. The basic norm of conduct that chief executive officers want to have firmly established is that they are impeccably honest. It goes a long way in helping when the administrative seas turn stormy.

Finally, good working relationships between governing boards and administrative officers result *when the chief executive officer gives honest feedback to the board about the board's performance.* The principle of feedback between supervisor and subordinates which we have highlighted in a number of instances in this book should be in effect right to the very top levels of the institution. It is only when board members recognize what is expected of them that they can begin to zero in on specific areas where they may be of most help to the institution.

A comment made by Peter Drucker perhaps best summarizes what the relationship should be between the governing board and the top management of an organization: "To make the Board of Directors a real organ of the enterprise rather than legal fiction; to define its functions clearly and to set definite objectives; to attract outstanding people and make them able and willing to contribute . . . are admittedly difficult. But it is one of the most important things the chief executive can do, and one of the major conditions for its own success in discharging its jobs."[43]

SUMMARY

This chapter has outlined six theoretical concepts which, if understood and implemented, can assist you in developing productive task-oriented groups. We learned that if a group is to be effective the task must be sharply defined and that procedural, critical thinking, and social norms of conduct must be established. We noted that cohesion is directly related to the perceived significance of the task; therefore, as a group leader you will want to ensure that the membership understands the importance of its deliberations. Finally, we noted that governing boards can play an important role in strengthening

[43] Ibid., p. 181.

the organization. This is particularly true when the relationship of the top management to the governing board has been well defined.

STUDY QUESTIONS

1. You have been asked to chair an important committee. There are eleven members appointed to the committee representing various vested interests. The topics you will be discussing have many emotive meanings for the membership. You question whether the issues that will be discussed can be approached calmly and objectively. You have three months—which you believe to be an unrealistic deadline—in which to submit your final report.
   a. List the *activities* you would undertake prior to the first meeting in order to prepare yourself for your leadership role.
   b. Determine a *strategy* through which you can bring objectivity to the discussions.
   c. What *evaluative criteria* might be used in determining whether your committee is effective? How should you determine these criteria? When should these criteria be used?

2. You have taken a position as the chief executive officer of a medium-size hospital. Historically the board of trustees of this hospital has met once or twice a year and has largely been a "rubber-stamp" for the proposals made by the former chief executive officer. Your goal is (a) to help the board of trustees become more knowledgeable about the problems confronting the institution and (b) to involve them in a long-range planning and development project. List the possible actions you might consider taking to help achieve your goal.

ADDITIONAL READING RESOURCES

CULBERTSON, RICHARD A., "The Governing Board and the Nursing Administrator: An Emerging Relationship," *Journal of Nursing Administration,* 9, no. 2 (February 1979), 11–13.

FAHLE, ROGER, "Adaptation to Environmental Change: The Board's Role," *Hospital and Health Services Administration,* 25, no. 1 (Winter 1980), 23–27.

FISHER, B. AUBREY, *Small Group Decision Making* (New York: McGraw Hill Book Company, 1980).

KAUFMAN, KENNETH, STEPHEN SHORTELL, SELWYN BECKER, and DUNCAN NEUHASER, "The Effects of Board Composition and Structure on

Hospital Performance," *Hospital and Health Services Administration,* 24, no. 1 (Winter 1979), 37–62.

KOVNEV, ANTHONY R., "Readings for the Chairperson of Your Board," *Health Care Management Review,* 4, no. 1 (Winter 1979), 55–57.

LEVY, LESLIE, "Reforming Board Reform," *Harvard Business Review,* January-February 1981, pp. 166–72.

"Task Forces: Reap Big Rewards at Small Costs," *Health Services Manager,* 13, no. 5 (May 1980), 3–5.

7

Competency: Understanding the Causes of Disruptive Conflict

Speak when you're angry—and you'll make the best speech you'll ever regret.—Lawrence J. Peter

I'm not smart. I try to observe. Millions saw the apple fall but Newton was the one who asked why.
—Bernard Baruch

OVERVIEW   The purpose of this chapter is to examine the concept of role and how role considerations influence interpersonal conflict. The thesis of this chapter is that, when there is role confusion, role insecurity, and lack of fulfillment in one's role, the likelihood of disruptive conflict increases. Upon completion of the chapter, the reader should be able to:

- Differentiate between constructive and disruptive conflict

- Describe a procedure that would diminish role confusion

- Differentiate between a role prescription and a role description

- Delineate the causes of defensive behavior

- Specify procedures that would diminish defensive behavior

- State the positive effects that accrue when systematic feedback is given

The word "conflict" stems from the Latin *conflictus* which is the act of striking together. *Webster's Third New International Dictionary* defines conflict as the "clash, competition, or mutual interference of opposing or incompatible forces or qualities" and as "an emotional state characterized by indecision, restlessness, uncertainty, and tension resulting from incompatible inner needs or drives of comparable intensity." Within the context of organizational behavior Kenneth Boulding's definition has particular relevance: "Conflict may be defined as a situation of competition in which the parties are *aware* of the incompatibility of potential future positions and in which each party *wishes* to occupy a position that is incompatible with the wishes of the other."[1]

As a starting point it should be recognized that conflict is endemic to most organizations. In every social structure there are occasions for conflict since members of the organization have differing perceptions concerning the organization's goals, values, priorities, and methods of operation. When there are scarce resources there is bound to be competition as various groups make claims to what they perceive to be their rightful base of support.

As we have noted health organizations exist in a conflict-prone environment. Hospitals are facing a multitude of issues, each of which creates proponents and opponents. Increased competition among hospitals for patients, unionization of personnel, turf battles between administrators and physicians and trustees, and the increasing militancy of various professional groups create a climate where mistrust, defensiveness, and conflict can quickly surface.

A climate of conflict also exists in public health settings. The goals of public health agencies may be a subject of heated debate depending upon the community in which the agency exists. Should public health agencies take aggressive positions on enviromental issues? Should they support abortion clinics? Should they give direct medical services to middle-class families? Should state health departments accept federal money to initiate public health projects with the realization that once the money is expended the project will probably go out of existence? There are few clear answers to such questions. Consequently, there are bound to be differing perceptions concerning the role of public health agencies. Such differing perceptions are bound to create conflict within agencies and among decision makers in the community.

Employees in health organizations often do not become involved in the philosophical battles being waged over public policy. They do, however, bear the brunt of the effects of whatever policies are adopted. Familiar work patterns are changed as new policies are implemented. Legislation requiring continuing education credits and/or credentialing means that experienced employees are mandated to attend classes and learn concepts that may or may

[1] Kenneth Boulding, *Conflict and Defense: A General Theory* (New York: Harper & Row, 1962), p. 5.

not be relevant to their work. The emergence of new personnel with new responsibilities often means that the roles of other employees change. The ultimate threat to employees comes when cost-containment measures are instituted that threaten their positions. Increasingly employees are not content to let themselves be buffeted by the winds of change without exerting their own influence. Such a decision places them squarely in the arena of conflict.

CONFLICT AND ROLE BEHAVIOR

The purpose of this chapter is to examine several primary causes of conflict within health organizations. A fundamental premise implicit in the following analysis is that organizational conflict is ultimately rooted in role considerations. While the impetus for conflict is multifaceted—involving such issues as changing priorities and the need for resource retrenchment—*the basic cause of conflict is uncertainty over what projected change might do to the roles of individuals in the organization.* Regardless of the reasons for such change, any change in role that is perceived as diminishing the importance of that role is bound to generate conflict. Therefore, if we are to understand organizational conflict it is necessary to examine the concept of role behavior.

Preliminary Considerations

Before turning attention to the topics of role confusion, role security, and role fulfillment, several introductory comments may be helpful. First, *conflict is not necessarily a negative factor in organizational growth.* John Dewey reportedly said that conflict is the gadfly of thought. It stirs us to observation and memory. It instigates to invention. It shocks us out of sheeplike passivity. Conflict is a sine qua non of reflection and ingenuity. Without creative conflict, organizational growth will be stunted for it is in the arena of conflict that new ideas, new ways of looking at old issues, and new methods for solving organizational problems emerge. As Robert Blake and Jane Mouton have noted:

> Differences are intrinsically valuable. They provide the rich possibility that alternatives and options will be discovered for better and poorer ways of responding to any particular situation. Preserving the privilege of having and expressing differences increases our chances of finding "best" solutions to the many dilemmas that arise in living. They also add the spice of variety and give zest to human pursuits.[2]

[2] Robert R. Blake and Jane Srygley Mouton, "The Fifth Achievement," in *Conflict Resolution through Communication,* ed. Fred Jandt (New York: Harper & Row, 1973), pp. 88–89.

Even though most of us would probably agree that conflict in and of itself is not necessarily negative, we also would agree that we would rather avoid it if possible. It is the rare person who enjoys being in the middle of conflict situations. One of the reasons why people tend to think of conflict in derogatory terms is that they dislike the disruptiveness that results when anger and hostility are expressed. While anger can be destructive, it should be remembered that the ability to constructively verbalize and vent frustrations is basic to a healthy personality. Some people direct their anger inward. They may be boiling mad but never say a word to another person. Such people often experience the brunt of their own anger in the guise of headaches, high blood pressure or insomnia. Other individuals may try to hold their anger in but eventually they explode with their frustrations —often in inappropriate situations— because the pressure is too intense. Anger should be viewed as a basic human emotion that needs to be controlled and used in a constructive manner. If our anger is faced and communicated openly, we can vent potentially destructive feelings before we become poisoned by them. Anger and its resulting cynicism must be dealt with or it can slowly but certainly erode our effectiveness.

As a starting consideration, therefore, it is important to differentiate disruptive conflict from creative conflict. Disruptive conflict might be defined as a climate of defensiveness that inhibits the individual, work unit, or organization from achieving its objectives. Creative conflict might be defined as an assertive leveling with others in order to negotiate and resolve differences of opinion.

A second preliminary consideration is that *conflict is usually personalized.* What appears to be a simple disagreement may have profound *personal* and *emotive* meanings for the respective parties. A dispute over hiring practices between the personnel officer and a department head may be a test case in which each is seeking to define each other's authority and influence. The tension between the nursing in-service director and a head nurse over what educational programs are appropriate for the coming year may, in reality, be over the issue of who has the most power in the nursing hierarchy.

The more serious the conflict, the greater the likelihood that the self-perceptions of those engaged in the conflict will be analyzed and altered. Conflicts generally arouse feelings of inadequacy. Who respects me? Who values my ideas? Who is seeking to diminish my authority? Who is trying to get ahead at my expense? To understand what is involved in a given conflict, we must focus not only on the surface issues, but also on what the surface issue represents *in personal terms* to each party. The old adage, "Don't take it personally," is inappropriate when it comes to diagnosing the causes of conflict. People engage in conflict precisely because they do take the issues personally. The ability to understand why it is that people are taking the issue personally is basic in determining the etiology of conflict.

A third preliminary consideration is that *disruptive conflict can dissipate an organization's vitality.* An individual has a finite amount of energy that can be expended in a given work day. Organizations that have numerous conflicts tend to dissipate the creative energy of employees. The psychological energy that could be given to realizing organizational objectives is often expended in plotting and executing private and not so private grievances. Work groups may cease to set demanding objectives and to experience the sense of achievement that comes when a challenging task has been realized. Instead, their energy is given to protecting the ego of the unit. Energy that is given to designing and executing self-protective stances is self-defeating for the entire organization.

In summary, conflict is not always harmful to the organization. When it is disruptive it must be successfully managed. The ability to successfully manage conflict will be dependent upon whether the administrator understands the etiology of the disruptive tensions.

Role Confusion

Problems within organizations frequently appear because of conflicting beliefs concerning the roles of employees. As Albert Wessen states, "Before an organization can function effectively, there must be clearly defined allocations of role and authority.[3]

The hospital has particular problems related to role confusion. Earl Koos found that patients are frequently disturbed by the many different employees who serve them. The patient who initially believes that the hospital is an organization that employs only three types of employees—doctors, nurses, and janitors—easily becomes frustrated when there is contact with people of diverse specialties. "It appears, for example, that the hospital's changing social structure—in which the old and relatively simple hierarchy of doctor-nurse-orderly-kitchen-maid has been replaced by including all manner of aids, technicians, floor cleaners, and so on—has created confusion and frustration for the patient and his family.[4]

One of the respondents in the Koos study stated his sense of frustration in the following way: "It was that I never knew exactly who did what for me . . . If I rang my bell, someone came and then said, 'I'll have so-and-so do that.' But maybe so-and-so never came, so I was just left to lie there.[5]

As employees have become professionalized in specific areas their role

[3] Albert F. Wessen, "Hospital Ideology and Communication Between Ward Personnel," in *Patients, Physicians, and Illness,* ed. Gartly Jaco (New York: Free Press, 1958), p. 448.

[4] Earl Koos, "Metropolis—What City People Think of Their Medical Service," in *Patients, Physicians, and Illness,* ed. Gartly Jaco (New York: Free Press, 1958), pp. 114–15.

[5] Ibid., p. 115.

has changed within the hospital. The nurse is no longer just a "nurse." She is a graduate nurse, a registered nurse, a professional nurse, a registered psychiatric nurse, etc. The different roles enacted by different personnel are not only confusing to the patients, but often are a source of frustration for the professional herself.

> . . . the profession of nursing and others have failed to lead out of this maze of confusing titles and have left the rest of the community on its own to figure things out. One has only to go into the hospital . . . and observe that almost anyone who wears a white uniform and is usually presumed to look like a nurse is dubbed "nurse." This creates so much confusion that in many hospitals those who are not nurses must defend themselves by frequent . . . exhortations that "I am not a nurse, I am a technician, dietician, etc."[6]

Not only is the patient confused with "just who does what around here," but other members of the healing team often are confused concerning the same manner. Dr. Jacob Halberstam states:

> When jobs are clearly defined, when each specialist knows exactly what he is to do in treating a patient, it is possible to reduce competition among members of related disciplines. . . . But in some settings, especially when responsibilities overlap, and the psychiatrist, the psychologists, and the psychiatric social worker may be working with the same patient, unless the responsibility and purpose of each is spelled out, there will be trouble. Frequently jealousies become so intense that professionals don't speak to each other.[7]

The evidence seems to indicate, as Dr. Halberstam noted, that professionals in the hospital setting are often unaware of the nature of their colleagues' work. A workshop was held at the University of Chicago with the purpose of discussing communication barriers among members of the health team. Stereotypes were singled out as a common cause for minunderstanding.

> Asked to give their impressions of another profession, workshop participants revealed that they as professionals shared with laymen some common images of other professionals—the nurse as Florence Nightingale, the pharmacist as the dispenser of pills, the physician as a god, the social worker as an arbiter of family troubles, and the nutritionist as a regulator of diets. It was quite evident from the workshop discussions that many specialists have not made their purposes and functions clear to their colleagues on the health team.[8]

[6] J.C. Jackson, "By Any Other Name," *Canadian Hospital,* 42 (October 1965), 78–79.
[7] Quoted in Helen Neal, *Better Communications for Better Health* (New York: Columbia University Press, 1962), pp. 57–58.
[8] Helen Neal, *Better Communications for Better Health* (New York: Columbia University Press, 1962), p. 59.

Role problems within health agencies can even be more complex than the role problems present within the hospital. This is particularly true of agencies that employ public health people and paraprofessionals. What is the role of a community health aid or a community health planner? What are the unique training and skills that the sanitarian, health educator, public health dentist, public health nurse practitioner, drug counselor, or biometrician bring to the agency? To repeat, As new health roles proliferate, there is increased confusion as to who does what for whom, in what setting, and with what authority. Whenever there are multiple roles being enacted for the benefit of the consumer there is the possibility and, indeed, the probability that we will misunderstand one another simply because we do not know what one another does.

As a health professional you may wish to examine how well acquainted you are with the roles being enacted within health organizations. The more you know about those roles, including the professional preparation needed to carry out the role and the knowledge and skills the employees have upon the completion of their education, the better you will be able to clarify for others their place within the organization. Employees who believe that the administration doesn't really know about the field they represent will often spend enormous amounts of energy in seeking to make their role credible. When their energy is focused on raising their personal credibility it is no longer available for meeting the goals that have been assigned to them. Because role confusion is a major problem for health professionals it is important that administrators carefully define—in conjunction with the employee—what the employee's precise role will be in the organization. Figure 7—1 demonstrates one way in which this can be undertaken. Note how the mandatory, allowable, and disallowed roles are carefully delineated.

Mandatory role activities are those that are basic to the employment of

Mandatory roles	*Allowable roles*	*Disallowed roles*
1. Will undertake home visits 30 hours per week.	1. Can take one course at the University per year.	1. Cannot work hours other than when the agency is open.
2. Will be on call one weekend per month.	2. Can participate in the teaching program of the prenatal clinic.	2. Cannot extend home visits to those families with incomes over $5,000 per year.
3. Will serve on committees taking not more than four hours per week.	3. Can, in conjunction with the Nutrition Department, assist in planning the August workshop on nutrition education.	3. Cannot privately consult with patients of the clinic and charge fees.
4. Will supervise three home health aids.	4. Can work one day a month with professional organizations.	
5. Will serve as the health department representative to the Metropolitan Health Board.		

Figure 7-1 Position: Community Health Nurse, Roseville Community Health Department.

the individual. These are the activities that must be done and that justify the individual's employment in the organization. The allowable role activities are those that the individual *may* choose. A person in housekeeping, for example, who has a special interest in children could select pediatrics if she was given a say in what department her responsibilities will be carried out. The disallowed role activities are those in which the employee cannot participate. If there are two departments that are closely related to one another in what they do for the patient, it is advisable to make clear the precise boundaries of their responsibilities. For example, health educators and social workers often have similar responsibilities. If a clear boundary line exists as to who does what, and for what purpose, it may diminish potential "infighting" between the units.

The advantages of clearly delineating the employee's role has advantages for both the supervisor and the subordinate. Such a process clearly lets the subordinate know that the administrator has knowledge of and appreciates the roles that the subordinate will be carrying out. The fact that the subordinates can negotiate part of their role gives them choices in their work. By stating what the subordinate is expected to do, there is a base line for future evaluation. Perhaps the biggest advantage, however, to delineating roles is that misunderstandings due to differences in perception about what the employee should be doing are prevented.

A corollary issue related to role emerges when the *role prescription* is different from the *role description*. The role prescription is the idealized role that the newly employed individual expects to have at work. The role description represents how the job actually is. Whenever there is a difference between the role prescription (how the individual would like to perceive the job) and the role description (how the job actually is), the likelihood of problems increases.

Consider the case of Jane Lostern who had just completed her Master of Public Health degree program in public health nursing. Her major emphasis was in pediatrics. As a pediatric nurse practitioner she developed a perception of what her role should be in the health care system. She felt, for example, that by being a nurse practitioner she should be able (1) to screen patients and to diagnose and treat certain illnesses, (2) to work cooperatively with a physician, recognizing and respecting each other's area of competency, and (3) to have the respect of mothers and fathers who bring their children to the clinic.

Upon her graduation she selected a nursing position with a group of pediatric physicians. The pediatricians hired her because they felt that she could be of help in educating patients and their parents in regard to treatment procedures that they had defined.

During the first week that Lostern was on the job she became aware that there were going to be problems. When the physician was diagnosing the patient's illness, the physician never asked for Jane's opinion nor did the physician delegate any meaningful work for Jane to do with the patient. When she suggested that she could screen the children before the physicians saw the child, there was considerable skepticism. However, one of the pediatricians agreed to try it. While most of the parents didn't seem to mind, several voiced to the physician their reservations about what the nurse was doing. This was deeply resented by the nurse practitioner.

The single greatest problem, however, was that Lostern simply didn't feel that she had the respect of the physicians in the clinic. She felt that they didn't appreciate her technical competence and were not making it possible for her to prove herself. Jane constantly pressed for them to change their ways, but the changes were few. As time passed, Jane's resentment grew, but there seemed to be little hope of having substantial changes made in her role as a nurse within the clinic.

The problems Jane Lostern experienced were due to the fact that the pediatricians and the pediatric nurse practitioner did not have a sound understanding of the role the pediatric nurse practitioner was to have in the clinic. Many new graduates find themselves in this predicament upon beginning their work. What they wished the role to be like turns out not to be the way it is. Newly employed physical therapist graduates may feel that most of the hours in the workday should be spent in working with patients; instead, they may find that many hours are spent filing forms. The health education specialist would like to spend the workday designing, implementing, and evaluating exciting new educational programs that would prevent health problems from emerging in the community. Instead, much of the workday is spent managing the film library and producing pamphlets wanted by the health officer. The nurse may expect, on the basis of considerable training in the psychosocial area, to be helping patients with personal and family problems; instead, the nurse finds that the patients often talk over such problems with their physician or clergyman.

Over the years I have tried to follow the careers of former students. Those individuals whom I see six months or a year after graduation and who are having difficulty making the transition between the student world and the professional world often have a similar complaint: "My work just isn't like I expected it to be."

To be certain, educators have a particular responsibility to educate individuals for the real job requirements. Nevertheless, the administrator who is hiring has a unique opportunity to prevent problems from occurring because of divergent role prescriptions. When the administrator stipulates what the role actually is, prospective employees can determine whether or not they want the job. This is not to suggest that the role cannot be altered to fit the unique talents and interests that a prospective employee brings to the work situation. It does suggest, however, that the administrator clearly defines what the work situation is so that the employee clearly understands the nature of the expectations.

In summary, the more clearly a role can be defined, the greater the likelihood that conflict will be avoided. When individuals are not clear as to what is expected of them, when they do not understand the responsibility and authority implicit in the roles of their colleagues, misunderstandings increase. By making the roles clear so that the prescription is the same as the description, the administrator helps to create an environment for dialogue.

Role Security

Individuals who are defensive represent a formidable challenge to health administrators. In any given day a significant portion of time can be invested in allaying the fears, resentment, and anxiety of individual employees who are defensive. Defensiveness results when an employee is not secure in his or her role. The greater the insecurity concerning the role, the greater the probability that the employee will be defensive. The work environment will also heighten or diminish the possibility of a defensive state. The administrator who feels confident within the confines of the administrative staff meetings may seldom appear defensive. However, when the administrator is subjugated to intense questioning by the county commissioners in front of members of the press, the symptoms of defensiveness may emerge.

Because defensiveness is present in conflict situations, it is important for the consciously competent administrator to know (1) the causes of defensive behavior, (2) the psychological conditions that result from being defensive, and (3) procedures for diminishing a defensive posture.

Causes of defensive behavior   Defensive behavior has been defined as "that behavior which occurs when an individual perceives threat or anticipates threat."[9] An employee feels defensive when he perceives that his "boundary" has been threatened. A "boundary" serves to define the area that an individual perceives as being distinctly his own. When a boundary is threatened there is conflict.

Individual employees can have their boundaries threatened whenever anyone trespasses over territory that they perceive as uniquely their own. We have observed how the emerging roles of health professionals need definition. Definition is needed partly because any new role can threaten the boundaries of an established role. Physicians, for example, often take a self-protective stance against a nurse practitioner because they feel that their traditional boundaries are being threatened.

Any action taken by a person that encroaches on the boundary of another person generates conflict. If the head of the housekeeping department enables the employees in housekeeping to leave work thirty minutes early on Christmas Eve, one can anticipate conflict with the head of personnel. "That was not her decision to make," could be the stance taken by the personnel

[9] Jack R. Gibb, "Defensive Communication," *Journal of Communication* xi, September 1961, pp. 141-48.

director. Note that the difference in opinion is not related to the issue of whether employees should leave thirty minutes early even though the resulting discussions could focus on that topic. Rather, the critical issue is that the director of housekeeping has threatened the boundary jurisdictions of the director of personnel.

Not only do individuals have boundaries but so do work groups, organizations, and communities. A health education unit in a health department could become defensive if the public health nurses embarked on an aggressive diabetes education program. This would be particularly true if the health education department was not consulted. Potential government grants and contracts can cause unhealthy competition between government agencies. Administrators of competing organizations may genuinely feel that their organization can best meet the specifications under which the grant or contract will be awarded. If one of the organizations has been the traditional recipient of government awards, any new agency competing for similar rewards will be viewed negatively. This is due to the fact that the new agency is threatening the boundaries of the old.

Communities can also be threatened when their boundaries are invaded by another group. Consider a county health department who, with good intentions, advocates a state law that would require a higher frequency of restaurant inspections in a given municipality. If the municipalities were not consulted or involved in the decision-making process they could well ask what right the county has in telling them how often they should inspect their own restaurants. The community's perceived boundary was threatened.

While the perceived threat to one's self (or to one's work unit) is the primary cause of defensive behavior, there are various "climates" of communication that tend to heighten an individual's defensive posture. An understanding of the causes of defensiveness must be rooted in an understanding of these defensive climates. Research undertaken by Jack Gibb suggests that there are six such climates: evaluation, control, strategy, neutrality, superiority, and certainty.[10]

The first defensive climate is what Gibb terms *evaluation orientation*. "Speech or other behavior which appears evaluative increases defensiveness. If by expression, manner of speech, tone of voice, or verbal content the sender seems to be evaluating or judging the listener, then the receiver goes on guard."[11] If you have been in a conversation and were struck by the fact that the other party was evaluating you, you probably became anxious. If you felt that the individual who was evaluating you was probably not doing so fairly (that is, if the person did not have the relevant information), your anxiety may have been increasingly heighted.

[10] Ibid., p. 142.
[11] Ibid.

Control orientation comes about when we feel that someone is trying to change an attitude, influence behavior, or restrict the field of activity. The effort to control is particularly aggravating, according to Gibb, when it is not carried out openly: "The degree to which attempts to control produce defensiveness depends upon the openness of the effort, for a suspicion that hidden motives exist heightens resistance."[12]

The basic reason why we become defensive when we feel that someone is trying to control is that we perceive that the other party feels we are inadequate. As Gibbs states, "That the speaker secretly views the listener as ignorant, unable to make his own decisions, uninformed, immature, unwise, or possessed of wrong or inadequate attitudes is a subconscious perception which gives the latter a valid base for defensive reactions."[13]

Strategy orientation comes about when we feel that we are being "set up" for something or when we feel that we do not know the real motives of the individual we are dealing with. An example of this may be the department head who works very independently and who seldom comes to your office for consultation. When that department head finally does come by the office, your natural reaction may be to be on guard because something undoubtedly must be up her sleeve!

If you ever have had the feeling that you don't know where you stand with your supervisor, you can probably understand why *neutrality orientation* can evoke defensive responses. We desire to be perceived as valued persons who are respected for what we can do and reinforced positively for our efforts. If we work for a supervisor who is detached from us, who never gives a word of appreciation, who doesn't affirm that we are a valuable employee of the organization, the chances are very good that our relationship with that supervisor will put us into a defensive posture.

Superiority orientation comes about when an individual clearly communicates her superiority to us. This orientation can be given in many different ways. If the supervisor does not ask for assistance from subordinates they will perceive that their ideas have little worth; if the supervisor insists on being called Ms., Mr., Mrs., or Dr. while calling subordinates by their first names, a status inequality is symbolized.

The sixth defensive climate that Gibb delineates is the *certainty orientation* created by those who are unwilling to learn from others. "The effects of dogmatism in producing defensiveness are well known. Those who seem to know the answers, who require no additional data, and who regard themselves as teachers rather than as coworkers tend to put others on guard."[14] The outside consultant, for example, who comes to an organization with all of the

[12] Ibid., p. 143.
[13] Ibid.
[14] Ibid., p. 145.

answers will probably not be accepted by the members of the organization. They may treat the consultant politely but long after the consultant has left, the recommendations will sit in an obscure file.

In summary, defensiveness emerges when individuals feel a threat to their inner world. The six communication climates that tend to heighten anxiety are evaluation, control, strategy, neutrality, superiority, and certainty.

Psychological conditions resulting from defensiveness   When confronted with a person who is defensive it is important to recognize that two factors will influence your conversation. First, the probability is high that the defensive individual's ability to listen will be diminished. If you try to reason with a defensive individual it is likely that only a fraction of what you are conveying will be heard and internalized. The reason for this is that the individual's psychological energy will be given to protecting his ego as opposed to understanding what you are saying.

The second factor that will influence your conversation with a defensive individual is related to the extent to which the person's defense mechanisms are activated. The individual who perceives a threat is compelled to defend himself. One way of doing this is to displace frustrations and anger on someone else. Therefore, a sanitarian doing inspection work may find that the reasons that are given for why a regulation has been ignored are "the insane amount of paper work," or "I don't have the staff resources," or "my subordinates are incompetent." The fault generally is displaced elsewhere.

Consider the following interchange between a hospital administrator and the building and grounds superintendent:

Administrator: Last time we discussed some of the areas where accidents could take place in our hospital.

Superintendent: Yes, I remember the discussion. You told me the lights in the parking lot were out and that railings need to be installed in the bathrooms in the old section of the building.

Administrator: Yes, and I think we also discussed that the third step on the second flight of stairs in the rear of the building is accident prone.

Superintendent: Yes, I remember that too.

Administrator: I thought our agreement was that you would do something about these problems before our next review.

Superintendent: [*At this point the superintendent communicates many messages nonverbally. His arms are crossed in a signal of defiance, he turns red, and possibly his jugular vein protrudes!*] Well, you know how it is. I have all of those year-end forms that you sent down that have to be filled out. Then my assistant, George, quit on me last week. And you know my other assistant—why, you can't depend on him for anything. You know, the other day I asked him to do a simple task like getting some new tools and he was gone for all day.

As you note, the problem is someone else's fault. In this case it is the fault of all of the forms, the assistant who quit, and the assistant who stayed on. Generally, whenever someone displaces frustration, responsibility for the problem will not be assumed.

Diminishing defensive behavior   There are several suggestions that may be of assistance to you in working with defensive individuals. First, try to *determine what it is that is making the individual anxious.* This is critical if you are going to be able to diminish the defensive behavior. Earlier we discussed six defensive climates that heighten defensiveness; for each of these climates there is a supportive climate that will diminish the defensiveness:

DEFENSIVE CLIMATES	SUPPORTIVE CLIMATES
1. Evaluation	1. Description
2. Control	2. Problem Orientation
3. Strategy	3. Spontaneity
4. Neutrality	4. Empathy
5. Superiority	5. Equality
6. Certainty	6. Provisionalism[15]

The key to diminishing defensiveness is to identify which climate is basically causing the defensive posture and to counter with a supportive climate. If evaluation is the perceived threat, a counter with *description* would be helpful. A "descriptive climate" might be defined as that orientation in which the sender of a message describes that which is perceived. Consider the example of a conversation held between a nursing service director and a head nurse. The reason for the interchange is that, on the previous night, three of the six registered nurses did not appear for work and there was a resulting staff shortage.

Example 1—Evaluation Climate: "Once again," states the nursing services director, "we were inadequately staffed on Two-North. I can't understand how in the world this happens on your floor so often."

Example 2—Descriptive Climate: "I noticed that during the past three weeks we have often not had adequate staff support on Two-North. I would presume that this is causing some problems for those nurses who are on duty and I was wondering how we should address the problem."

[15] Ibid., p. 145.

As you can readily see, Example 1 would increase the defensiveness of the head nurse. There is an implied evaluation—possibly an unfair evaluation—that the head nurse is at fault. In Example 2, however, the nursing service director is simply describing what may be a problem and is asking for assistance on how to solve it.

If it can be determined that a *control orientation* is causing defensiveness, the way in which to counter this is to use a *problem orientation*. You will recall that a control orientation is one in which an individual is bombarded with a persuasive message that is designed to elicit change.

> Problem orientation, on the other hand, is the antithesis of persuasion. When the sender communicates a desire to collaborate in defining a mutual problem and in seeking its solution, he tends to create the same problem orientation in the listener, and of greater importance, he implies that he has no predetermined solution, attitude, or method to impose.[16]

A *spontaneous orientation* is the antidote to a *strategy orientation*. "Spontaneity" in this context might be thought of as the revealing of the motivations which are behind a request. Instead of communicating in such a way that the hearer feels that she is being manipulated to do something, a clear, forthright statement as to the reasons for the request will generally help the other party in understanding what is requested and the rationale for the request. It will also diminish defensive behavior.

If you find that your subordinates are guarded when they talk with you or if you find that they seldom reveal what it is they are thinking, the chances are good that the defensiveness which you perceive may be rooted in your *neutrality orientation* towards them. You will recall that neutrality emerges when the supervisor is somewhat detached from subordinates or when there is little affirmation and positive reinforcement of the subordinate. The way to counter such defensiveness is with *empathy*.

> Communication that conveys empathy for the feelings and respect for the worth of the listener . . . is particularly supportive and defense reducing. Reassurance results when a message indicates that the speaker indentifies himself with the listener's problems, shares his feelings, and accepts his emotional reactions at face value.[17]

Superiority and *certainty orientations* are closely linked to one another. Note how the superiority and certainty come through in the following example: "We don't need a county hospital," said the city commissioner. "I've been around here for forty years and have served on this council for twenty and I can tell you that the taxpayers will never stand for a multimillion dollar

[16] Ibid., p. 146.
[17] Ibid., p. 147.

extravaganza. You commissioners who support it should be the ones to pay for it.''

Equality and *provisionalism* are the supportive climates that diminish the defensiveness that emerges from superiority and certainty. Equality is reflected in communication that emphasizes that the sender is willing to enter into participative planning with the hearer in a climate of mutual respect and trust. Provisionalism is reflected in communication that tends to emphasize that the sender is investigating issues rather than taking sides on them, is concerned with solving rather than debating, and is willing to experiment and explore with others the feasibility of various alternatives. Note how equality and provisionalism can be seen in the following example: ''There are a wide variety of beliefs amongst the city commissioners as to whether we need a new county hospital. I respect the views of those who definitely believe that such a structure should be built. I, however, have serious reservations and before making a final decision would appreciate it if we could discuss several alternative approaches.''

The second suggestion for diminishing defensive behavior is to *remember that the defensive person does not listen well, and in all likelihood has a need to vent frustrations and anger.* Therefore, it may be wise for you to permit such venting and, in so doing, to allow the person to relieve anxiety. By letting the other individual express strong feelings, you may receive clues as to the nature of the threat that the individual is perceiving. Since the defensive person does not listen well, it is important to limit what you say until you are certain that the individual is, in fact, listening to your ideas and suggestions. This may come about minutes, hours, days, or even months later. If you must communicate information to the defensive individual and if you perceive that he or she is not listening, your best results will come if you verbally discuss your concerns and place them in writing. After the interview is over, the defensive person will read what you have stated. In a calmer atmosphere your messages may be listened to.

The third suggestion, and perhaps the most important, is to *control your own anxiety when dealing with a defensive person.* Defensiveness begets defensiveness. When you meet someone who is ''uptight,'' and if you feel that their uptightness is due to something that they perceive in you, your natural reaction is to respond in a similar way. However, the more you can remain calm and collected while trying to understand and empathize with what is being stated, the better you will be in working through the defensive posture to a more constructive climate. Remember, your own ability to listen, to perceive the source of threat, and to respond in a supportive way will greatly determine whether the defensive behavior will be destructive.

In summary, defensiveness is a human reaction that results when a threat is perceived by someone who is not secure in his or her role. Communication climates that elicit defensive behavior need to be countered with climates of support. If it is recognized that defensiveness causes defensiveness, if defensiveness is countered by diminishing the magnitude of the threat, and if supportive climates of communication are utilized, defensiveness can be diminished.

Role Fulfillment and the Need for Feedback

Earlier, the challenge of building a humane work environment was referred to as one of the critical challenges facing administrators. It was noted that the feelings of alienation lead to what Camus referred to as a "soulless environment." It was Abraham Maslow who perhaps better than anyone else pinpointed the needs people have and how they influence human behavior.[18] Maslow postulated that there are five human needs in ascending hierarchical order:

—Need for self-actualization
—Need for esteem
—Need for belongingness and love
—Safety needs
—Physiological needs

Physiological needs refer to food, warmth, shelter, water, sleep, and other bodily needs. When their physiological needs have been met, human beings then seek to satisfy safety needs. Safety needs include both physical and emotional security. When safety needs have been met, the need for belongingness and love becomes important. While physiological and safety needs are centered within oneself, the need for belongingness and love is a social need—the need for other people. It is the feeling that one belongs to a larger community of individuals. It implies both the giving and the receiving of affection and concern. When one's need to be in relation to others has been met, esteem becomes an important need. The need for esteem refers to the need to feel a sense of self-respect and respect from others. When all the lower needs have been met, one is free to strive after the highest need, the need for self-actualization. Self-actualization refers to the need to realize one's potential. It may be helpful to think of self-actualization as a sense of achievement in one's life.

The extent to which people find their existence meaningful is correlated with how well the above needs are met. The worker who is most fulfilled in his job is one who feels a sense of security, belonging, respect, and achievement. Your own work experience probably verifies this. If you think for a moment about when you were most content and pleased about your work, it probably came at the time that your human needs were being met.

[18] Abraham Maslow, *Motivation and Personality,* 2nd ed. (New York: Harper & Row, 1970), pp. 1-62.

One of the most critical questions, therefore, that an administrator at any level needs to ask is "How do I go about meeting these very dynamic needs of employees?" On the surface many suggestions come to mind. We can assist employees in meeting their security needs by keeping them informed of what is happening and what they might be doing in the future. It may be possible to occasionally socialize with employees in order to help bring about a sense of cohesiveness. In addition, the esteem needs can be partially met by recognizing and publicizing the achievements that individual employees have attained.

While suggestions such as these may be useful, the consciously competent manager cannot leave to chance that these dynamic human needs will be met. A system needs to be built into each unit of the organization to bring to the surface the private needs of workers and put into motion procedures to meet those needs. The system advocated in this chapter is related to the concept of *feedback*.

The concept of "feedback" is a critical aspect of current management thought. While feedback is not a panacea for meeting the security, belonging, esteem, and achievement needs of workers, when pragmatically implemented it has a direct bearing on meeting such needs and resolving the problems and tensions that result when such needs are not met.

In its purest form, feedback is the process of adjusting future actions based upon information about past performance.[19] Many applications of the idea can be found in medical practice. Assessing the daily exercise patterns of a middle-aged businessman will give the physician a basis for advising the eager jogger concerning his exercise routine. A physical therapist who has given instructions to a patient may question the patient in order to determine whether the instructions are clearly understood.

Feedback, however, is more than adjusting future actions on the basis of past performance. It involves making a judgment about someone's actions and then informing the individual of that judgment. It means rewarding a person for work well done as well as informing a person about work that was not up to the desired standard of quality.

There are three types of feedback: positive, negative, and problem-centered feedback. *Positive feedback* is informing employees that their work and presence in the organization is valued. A hand-written note from the hospital administrator to the chairman of a hospital committee, thanking him for the work that was done in preparing a committee report, is one example of straightforward positive feedback.

Negative feedback is the stating of a derogatory judgment concerning a person's behavior without offering any assistance to resolve the perceived difficulty. "We cannot tolerate your negativism," or "We have more complaints

[19] W. Warren Haynes and Joseph L. Massie, *Management, Analysis and Cases* (Englewood Cliffs, N.J.: Prentice-Hall, Inc., 1969), p. 325.

from your floor than any other," illustrate negative feedback. While there may be times that such pointed comments are needed, this "parent-child" interaction should rarely be utilized.

Problem-centered feedback might be defined as interaction that focuses on negative behavior but in a manner that seeks to find a solution to the problems caused by such behavior. Note how the following examples focus on tangible problems, but in a way that hostilities would be blunted.

> *Example 1:* "I think you are aware that we have received a number of complaints from patients concerning the care they have received while on Two-North. I am wondering if sometime next week we could find time to discuss the problems and determine some possible solutions. When might be a good time for us to meet?"

> *Example 2:* "Mrs. McDonald, you have voiced a number of complaints concerning the new charting system. Would you have time tomorrow to talk about your concerns? It's important that we develop the best possible system, and I would like your ideas."

Because of the multiple demands made on administrators, the feedback function of management can easily be deferred. It is not uncommon to hear an administrator say, "Well, I know I should give them more help with their frustrations, but where in the world am I going to find time?" It is common for administrators to get so involved with the few individuals who are having problems that those who are doing their work well are not recognized for their efforts. You have probably known an employee who year after year did high-quality work but then gradually allowed the quality to diminish. In all likelihood if you were to study that situation you would find that the employee feels that since the high-quality work was not appreciated there was no point in investing effort to maintain high standards.

The competent health administrator should give feedback to employees on a regularly scheduled basis. If the administrator does not reinforce quality work, the quality may begin to slip ("Who cares anyway?"). If the administrator does not periodically discuss work-related problems, employees may feel isolated and alone with issues that they cannot individually resolve. In order to give valid feedback it is necessary for the administrator to have knowledge in four areas:

1. Were the objectives accomplished? Were they accomplished by the designated deadline?
2. What unresolved work problems surfaced as the objectives were being accomplished?

3. Are there suggestions as to how similar objectives could be more effectively and efficiently realized in the future?
4. How do subordinates think and feel about their jobs, their associates, their organization?

The first three areas deal primarily with work-related matters about which the alert administrator should be informed. The fourth area is related to the subordinates' personal feelings and attitudes about work. Unfortunately, the fourth area is often neglected. It is in this area, however, that one finds misunderstandings, disagreements, and personality conflicts. While this area is often difficult to deal with, it is a critical area if the administrator is to get the necessary information on which to give the subordinate feedback. If valid information is retrieved in each of four areas, the thoughtful administrator will be in a better position to give subordinates assistance on work-related problems as well as an evaluation of their contributions to the organization.

Benefits of feedback   If supervisors give feedback on a regular basis to subordinates, what benefits could one anticipate? First, *there would be increased respect between the supervisor and subordinate.* Supervisors who become helpfully involved in work-related problems tend to be highly valued and respected. Supervisors who remain aloof and who let subordinates "sink or swim" tend not to be highly valued. The administrator who finds it difficult to show appreciation for credible performance by subordinates will not be as highly valued as the one who gives positive reinforcement.

Feedback between supervisor and subordinate creates a climate of trust in which individuals know where they stand and know that "when the chips are down" they can receive the assistance they need. Within the context of groups, individuals who participate readily and respond to comments and suggestions made by other individuals will also be more highly valued than those who do not. Members of groups who have a high rate of participation and a low rate of feedback are not as highly regarded by their peers as those who have a high rate of participation and a high rate of feedback.[20]

A second benefit that accrues when there is feedback is that *misunderstandings decrease.* Administrators have two sets of problems that relate to internal organizational communication. The first problem is related to the retrieval of accurate and complete information from subordinates. Chris Argyris has realistically described the business executive who becomes more and more isolated from staff members. The executive is increasingly alone,

---

[20] Dean C. Barnlund, *Interpersonal Communication Survey and Studies* (Boston: Houghton Mifflin, 1968), p. 230.

wondering who is and who is not stating the facts.[21] As W. Charles Redding notes:

> People in the organization find it increasingly difficult to "level" with each other; anxiety abounds; as a result, communication becomes more and more divorced from its true function of describing the real state of affairs. Some recent research conducted in actual business organizations . . . seems to substantiate this gloomy view. For example, Read's study indicates that those middle managers who express the strongest aspiration toward promotion in the company are the ones who communicate least accurately with their immediate superiors. This tendency was noted in his research even when a high degree of interpersonal trust and confidence existed between the superior and subordinate.[22]

The ability to obtain accurate and complete information is not an idle challenge for most administrators.

A second problem confronting all supervisors is to make their instructions clearly understood by the recipients of those instructions. Often instructions have to be transmitted through various people and positions. As the instructions are sent, they can become distorted *in the direction that is most favorable to the receiver.* When the instructions are not followed the typical response is, "But I told him. . . ." Obviously what was clear to the supervisor was not clear to the subordinate. The net result is a misunderstanding.

Systematic feedback conferences can alleviate the problems of misunderstandings associated with both problems. Subordinates generally do not level with supervisors unless the supervisor clearly sets an environment for such leveling. When an ãdministrator sends messages that demonstrate an attitude of support, and when those messages are coupled with an attempt to retrieve positive *and* negative information, the probability increases that subordinates will send reliable information. The establishment of a psychologically safe working environment where information can be transmitted without fear of drastic and unfair adverse consequences is critical if the unit is to function effectively. In addition, if the feedback conferences are perceived by the subordinate as helpful, instructions that are not clear or that need further elaboration will be verbalized by the subordinate. In organizations where there are limited opportunities for feedback, employees tend not to question instructions. This often holds true even when the employees do not understand the instructions. The fear of looking "dumb" or "uninformed" is often so great that, unless there are opportunities for open discussion, employees would rather take their chances and hope that they will execute the instructions cor-

[21] Chris Argyris, *Personality and Organization* (New York: Harper & Row, 1957), p. 157.
[22] Charles Redding and George Sanborn, eds., *Business and Industrial Communication* (New York: Harper & Row, 1964), p. 54.

rectly. Unfortunately, the results of such actions can have unfavorable consequences for the organization.

A third benefit that accrues when feedback is systematically given to subordinates is related to *the employee's self-concept.* The supervisor is a significant person in a subordinate's life. The immediate supervisor has a very important and powerful role in shaping an employee's self-concept and self-confidence. Research on feedback demonstrates that the lack of feedback will tend to foster low confidence and hostility. Conversely, when there is open, direct, and supportive feedback from the supervisor, the employee's confidence tends to increase.[23] Feedback also influences the employee's valuation of his role. If there is little supportive feedback that would enable the employee to meet his needs for belonging, respect, and achievement, the employee will tend to diminish the importance of his role.[24] Once again, over time the quality of the employee's work will probably decrease.

In summary, it is clear that tangible, specific benefits accrue to the organization when feedback is given. It should be noted, however, that there are specific costs that accrue when a systematic feedback system is operating within an organization.

Costs of feedback   An important cost consideration is the fact that the giving of feedback takes an investment of time. Leavit and Mueller found that, as opportunities for feedback increase, the amount of time necessary for the completion of tasks also increases.[25] This is due to the fact that instructions will be clarified and perhaps questioned, problems with tasks will be discussed, and areas of discussion that would be ignored under zero feedback conditions will be brought into the open. All of this takes an investment of time and effort.

There are also personal costs that should be considered before implementing a systematic feedback program. An administrator takes risks when the communication system of an organization is opened to the type of interaction on which we have been focusing. One risk is that the administrator may learn that managerial practices are less effective than intended. For example, it may be found that instructions believed to be clear are not received as such by the members of the unit. Problems may also surface that were obscure or not known.

Perhaps the greatest risk that administrators face when implementing a formal feedback program is that judgments and decisions may come under

---

[23] William Brooks, *Speech Communication* (Dubuque, Iowa: Wm. C. Brown, 1971), p. 96.

[24] John R. Wenburg and William W. Wilmont, *The Personal Communication Process* (New York: John Wiley, 1973), pp. 129–30.

[25] Ibid., p. 134.

question by subordinates. Decisions that traditionally were made solely by the administrator stand the risk of being altered when others are consulted. Hopefully, the altered decision will be the best decision, but it will probably be different from the one that the administrator originally made. Whenever feedback is allowed, one runs the risk of decision alteration.[26]

While there are costs in implementing and carrying out a systematic feedback program, the benefits both to the individual and to the organization seem to outweigh those expenses. The human needs for security, belonging, respect, and achievement are partially met through such communication. Decreased misunderstandings and increased employee effectiveness also accrue from such interaction. In brief, the benefits from such practices appear to be well worth the investment of time and effort.

SUMMARY

This chapter has suggested that many organizational conflicts have their etiology in role considerations. An employee's role should be clearly defined so that the possibility for misunderstanding is diminished. When the role prescription is congruent with the role description, communication problems are minimized. Communication problems resulting from defensive behavior are also minimized when individuals feel secure in their roles. The utilization of supportive climates of communication as opposed to defensive climates minimizes defensive and self-protective stances. Finally, systematic feedback helps to create a sense of fulfillment in one's role. Feedback tends to heighten the respect between supervisors and subordinates and improves the quality of the communication between them.

STUDY QUESTIONS

1. As a newly appointed chief executive officer, you note that your organization has a once-a-year performance review program. Department heads have informed you that the program is largely ineffective and looked upon as a "joke" by most employees. Your goal during the coming year is to institute an effective feedback system so that every employee is aware of how their performance is being evaluated.
   a. How would you institute a regularly scheduled feedback program?
   b. Is it important to train department heads in how to give positive and problem-oriented feedback? What might be the major topics that should be discussed in such a training program?
   c. Most newly instituted performance review sessions are perceived by employees to be a threat. What might you do to diminish that threat?

[26] Ibid.

    d. List the criteria by which you will evaluate whether or not the feedback system is increasing employee productivity and morale.

2. A fifty-six year-old department head, whom you are supervising, bursts into your office waving a memorandum that you sent to him the previous day. His face is flushed and a tone of anger underlies his words. "I've worked in this place for twenty-six years. And for twenty-six years we have had meager budgets, poor equipment, and poorly trained personnel. And then you keep telling me to do more, more, and more. I tell you this place is like a zoo. Always do more on less and less. When are you executive types going to realize that there is a limit to what we can do?"

    a. Diagnose the possible causes for this type of behavior. Review Maslow's hierarchy of needs as you make your diagnoses.

    b. What problems in your administrative style may have precipitated this conversation?

    c. How would you diminish the defensive behavior of this department head?

ADDITIONAL READING RESOURCES

ALPANDER, GUVENC C., "Role Clarity and Performance Effectiveness," *Hospital and Health Services Administration,* 24, no. 1 (Winter 1979), 11–24.

DOOLEY, SUSAN L., and JAN HAUBEN, "From Staff Nurse to Head Nurse: A Trying Transition," *Journal of Nursing Administration,* 9, no. 4 (April 1979), 18–22.

FILLEY, ALAN C., *Interpersonal Conflict Resolution.* Glenview, Ill.: Scott, Foresman, 1975. Pp. 21–30.

LEVINSON, HARRY, "Asinine Attitudes toward Motivation," *Harvard Business Review,* January-February 1973, pp. 18–26.

MOORE, TERENCE, and DUANE WOOD, "Power and the Hospital Executive," *Hospital and Health Services Administration,* 24, no. 2 (Spring 1979), 30–41.

8

Competency: Resolving Disruptive Organizational Conflict

I cannot give you the formula for success, but I can give you the formula for failure, which is: Try to please everybody.—Herbert Bayard Swope

OVERVIEW The purpose of this chapter is to delineate methods that can be used in managing disruptive interpersonal, intragroup, and interdepartmental conflict. Upon completion of this chapter the reader should be able to:

- Differentiate win-lose, lose-lose, and win-win strategies of conflict resolution

- Discuss five approaches to conflict situations: avoidance, forcing smoothing, compromising, and confrontation

- Define communication techniques that can assist in clarifying the meaning of messages

- Define three problem-solving methods

One of our graduating students came by the office to say goodbye. In the course of the conversation several thought-provoking observations were made about an independent study program that she undertook in a community health clinic. This particular clinic has had a history of turmoil due to misunderstandings and disagreements between staff members and between the administrator of the clinic and the heads of several of the departments. "You know," she said, "before I became involved at the clinic I was certainly naive. I really thought that the major interest and concern of health professionals was the patient! But what I found out is that most of the discussions among staff members revolve around office politics. I never would have imagined that the concept of the 'health team' which we discussed so often in class is so far removed from the way things really are out there. So many professionals seem to spend their energies protecting themselves and their departments." She went on to say that three individuals in the clinic submitted their resignations during the previous week due to intense intrastaff conflict. Other employees were withdrawing into their departmental enclaves hoping that the tensions would dissipate.

As I was listening to the description of the problems the student had experienced it became apparent that she was coming to an important understanding about organizations and the way they function. All organizations have conflict; in fact, conflict is an inherent factor in the functioning of an organized system. Conflict is not an aberration in organizations; rather, it is one of the variables that must be adroitly managed if the productivity and morale of workers are not to be crippled. As Richard Beckhard has noted, "One of the major obstacles to effective organizations is the amount of dysfunctional energy spent in inappropriate competition—energy that is not, therefore, available for the accomplishment of tasks."[1] Beckhard states that if all of the energy that is used by one group of individuals to "get another group"and vice versa was available to improve organizational output, productivity in most organizations would increase tremendously.

The purpose of this chapter is to discuss various methods that can be used in successfully managing disruptive interpersonal, intragroup, and interdepartmental conflicts. At the outset, it is important to distinguish between strategic approaches and tactical approaches. *Strategic* mechanisms might be defined as anticipatory devices that recognize the potential for disruptive conflict in advance and attempt to structure situations to minimize anticipated harmful confrontations. In the previous chapter an effort was made to outline several strategic mechanisms. The clear definition of roles coupled with the giving of systematic feedback on performance are strategic mechanisms that increase the likelihood that disruptive conflict can be anticipated and, to a large extent, prevented. In this chapter attention will be focused on *tactical*

[1] Richard Beckhard, *Organization Development: Strategies and Models* (Reading, Mass.: Addison-Wesley, 1969), p. 14.

approaches to conflict. Tactical approaches might be defined as mechanisms that are designed to diffuse, manage, and resolve disruptive conflict once it has become apparent.[2] The discussion of tactical approaches will begin with a description of win-lose, lose-lose, and win-win strategies. The remainder of the chapter will focus on attitudes and behaviors that need to be evident if win-win strategies are to be effective.

WIN-LOSE, LOSE-LOSE, AND WIN-WIN STRATEGIES

In a thoughtfully written book concerning interpersonal conflict resolution, Alan C. Filley suggests three strategies that are commonly used in dealing with conflict situations: the win-lose strategy, the lose-lose strategy, and the win-win strategy.[3] The *win-lose strategy* is exemplified in the voting patterns that take place in committee meetings where the majority wins and the minority loses. If an individual or a small group of individuals within a committee consistently has the fewest votes they become the perennial losers. When the losses are perceived as personal defeats, majority rule can become a punishing experience for the members of the minority.

Autocratic administrators who make decisions without consulting subordinates may also exemplify a win-lose orientation towards conflict situations. This is particularly true when the questioning of administrative actions is perceived as a threat to administrative authority. In such a situation differences of opinion will seldom be considered on their own merit. The net result is that administrators may "win" because of the authority vested in their positions; the organization, however, will "lose" if controversies are not adequately resolved.

Staff members strive to cope with a win-lose administrator in ways that are generally unproductive for the organization. They may spend inordinate amounts of energy discussing strategies for dealing with the supervisor's win-lose style. They may decide to communicate as little as possible with the administrator and thereby attempt to avoid situations where they may lose. If a decision is made by the staff to limit communication with the administrator, emerging problems may not be dealt with and may grow to resemble organizational time bombs waiting to explode. The intent of such a strategy is the mistaken belief that the administrator will take the brunt of the blast. Unfortunately, when this approach is taken everyone seems to lose. The administrator loses because problems do not become apparent until it is too late to do anything about them; the staff loses because the administrator invariably

---

[2] David Leslie, "Conflict Management in the Academy: An Exploration of the Issues," Journal of Higher Education, 43, no. 9 (December 1972), pp. 14–19.

[3] Alan C. Filley, *Interpersonal Conflict Resolution* (Glenview, Ill.: Scott, Foresman, 1975), pp. 21–29.

blames them for the problems; the organization loses because energy that would normally be available for constructive problem solving is dissipated in intraorganizational warfare.

A second strategy described by Filley is the *lose-lose strategy*. This method is "so named because neither side really accomplishes what it wants or alternately, each side only gets part of what it wants. Lose-lose methods are based on the assumption that half a loaf is better than none, and avoidance of conflict is preferable to personal confrontation on an issue."[4]

An example of the lose-lose approach to conflict situations can be seen when two individuals attempt to resolve a mutually shared problem in the following way: Each individual has an "ideal" solution to the problem in mind but knows that the solution he favors would not be acceptable to the other party. Therefore, in order to avoid disagreement and conflict, each comes to the meeting with a solution that he knows the other party will immediately accept. They agree on a compromise solution that neither party feels particularly good about. Neither party won, but at least there were no disruptive tensions.

A lose-lose approach to conflict situations does have some merit and should not be dismissed as an entirely inappropriate way of managing conflict. Individuals who use this approach are often approachable simply because they want to find an accommodation. Solutions are, in fact, agreed to and, even though they may not be enthusiastically greeted by the participants, they may be effective in diminishing the negative effects of a problem.

The primary shortcoming of a lose-lose method is that participants do not have a strong commitment to solutions that are looked upon as organizational compromises. "It was the best decision under the circumstances" is a frequent comment made by participants. If there is little commitment to the solution it may be ineffective in dealing with the problem. When this happens the compromise solution will become known as "just one other approach which didn't work."

Filley notes that there are some common characteristics of the win-lose and lose-lose strategies. Each method makes a clear distinction between the parties, rather than providing a we-versus-the-problem orientation. Attention is focused on personalities rather than on defining the scope of the problem and finding solutions. Each party tends to see the issue from his own perspective rather than attempt to define the problem in terms of mutual needs. Because of these characteristics, win-lose and lose-lose approaches to conflict situations may accentuate interpersonal tensions. Since workable solutions are not found, there may be a tendency to blame one another when the inadequacies of the solutions become apparent.

The primary goal of a *win-win strategy* for conflict resolution is to find solutions to organizational problems that will have high quality and high ac-

[4] Ibid., p. 23.

ceptance. If this goal is to be realized, several values need to be integrated into the patterns of administration. The first value is related to the administrator's belief that it is possible to find solutions that will, in fact, have high quality and high acceptance. This value implies that the administrator is willing to look at the goals, motivations, and needs that other individuals bring to the conflict situation. It implies a realization that whether a defined solution satisfactorily resolves a given problem will be determined by the commitment each party feels toward the solution. Therefore, the ability to find solutions that will obtain a high degree of commitment is a necessary prerequisite if the solution is to be maximally effective.

The second value that a win-win administrator must support is related to a willingness to foster honest communication. The administrator who has this value is saying, "It is our collective responsibility to be open and honest about facts, opinions, and feelings."[5] When individuals believe that they are receiving only partial information concerning a problem, they become defensive. When an individual is evasive concerning the reasons why a position is so strongly advocated, distrust tends to arise. Conversely, honesty begets honesty. When an individual can verbalize her feelings, motivations, and perceptions, others in the group generally follow that norm. The result is that the problems can often be more sharply defined and the critical issues openly discussed. It is immensely difficult to find solutions to problems unless one has adequate information. As Norbert Wiener has stated, "The process of receiving and of using information is the process of our adjusting to the contingencies of the outer environment, and of our living effectively within that environment.[6] An administrative pattern that accentuates open communication can provide vital information that is needed in order to adequately confront the problem.

A third value basic to win-win approaches is rooted in a strong conviction that serious problems are best resolved when well-defined process-oriented decision-making methods are utilized. To begin discussion of a serious problem without a method through which defensiveness can be diminished often results in heightened anxiety and hostility. The administrator who values problem-solving methods is saying in effect, "I will control the process by which we arrive at agreement, but I will not dictate the content of our meeting." A problem-solving methodology that is defined, agreed to, and implemented increases the probability that defensiveness can be diminished and that creative solutions can emerge.

How should the above values be reflected in an administrator's style? If win-win orientations are to become integrated into the daily patterns of ad-

---

[5] Ibid., p. 27.

[6] Norbert Wiener, *The Human Use of Human Beings* (New York: Avon Books, 1950), p. 27.

ministration, three conflict perspectives need to be understood and applied to emerging problems. These conflict perspectives involve a willingness (1) to adopt and practice a confrontation style of approaching and managing conflict, (2) to invest effort in helping others clarify the meaning of messages, and (3) to follow systematic processes in order to arrive at high-quality solutions that bring about high acceptance.

Conflict Perspective 1: A win-win orientation is facilitated by a confrontive style in managing interpersonal problems.

Everyone has a style in approaching—or avoiding—conflict producing situations. If you think a moment about individuals with whom you work you can probably easily recognize individuals who are open and direct concerning their perception of organizational problems. Other individuals probably come to mind who seldom share their perceptions.

Some individuals are classic "gunnysackers." A gunnysacker is one who has grievances, but instead of doing anything about the grievances places them into his "sack." At times the sack gets so heavy that it bursts. When this happens, the whole load is dropped. If you have had the experience of someone reacting negatively and in inappropriate ways to a comment that normally would not provoke any type of an outburst, the chances are great that you are confronting a gunnysacker. The sack was full and running over and some minor comment caused the contents to emerge—usually with intense feeling.

Other individuals cope with conflict situations by communicating with others of like mind in a manner that might be defined as "ain't-it-awful." Ain't-it-awful individuals delight in telling how bad things are in the organization. Often a "poor me" attitude permeates the conversation. It is interesting to note that ain't-it-awful types can generally be found having coffee with one another or eating together at lunch time! Individuals who have differing points of view are generally not welcomed in the group. Ain't-it-awful individuals seldom confront the problems in a constructive manner. They defend their inaction with the belief that "it wouldn't do any good" to try and do something constructive about their complaints.

Other individuals employ a "red-crossing" technique to emerging problems. A red-crosser is an individual who applies a minute band-aid to a gaping wound. A red-crosser wants to live in an imaginative world in which everybody is happy: "Let's quit our bickering." "Let's not divide our own house." "Come on, we don't have it so bad." "Sure there are problems but just think about all the good things we have going for us." The red-crosser does not want to deal with emerging problems. Unfortunately for the red-crosser, while it is possible to deny the reality of the problems temporarily, the difficulty seldom goes away. At a later time and often in a different form the problem will again emerge.

Five common managerial styles   Robert Blake and Jane Mouton have delineated five managerial styles, each of which has its own values, attitudes, and behaviors that impinge on the way in which conflict is seen.[7] I would like to discuss each style, utilizing R. J. Burke's classification system: withdrawing, smoothing, compromising, forcing, and confronting.[8]

Withdrawing. The first style of relating to conflict situations is to withdraw. For the person who withdraws, it is easier to refrain from initiating action rather than dissenting and perhaps be forced to retreat at a later point in time.[9] The person who withdraws does so in various ways. The person may become ill at the time of a confrontation meeting or may have "inadvertently scheduled another meeting." If a disturbing memo is received, the answer is deferred or it is filed away and forgotten. If someone raises a question about the memo, the individual may say "Sorry, I've not received it," or "I haven't had a chance to get to it." Blake and Mouton suggest that when the individual cannot withdraw, the approach that is often taken is to maintain strict neutrality by not voicing any personal opinion.[10] Maintaining neutrality can be done by communicating in safe ways with comments like "I'll have to study the matter at greater length," or "I can see John's point of view, but I can also see Mary's. I just don't know which way to vote on this matter." Needing time in order to study the problem in depth is a common communication tactic utilized by the withdrawer.

Why does the individual respond by withdrawing? One reason is that the individual believes that the safest way to manage explosive situations is to not become involved. This opinion is held firmly by individuals who have involved themselves in win-lose conflict situations and have repeatedly found themselves on the negative end of the negotiations. If perceived defeats were humiliating and if there are significant regrets over what happened, the individual may resolve to never again be drawn into the open over anything.

It is self-defeating for an individual to repeatedly withdraw from conflict situations because withdrawal means that the individual's creativity and productive ideas are seldom verbalized and hence seldom available to the organization. As their years of withdrawing continue, withdrawers may come to the office to "put in their time," but their real world is somewhere else—perhaps at the lake or the golf course or fantasizing about how retirement will be spent. Intradepartmental relationships particularly suffer whenever an individual withdraws. If staff members withdraw into their own little personal enclave, the supervisor will develop hostilities because it

[7] Robert Blake and Jane Mouton, *The Managerial Grid* (Houston: Gulf Publishing Co., 1964).

[8] R. J. Burke, "Methods of Resolving Superior-Subordinate Conflict," *Organizational Behavior and Human Performance* 5 (1970), pp. 393–411.

[9] Bill Feltner and David Goodsell, "The Academic Dean and Conflict Management," *The Journal of Higher Education,* 43, no. 9 (December, 1972), 694.

[10] Blake and Mouton, *Managerial Grid,* p. 94.

becomes difficult to know what a staff member is thinking, feeling, and doing. If the supervisor withdraws from conflict situations, staff members will become frustrated because problems are not dealt with in a rational manner. In short, everyone loses when even one member of a department uses a withdrawing style of conflict resolution.

Smoothing. A second approach to conflict resolution is to smooth over the differences of opinion in conflict-producing situations. Blake and Mouton suggest that the individual with this style wishes to avoid disagreement, negative emotions, rejection, and frustration. The emphasis of the smoother is to accentuate the positive emotions by saying something like "Well, I know that we have our difficulties, but look at all the good things we are doing." Or the comment might be "Let us not fight in our department—if we start disagreeing with each other we will be no better off than anybody else around here." The administrator who operates under a smoothing orientation "is very much concerned about his own acceptance. Unable to use stern and harsh methods of having his wishes acted upon by subordinates, this supervisor is likely to appeal to feelings and to reason. But the insecurity behind his own adjustment is likely to show through. As a result, and after brief efforts at reasoning, recognition through appeasement is the likely next quick step."[11]

Individuals who smooth over conflict situations have a low tolerance for disagreements and the expression of negative emotions. Conflicts, they reason, hurt people and therefore they should be avoided. No situation is so bad that it should cause differences of opinion that are hurtful. In short, the intent of the smoother is to conscientiously do his job but not to become involved in the politics of an organization. Blake and Mouton further describe this approach:

> People are likely to be cajoled and coaxed into agreement by looking at how good things are, relative to how bad they might be—accentuating the positive and eliminating the negative, in other words. At a superficial plane, the mental attitude is that "every cloud has a silver lining," or "everyday, in every way, things are getting better and better," "a person should count his many blessings and name them one by one." When conflict does appear, the approach which is taken is, "Let's come together on those things that we can agree on and not fight one another on those matters that do not seem to be resolvable." The please "Don't say anything if you can't say something nice" comes through loud and clear.[12]

Administrators who have a smoothing style use varying strategies to avoid conflict. One strategy is to "kill your employees with kindness" so that they dare not bring up disagreeable issues. Dealing with the problem at some later date "when people's emotions aren't so high" is yet another way of smoothing over an emerging problem.

[11] Ibid. p. 66.
[12] Ibid. p. 67.

Unfortunately, this approach does not result in the happy, cohesive department that the supervisor would like to have. Employees are frustrated because issues are not dealt with. They are also frustrated because the supervisor is generally "such a nice guy." Thus, it becomes quite difficult to become angry with the supervisor even though the department may be seething with issues and problems that are in need of resolution.

Compromising. The basis of the compromise approach to conflict is the belief that administration is the art of compromise. The compromiser seeks to find a middle position where all parties feel relatively comfortable. The emphasis in the negotiations is to find "common ground" and to probe to see how much territory each individual may be willing to give up in order to achieve their ends. Alan Filley describes this style as follows:

> The [compromise] person enjoys the maneuvering required to resolve conflict and will actively seek to find some strong middle ground between two extreme positions. He may vacillate between expressing anger and then trying to smooth things over and may seek to use voting or rules as a way of avoiding direct confrontation on the issues. If he is confronted with a serious disagreement, he will suggest some mechanism for finding a "workable" solution (such as voting or trading rather than working out the disagreement) in order to find the best solution.[13]

The compromise style can be effective in given situations. The administrator with this style recognizes that conflict is inevitable in complex organizations and therefore it is dealt with. The compromise individual is generally open to discussion of issues and will carefully analyze the strengths and limitations or proposals that may produce conflict.

When this approach to conflict is practiced by an administrator, multiple problems emerge for staff members who are direct and confrontive. The subordinate who likes to deal with conflict situations by defining the best possible solution will find that such an orientation will not be looked upon with favor by the administrator. The solutions that are suggested by the subordinate may be seen as "too far out," "not realistic," "will never work around here." Consequently, the subordinate receives very little positive reinforcement for creativity. The internal frustration felt by the subordinate can either drive her out of the organization, or force her to adopt a more compromising approach to conflict situations. The net result will be that the solutions that the subordinate subsequently suggests will not creatively solve the complex problems facing the unit and will generate little internal reward for the subordinate. The administrator may be pleased with the "practical solution" but the organization may lose the one solution that could have creatively and competently resolved the problem.

[13] Alan Filley, *Interpersonal Conflict Resolution*, p. 52.

When a subordinate practices a compromise orientation toward conflict, administrators who are direct and confrontive in their approach tend to discount the subordinate's opinions. A subordinate who routinely compromises is perceived as being so tentative that it is possible for her to shift without even being wrong or inconsistent. The subordinate will often try to balance the positive against the negative, a strength with a weakness. The net result of this type of communication behavior is that administrators come to see the subordinate as lacking character, integrity, and internal strength.[14]

The most basic limitation of a compromise approach is that it focuses on finding equitable solutions rather than determining the best possible solution for a problem. Since the emphasis is on compromise, effort is usually not expended in examining the quality of the solution but rather on how individuals will accept the solution. Therefore, creative solutions, which may in themselves generate conflict, are often eliminated in favor of less sound solutions that are perceived as being politically viable.

Forcing. The "forcing" style of managing conflict is characterized by attempts to meet one's own goals at all costs without concern for the needs or the acceptance of others.[15] Losing is associated with reduced status, weakness, and the loss of self-image. Winning, on the other hand, gives the individual a sense of exhilaration and achievement. There is no doubt in the mind of the forcer concerning the correctness of his position. Because there is no doubt, anger and frustration are expressed towards others who disagree. The main purpose of any resulting argument is to win and have others agree with the point of view that is being advocated.

The forcing approach to conflict management can create immense problems for an organization over a period of time. Because conflict is suppressed, issues that need thorough discussion are generally not raised. When they are raised, defenses will be heightened due to the fear among co-workers that "once we get into it we really will be in for a fight." Since conflict is personalized the issues are seldom dealt with objectively. If administrators use their authority and power to obtain acceptance of their ideas, subordinates will usually lose even if they make an exceptionally good case. After continued losses, subordinates may begin to say, "What the heck, it's no use. The boss will never listen." Subsequently, a superficial tranquility may permeate the atmosphere of the office; underneath, however, hostility abounds because the environment is not conducive to collaborative problem solving.

Confronting. The confrontive problem-solving approach to managing conflict begins with a philosophical perspective: Conflict is an inherent part of organizational life. Because it is an inherent aspect to all organizations, ongoing conflict resolution processes must be developed, implemented, and

---

[14] Blake and Mouton, *Managerial Grid,* p. 125.
[15] Filley, *Interpersonal Conflict Resolution,* p. 51.

periodically evaluated. The confrontive problem solver not only believes that conflict is inevitable but that conflict can be a creative force in surfacing issues and bringing about constructive change in the organization.

According to Filley, individuals with a confrontive problem-solving approach to conflict will actively seek to satisfy their own goals as well as the goals of others. The confrontive problem solver

> (1) sees conflict as natural and helpful, even leading to a more creative solution if handled properly; (2) evidences trust and candidness with others and recognizes the legitimacy of feelings in arriving at decisions; (3) feels that the attitudes and positions of everyone need to be aired and recognizes that when conflict is resolved to the satisfaction of all, commitment to the solution is likely; (4) sees everyone as having an equal role in resolving conflict, views the opinions of everyone as equally legitimate; and (5) does not sacrifice anyone simply for the good of the group.[16]

The net result of a confronting style is that problems are constructively dealt with. Members of the working unit are willing to share both positive and negative information with their supervisor. Information is not hoarded by one party and used at strategic moments in order to advance a parochial point of view; rather, it is shared because members of the working unit recognize their interdependence and the necessity of working together if the goals of the unit are to be realized. Because conflict-producing problems are seen as legitimate and normal occurrences, a sense of openness and support for one another emerges within the working unit. The elusive concept of the "management team" begins to become a reality because of the mutual commitment to achieving agreed upon goals, and because the working environment is one in which collaboration rather than competition is rewarded.

As might be anticipated from the above description, the confrontation problem-solving approach generally is the most effective approach. Lawrence and Lorsch investigated six organizations to determine the effects of confrontation (win-win methods), forcing (resorting to authority or coercion), and smoothing (agreeing on an intellectual or a nonthreatening level). On the basis of their research they concluded that the two highest-performing organizations used confrontation to a more extensive degree than did the other four organizations being studied, and that the next two organizations, in order of performance, used confrontation more than the lowest two.[17] R. J. Burke asked seventy-four managers to describe the way they and their immediate supervisors dealt with conflicts. His research utilized the five descriptive categories we have delineated.

[16] Ibid., p. 52.
[17] Cited in Filley, *Interpersonal Conflict Resolution,* p. 30.

Supervisors who were effective in resolving conflict used the methods in the following order: (1) confrontation, (2) smoothing, (3) compromise, (4) forcing, and (5) withdrawal. The least effective supervisors used instead: (1) confrontation, (2) forcing, (3) withdrawal, (4) smoothing, and (5) compromise. Confrontation is reported most frequently in the less effective group as well as the more effective group; however, the frequent use of forcing is not.[18]

It therefore appears that one's secondary method is very important in resolving interpersonal conflict.

In general, the confrontive problem-solving approaches to conflict are most effective. The style that should be utilized in a given conflict situation will, however, depend upon a number of variables including the type of issue being discussed, the approach towards conflict taken by the other individuals involved, and the desired outcomes. It is conceivable that in some situations a style other than direct confrontation might be desirable. For example, a supervisor may adopt a smoothing approach to conflict when staff members ask for a change in an office procedure. The supervisor may well reason that such a change, while a potential minor inconvenience, will result in more harmonious working conditions for the employees. Since the issue has relatively little consequence in realizing the goals of the organization, the supervisor may well acquiesce in the interests of maintaining high morale in the working unit. However, if the requested change in office procedure has implications for the overall effectiveness of the department, a confrontive problem-solving approach would be warranted.

Conflict Perspective 2: A win-win orientation is facilitated when effort is given to helping others clarify their messages.

Acknowledging experience and reflecting feelings are helpful interpersonal skills. However, they are not tricks or gimmicks. Nor can they be used mechanically. They are helpful only within a context of concern and respect. In human relations, the agents of help are never solely the techniques, but the person who employs them. Without compassion and authenticity, techniques fail.[19]

One of the most important characteristics of individuals who are effective at resolving interpersonal conflict is that they have the interest and the ability to clarify the meanings behind the words that others speak. This is not a small talent nor an insignificant task. Because efforts are not often given to clarifying the meaning of words, multiple misunderstandings abound in many

[18] Cited in Filley, *Interpersonal Conflict Resolution,* p. 31.
[19] R. Wayne Pace and Robert R. Boven, *The Human Transaction* (Glenview, Ill., Scott, Foresman, 1973), p. 198.

organizations. The often-heard statement, "But, I thought I told them . . . ," is symbolic that the meanings behind the words were not understood.

There is ample evidence that individuals bring a set of attitudes, beliefs, and values to any given communication situation. A single event, particularly if it is conflict producing, will be seen from multiple perspectives by individuals who view the same situation. We seldom see the same event from the same perspective. Our construction of reality is highly personal and is unique to our own attitudes, beliefs, and values.

An illustration of how attitudes shape our perceptions is found in a well-known case study conducted in the aftermath of a football game between Dartmouth and Princeton. The football game, which touched off a spectacular sequence of events, is described by A. H. Hastorf and H. Cantril:

> A few minutes after the opening kickoff, it became apparent that the game was going to be a rough one. The referees were kept busy blowing their whistles and penalizing both sides. In the second quarter a Princeton player was taken off the field with a broken leg. Tempers flared both during and after the game. The official statistics of the game, which Princeton won, showed that Dartmouth was penalized 70 yards, Princeton 25, not counting more than a few plays in which both sides were penalized.[20]

After the game was completed, spectators loyal to their respective universities hurled insults and accusations at the opposing team, blaming them for the penalties, injuries, and combative conduct. Upon the completion of the game, Hastorf and Cantril requested students from the respective schools to fill out a questionnaire after they saw a film of the game.

> The reports were so divergent that it seemed each side witnessed separate events. For example, Princeton students who watched the film "saw" the Dartmouth team commit over twice the number of infractions reported by the Dartmouth students. Spectators from the respective teams "saw" more than twice the number of "flagrant" violations made by the members of the opposing team. The "same" sensory impingements emanating from the football field, transmitted through the visual mechanism to the brain, obviously gave rise to different experiences in different people. The significances assumed by different happenings for different people depend in large part on the purposes people bring to the occasion and the assumptions they have of the purposes and probable behavior of other people involved. . . .

> It is inaccurate and misleading to say that different people have different "attitudes" concerning the same "thing." For the "thing" simply is not the same for different people whether the "thing" is a football game, a presidential candidate, Communism, or spinach. We do not simply "react to" a happening or to some impingement from the environment in a determined way (except in a

[20] A. H. Hastorf and H. Cantril, "They Saw a Game: A Case Study," *Journal of Abnormal and Social Psychology,* 49 (1954), 129–34.

behavior that has become reflecting or habitual). We behave according to what we bring to the occasion, and what each of us brings to the occasion is more or less unique.[21]

An administrator who starts with the belief that an event viewed by two or more people will be seen the same way will ultimately become frustrated in communication situations. Statements such as "They were at the meeting, weren't they?" or "They heard what I told them; I certainly repeated those instructions enough" reflect a belief that others should see the same event in the same way that the sender of the message views the situation. Such congruity in perceptions seldom takes place. What we see and what we hear are greatly influenced by our emotional state, past experiences, and the expectations we bring to a given situation.

Because individuals see communication events from multiple perspectives, the effective resolution of conflict can only be undertaken when individuals involved in the conflict invest energy in seeking to understand one another's point of view. In the idiom of the day, it is important to understand "where they're coming from." The ability to determine the perspective of the individuals with whom you are working—including their attitudes, beliefs, and values about a conflict situation—is critical if progress is to be made in resolving tensions.

Reflecting content and feeling   How does one determine the mental set of individuals towards a given situation? How does one probe in such a way that the other individual's perspective on a problem can be clearly seen? One clarifies messages by periodically reflecting back to the sender the content and the feeling of what is being heard in the conversation.

> Reflecting the *content* of a message represents the interpreter's attempt to clarify by repeating to the source the same statement (the same literal meaning) uttered by the latter. This type of response permits the source to hear and mull over what he or she has just said. Hearing the utterance from a different source often provides sufficient motivation to think through the validity of the comment.[22]

For example, if the personnel director states to the administrator "I think everyone in the hospital should have a 5 percent raise for this next year," the administrator may respond by saying, "I take it then that you believe that custodians, civil service staff, and department heads should all receive the same 5 percent increase. Is that correct?" The administrator's reflection of the statement made by the personnel director can help to clarify in the personnel director's mind the implications of what he has said. The technique is also

[21] Ibid., p. 133.
[22] Pace and Boven, *Human Transaction,* p. 191.

a good check in determining whether the reflector has heard the source correctly.

The reflection of *feelings* consists of expressing back to the source latent meanings, connotative meanings, and vocal tones that seemed to imply feelings of which the source may not be entirely conscious.[23] If you heard the above statement concerning the 5 percent raise you may wish to feed back perceptions such as: "You seem comfortable with the 5 percent figure. Are you?" or "You seem to feel rather strongly that raises should be uniform for this next year. Is that correct?" Once again, by reflecting what it is that you are hearing, you make it possible to uncover the latent meanings of the messages—meanings that may help to clarify the other person's point of view.

Research has demonstrated that feeding back to an individual what he or she has stated will elicit statements of the kind being reflected. William Verplank discovered "that both reflecting and agreeing with statements influenced the rate at which speakers stated opinions; the subjects increased the number of opinion statements they made when reinforced by statements of reflection and agreement."[24] In brief, the ability to feed back what it is that one is hearing provides avenues for clarifying due to the fact that the other person will make additional statements.

Summarizing   In order to understand one another, not only is it important to reflect what it is that one is hearing, but it is essential that there be a summary statement at the conclusion of each interview. A concluding statement, such as the following one, can help to ensure that the conclusions arrived at are mutually shared: "I will talk to Mrs. Smit and obtain her opinions about what to do concerning the problems of the new charting system. In the meantime, you are going to call Mr. Pierson at Shalom Hospital to see how they managed their new system. We will then meet at the beginning of next week and see what we might recommend in resolving those charting difficulties. Is that agreeable with you?" Such a summary ensures that the mutual expectations are clearly known to each party. Many communication problems can be prevented if the outcomes of a meeting are restated and clarifed in a simple summary.

The techniques of restating and summarizing may seem simple and easy to use. Such techniques *are* easy to implement, providing there is a highly conscious desire to use clarification procedures in interview situations. When clarification techniques are implemented, the rewards are immediate. The quantity of information as well as the quality of that information improves. Agreements arrived at are more than affirmative nods of the head for there is a mutual understanding of the meanings of the agreements. Finally, when

[23] Ibid.

[24] William S. Verplanck, "The Control of the Content of Conversation: Reinforcement of Statements of Opinion" *Journal of Abnormal and Social Psychology,* 51 (1955), pp. 668–76.

clarification procedures are utilized, communication miunderstandings are pinpointed in the early phases of discussion rather than emerging at a later point in time.

Conflict Perspective 3: A win-win orientation is facilitated by the use of problem-solving methods.

Once a decision has been made to confront a conflict situation, thought should be given to whether a problem-solving process should be used. A problem-solving process might be defined as a structured, step-by-step approach that enables participants to identify the nature of the problem and to suggest various solutions that will resolve the perceived difficulties.

Some individuals do not like the idea of using a structured process in helping solve interpersonal problems. I have known administrators who rebel at the thought of "getting all tangled up in a process when you can usually get things straightened out by simply talking it out." There is evidence that a direct, unstructured approach may be effective simply because the broaching of a subject tends to diminish the hostility between individuals. Alan Filley has noted:

> Common association between two parties, even though it may not be judged positively or negatively, may induce positive feelings between them in a problem solving situation. One method to increase mutuality is simply to increase interaction. While we have already seen that interaction can lead to some forms of conflict, there is also evidence that it leads to cohesion between the parties.[25]

While some may prefer an unstructured discussion about a problem, others prefer a process that will help to diminish hostility and create a climate where rational discussions can occur. Structured problem-solving methods can help in pinpointing the precise causes of interpersonal difficulties and in identifying creative solutions to mutually shared problems. I have found that the more complex and emotive the problem, the more helpful it is to use a structured process. The following paragraphs will focus on three methods that can be used in one-to-one, intradepartmental, and interdepartmental settings.

Managing one-to-one conflict situations   A five-step problem-solving method is preceded by the asking of two critical questions:

1. Is it possible, at the present time, to resolve the conflict situation in a way that will be satisfactory to all parties?
2. What environment can best facilitate the discussion of the issues?

[25] Filley, *Interpersonal Conflict Resolution,* p. 103.

The first question seeks to determine whether, *at the present time,* it is possible to engage in collaborative problem solving. The timing factor in conflict resolution appears to be a critical variable that will affect negotiated outcomes. There are specific time periods in which both parties are amenable to discussing their problems and there are time sequences in which both parties, because of their attitudes, beliefs, and emotive involvement with the problem, would not be able to engage in collaborative problem solving.

Individuals are most amenable to resolving their problems when their level of discomfort concerning the problem is so great that they have trouble thinking about anything else but the problem. An individual who is heavily invested in a problem will often welcome initiatives designed to alleviate the dissonance. If, for example, an administrator hears through the grapevine that a staff member is continually making reference to a particular grievance, the time might be right for a problem-solving interview. Individuals will also be amenable to problem-solving initiatives if they see a way through which they might be able to win more than they will lose. Individuals dread any conflict resolution effort if they feel that the conversation will only result in them giving up more than they gain. Finally, a critical time for problem solving comes when the organization's effectiveness is eroding because of a conflict situation within the staff. Some problems, if left unattended, will only compound. Such difficulties should be confronted in an expeditious manner.

The answer to the second question, where the meeting should be held, is a significant factor in resolving difficult interpersonal conflicts. While discussion of day-to-day problems can be effectively carried out in the office of either the supervisor or the subordinate, a confrontation relative to a divisive issue might best be undertaken in a neutral setting. An office of a supervisor can intimidate employees to the point where they may not be willing to openly share their attitudes and beliefs about the problem. On the other hand, a neutral setting might provide an environment where defensiveness can be diminished and where interruptions are nonexistent.

Not only should one carefully select the place where problem solving can best be accomplished but it is equally important to allocate sufficient time to work through difficult situations. To allot thirty minutes to an employee who has been seething with a problem for months is to do an injustice to both the employee and the problem. Conflict resolution usually involves an immense amount of time and energy. Relying on a short conference to deal with a serious problem might result in additional frustration. In view of this you may find it helpful to schedule three or four meetings for the discussion of a serious issue. When you as an administrator budget adequate time for the discussion of a problem, you are signaling your perceptions concerning the importance of the problem and your intent to find satsifactory resolutions.

After the two preliminary questions have been satisfactorily answered a meeting should be scheduled. *The first step of the one-to-one process is to focus on the definition of the problem.* Careful attention should be given to whether one is dealing with the *overt* or the *covert* problem. The overt problem represents the symptoms of the conflict while the covert problem represents a precise variable that is causing the conflict.

In our culture we often become so preoccupied with finding solutions that adequate effort is not given to separating symptoms of a problem from the problem itself. For example, a dispute between the nursing director and in-service training coordinator may appear to be a difference of opinion as to the nature of the educational programs that the hospital is offering. In reality the conflict over the educational programs (the overt problem) may be masking a more basic issue—that is, who has control over the educational programs (the covert problem). In this instance a great deal of time might be spent in discussing symptoms (should we offer educational programs for diabetics or should we offer parent effectiveness classes?) rather than addressing the key issue of control. Only when the substantive issue is addressed can meaningful strides be made toward resolving the interpersonal conflicts.

The importance of differentiating overt and covert problems can be illustrated with the following example. A director of school of nursing called a management consultant and discussed with him the problems that the school was facing. The essence of the conversation was that the school's faculty was riddled with dissension, bickering, and internal disputes. Morale was very low and the director feared that the productivity of the faculty was being negatively influenced by the intrafaculty disagreements. She asked the consultant to conduct a one-day workshop with the faculty that would have as its basic purpose the resolution of their conflicts. A date was set and most of the faculty came to the workshop.

At the conclusion of the day, the consultant was able to isolate what he thought were the problems: (1) faculty workloads were too heavy; (2) there wasn't enough opportunity for professional advancement; and (3) too much time was spent on faculty committees. Specific solutions were outlined and it was agreed that they would be immediately implemented.

The consultant went home at the end of the day feeling good about the workshop. Unfortunately, one month later the director called to say that "Ever since that workshop took place things have gone downhill." That was not the type of feedback the consultant was hoping to receive!

The consultant decided to initiate a different strategy in order to define the covert problems. He interviewed each of the faculty members individually. Almost without exception each faculty member informed him that the workshop did not deal with the real issues that were causing their problems. "Everyone was apprehensive about that workshop and it prohibited us from communicating honestly with one another," said one faculty member. "Those problems which we defined are irritants, but they are not our main problem." The real issue had to do with the relationship between the director of the school and the members of the faculty.

The director was a very strong and opinionated individual who did not tolerate disagreement. There was very little positive feedback given by the director to the members of the faculty. Consequently many of them wondered where they stood and whether they would be invited back next year.

The faculty, on the other hand, abdicated academic planning to the director and, when things didn't go the way they liked, would seldom discuss their perceptions with the director. The faculty delighted in playing "ain't-it-awful," but seldom would they openly and honestly share their perceptions with the director.

A second workshop was held and, although it was painful for the participants to focus on the problem, they were able to define the relationship issues that were negatively affecting the organization. The process that followed was tedious and defensiveness often flared. Nevertheless, by the conclusion of the second workshop everyone agreed that "at the very least, we are working on the true problem."

As can be seen in the above example, the complaints about teaching loads and committee assignments were really the symptoms of a problem that had not been correctly identified. Only after diligent questioning on a one-to-one basis was the critical issue correctly identified.

There is no easy way to determine whether one is dealing with symptoms or the problem itself in conflict situations. However, by being aware of the differences between overt and covert problems, by reflecting back what was heard, and by insisting upon honest confrontation with one another, the likelihood improves that the etiology of the problem will be discovered.

The second step in a one-to-one process is to list potential solutions to the problem. This is often referred to as the "brainstorming" phase of problem solving. In this step each person lists possible solutions that would help resolve the difficulty. Creative free association should be encouraged. "Wild ideas," which perhaps will later need to be tamed, should be requested. At the completion of this phase, four to six solutions should be placed in writing so as not to be lost in subsequent discussion.

Pausing between steps 2 and 3 is often helpful to the entire process. Expectations and positive feelings are generally quite high after the completion of step 2. It is not uncommon for individuals to say after completing step 2, "You know, I think we are beginning to get somewhere." Comments such as this mean that defensiveness is being lowered and individuals are beginning to believe that resolutions can be found.

In the third step, efforts are made to evaluate each of the solutions. This should be done systematically by first evaluating the strengths and then the weaknesses of each solution. Sometimes it is helpful to write each solution on a flip chart with the strengths and limitations carefully delineated. After this has been completed it is usually possible to identify the solution that has the most strengths and the fewest limitations. When one of the solutions is clearly seen as desirable, a sigh of relief and a sense of accomplishment is felt by each member of the group. Because each individual has given input into the process a feeling of ownership about the solution becomes apparent.

At times, however, the best solution does not become apparent. When this happens it is best to evaluate once again and to define the strengths and weaknesses of each of the solutions more carefully. After this has been completed, agreement should be reached on those solutions that are clearly unsatisfactory. Unsatisfactory solutions should be discarded so that only two or three solutions remain. Further discussion should seek to gain closure concerning the viability of each of the remaining solutions.

In the fourth step, effort is given to determine how the solution can be implemented. Written agreements should be arrived at to ensure that there is a common understanding about what is to be done to resolve the problem. The agreement should be *clear* (understandable to all and containing no vague words), *scheduled* (date stipulated as to when the solution will be implemented), *measurable* (everyone should be able to determine whether the solution has been effective), and the *end result specified.* An example of this is seen in the following:

> By November 30, the patient education department will have written a five-page document explaining to parents of cleft children the following: (a) nutritional problems associated with cleft anomalies, (b) feeding procedures prior to surgery, and (c) resources available to assist the parents. Mrs. Mary Peter, Director of Patient Education, and Dr. Michael Broson, Chief of Pediatrics, will have responsibility for writing this pamphlet. The pamphlet will be given to parents within the first week of the child's birth in order to assist the parents in managing the child's dietary patterns.

By stipulating who is responsible for what and by what date, the written agreement ensures that expectations are understood. Such carefully written solutions increase the likelihood that the proposed solution will, in fact, resolve the problem.

In dealing with a complex problem, particularly if there have been strong feelings about the problem, it is wise to periodically check to make certain that the agreed upon solution has been adequately put into effect, to determine whether the people who are affected are satisfied with the effects of the solution, and to resolve problems that may arise out of the implementation of the solution. One of the interesting facts about resolving organizational problems is that any new solution designed to alleviate an old problem usually creates new problems. By recognizing that new solutions will cause problems and by dealing with the emerging new problems as they arise, you will be able to help guarantee that the agreed upon solution is resolving the perceived difficulties.

In the fifth and final step, effort is focused on determining how the solution will be evaluated. If possible, written criteria of evaluation should be stipulated. It is also important to set a date as to when the evaluation will take place and to determine who the evaluator will be. Figure 8–1 summarizes the five-step process; Figure 8–2 illustrates possible solutions to a financial problem confronting the educational department of a hospital.

A basic goal in working through the five-step problem-solving process is to discuss the problem in such a manner that the self-respect of the other individual is strengthened and not diminished. You will recall that every individual has certain basic needs that influence how he or she functions in an organization. When these needs are satisfactorily realized, the individual's self-respect is strengthened. When these needs are not being met, you can expect behavior that seeks to fulfill such needs. In any meeting it is prudent to remember that all discussion will impinge upon the psychological state of participants. The three human needs that frequently seek fulfillment in problem-solving meetings are the following:

Step 1: What is the problem? Are we dealing with the symptoms of the problem, or the problem itself?

Step 2: What potential solutions are there to the identified problem?

Step 3: What are the strengths and weaknesses of each solution?

Step 4: How will the solution be implemented? Is the solution clear, scheduled, measurable and does it have its intended results specified?

Step 5: How will the solution be evaluated? Who will evaluate the effectiveness of the solution?

Figure 8-1   A process for resolving interpersonal conflict.

Step 1: Define the problem.

To meet the needs of prospective parents in Glenville, prenatal classes should be expanded by 25 percent by July 1. However, because of financial constraints the budget for prenatal classes is scheduled to be reduced by 15 percent effective July 1.

Step 2: List possible solutions.

a. Cut the prenatal classes from 45 to 30 per year.

b. Continue to offer 45 prenatal classes for this fiscal year but reduce the number of participants by 35 percent.

c. Determine whether it would be possible to offer joint prenatal classes with Hanover Hospital. By combining resources and using the hospital's facilities, it would be possible to offer more classes to a greater number of prospective parents.

d. Request the Westside Foundation to donate $5,000 to carry on the prenatal classes. Such funding would permit the number of classes to be expanded by 25 percent.

e. Request the administration to cut back the financial support of the diabetes education program by 30 percent and use such funds for an expanded prenatal program.

Step 3: Evaluate solutions (strengths and limitations). Determine the best solution.

Step 4: Define how the solution will be implemented.

Step 5: Define how the solution will be evaluated.

Figure 8-2   Example of a problem-solving process.

1. The need for security—"Is my job in jeopardy?"
2. The need to belong—"Am I still part of the team?"
3. The need for respect—"In spite of the problem, am
   I still respected for what I can do?"

The sooner one is able to meet these needs, the better the individual will be able to objectively focus on the problem. Statements such as the following, if genuinely made, represent one attempt to strengthen a person's self-respect:

> "Well, I think that the procedures we have just outlined should help to solve the problems we have been having. Before you go, I do want you to know, Jane, that while we may occasionally differ, I am still very glad that we are working together."

> "Mark, when problems have come up on our floor I have often asked for your advice and suggestions. Again I am in need of your assistance if we are to solve yesterday's staffing problems."

In the first example the supervisor, in her concluding remarks, is seeking to affirm that while they may disagree with one another, the supervisor is indeed appreciative that they are "on the same team." In the second example, the supervisor is seeking to meet the subordinate's need for self-respect by simply saying, "I would appreciate your point of view." The type of sensitivity reflected in the above statements cannot help but create a climate for good interpersonal relationships within the organization.

One last comment should be made in regard to the process of resolving one-to-one communication problems. Any emotional encounter between two persons generally results in a period of introspective analysis on the part of those involved. "Did I say too much?" "Did she really mean that she appreciated my criticism of her leadership?" "Will she really follow through on what we decided?" Such anxieties can be allayed by following through on whatever outcomes may have resulted from the interview. An effective administrator is one who tries to keep the staff informed about changes and developments in a department that result from a problem-solving session. This is particularly true when an administrator agrees to take responsibility to implement a decision. If for some reason or another, the outcomes of the interview cannot be implemented as readily as possible, a simple note or comment to the involved staff member will alleviate fears that the interview was not taken seriously.

Managing intradepartmental conflict   The management of conflict within a department often takes the wisdom of a Solomon. In any given work day conflicts can spring forth from multiple sources. Subordinates may argue among themselves or may align themselves against a policy that you want to implement. Consumers may criticize you for events over which you do not have direct control. Staff members may have different priorities as compared with yours and may argue for their interests without understanding how their positions will influence others in the organization. In brief, health administrators exist in a climate where differences of opinion and conflicts frequently emerge.

It is important that administrators have ongoing processes to deal with emerging conflicts. Problems that are unique to one subordinate can probably be dealt with individually, using a process such as the one which was previously discussed. However, when there are multiple problems confronting a department involving most of the staff members, a different process is warranted.

Figure 8-3 outlines one intradepartmental problem-solving process. Your use of this process should be modified to fit into your needs, expectations, and goals.

In the first step, the issue areas are delineated. All departments have issues that need periodic examination and resolution. As a general rule, every department should probably set aside time at least twice a year in which issues can be constructively aired. The fall is often an ideal time for a one or two-day retreat for the purposes of identifying such issues and to initiate work on them.

If such a retreat seems desirable, the first several hours should be spent in identifying the critical problems confronting the department. One way of making such an identification is by having individuals list, while working independently, the major issues that they feel need to be discussed. Approximately twenty to thirty minutes should be given to this phase of the problem-solving process.

In the second step, an effort is made to obtain group consensus concerning the relative importance of the identified issues. After each individual has submitted a list of central issues, all responses should be pooled on a flip chart or blackboard. After the issues have been listed, a brief discussion of each issue should be initiated. Generally not more than five minutes of discussion per issue should be allocated for this initial discussion phase. The basic intent

Step 1: Individual members work independently in listing issues that affect their department

Step 2: a. Individual perceptions are listed on blackboard
        b. Group rank orders the issues in order of importance

Step 3: Potential solutions listed for most critical problem

Step 4: Evaluation of solutions

Step 5: Delineation of ways to implement the solution

Figure 8-3   An intradepartmental conflict resolution process.

of this brief discussion is to gain a preliminary understanding of the nature of the issue that is before the group.

After the five-minute discussion on each issue, each group member is requested to determine what they consider to be the top three issues confronting the department. After they have had some time to think about this a vote is taken on each issue. Each member of the group has three votes which can be cast for the three issues that they believe are most important. At the conclusion of this phase of the exercise you will be able to rank order what the group perceives to be the three most critical issues confronting the department.

It should be noted that this process often results in strengthening the cohesiveness of a department. When the members of a unit feel that constructive steps are being taken to address the critical issues of a department, morale generally increases. When the supervisor communicates through the use of such a process that there is a genuine interest in finding solutions to complex problems, the respect of staff for that supervisor also increases. When employees feel that substantive progress is actually being made on problems they consider to be important, intraoffice communication becomes more frequent, and the quality generally improves.

In the third step, effort is made to find solutions to the identified problems. If your department is large (over eight members) you may wish to divide the large group into several small groups of four or five members. The assignment is to list all the *potential* solutions to the problem that the group decides to address. Make clear in your instructions that, in this step, no effort will be made to evaluate the solutions. If you are brainstorming in a large group, the recorder should list each solution on the blackboard. If a large group is subdivided into small working groups, they should return to the large group after approximately thirty to sixty minutes and have their solutions placed on a blackboard.

With a list of potential solutions now placed on the blackboard, your role is to help the group through *the fourth step, which is to evaluate each of the solutions.* The key to being successful in this step is to evaluate the solutions systematically. Each solution should be evaluated for its strengths and its limitations. The strengths and limitations should be listed of a flip chart or a blackboard.

After each solution has been discussed, one or two solutions will generally emerge as being most viable. If one solution is not clearly the most effective, further discussion of the strengths and weaknesses of two or three remaining solutions should be discussed.

In the fifth and final step, discussion should focus on possible ways to implement the solution. After the most viable solution has been delineated, it is important for the group to spend considerable effort deciding how the solution should be implemented. Oftentimes groups are so relieved that they were able to get consensus on a solution that this last stage is lost. Therefore, it is important that you, as the group facilitator, clearly allocate necessary time to discuss who will be responsible for what and by what dates. After the meeting has been concluded, the agreed upon implementation steps should be written and circulated to the members of the department. It is important to make certain the solution is clear, measurable, and scheduled, and that the desired result is specified.

The above process is not without its pitfalls. The administrator must be willing to let the members of a department work collectively on those problems that affect them if this process is to be successful. Some administrators would suggest that there is too high a risk of getting solutions that are not compatible with the administrator's perceptions of the department. If this is true in your case, you may want to outline for the department those issues that are "off limits" and therefore not open for discussion. Examples of possible "off limits" areas might be wage issues, policies that cannot be renegotiated, and personality conflicts with individuals outside of the department. If there are certain off-limit areas, it becomes very important to define such areas *prior* to the start of the meeting.

One criticism that is made of the above process is that it is difficult for an administrator to be an objective facilitator of the group discussion. This is due to the fact that most departmental problems are so intertwined with the administrator that it is impossible for the administator to objectively lead a problem-solving meeting. If you feel that you can discuss the problems with a fair amount of objectivity and can constructively listen to the comments put forth by the members of the unit, you should give leadership to this process. If you feel, on the other hand, that such objectivity would be difficult or impossible, you would be advised to ask someone else to facilitate the group meeting. Your choice of facilitator should be agreeable with the members of the work group. The two key characteristics of any potential group leader should be (1) their desire to be objective, and (2) their willingness to follow a systematic process in discovering workable solutions.

Managing interdepartmental conflict   The resolution of problems between two groups represents an immense challenge to administrators. Interdepartmental conflicts are often of a long-standing nature. Misunderstandings, disagreements, and the sending of incomplete or inaccurate messages between departments can result in a complex set of problems that defy easy solutions. When misunderstandings and disagreements are coupled with personalities who have a direct ego involvement in the difficulty, the challenge to resolve the problems becomes immense.

While the challenge to resolve interdepartmental difficulties is great, interdepartmental problems must be brought into a manageable focus if the organization's goals are to be realized. Problems between administrators and the medical staff, therapy departments and the nursing staff, or personnel department employees and department heads can evolve to the point that the care of patients is affected. In the public sector interdepartmental conflicts can seriously erode the organization's ability to respond adequately to the needs of consumers.

A problem-solving method delineated by Warren Bennis is particularly helpful in resolving interdepartmental conflict.[26] Bennis describes a conference which Chris Argyris and he led. The conference was for the top-echelon administrative officers in the U.S. State Department and Foreign Service officers. Argyris and Bennis charged each group to answer the following questions:

1. What qualities best describe our group?
2. What qualities best describe the other group?
3. What qualities do we predict the other group would assign to us?

Each group met in a separate room and were asked to develop a list of words or phrases that would summarize their answers. The results were as follows:

The Foreign Service officers saw themselves as:

1. Reflective
2. Qualitative
3. Humanistic, subjective
4. Cultural, broad interests
5. Generalizers
6. Intercultural sensitivity
7. Detached from personal conflicts

The Foreign Service officers saw the administrative officers as:

1. Doers and implementers
2. Quantitative
3. Decisive and forceful
4. Noncultural
5. Limited goals
6. Jealous of us
7. Interested in form more than substance
8. Wave of the future! (exclamation mark theirs)
9. Drones but necessary evils

[26] Warren Bennis, *Organization Development: Its Nature, Origins and Prospects* (Reading, Mass.: Addison-Wesley, 1969), pp. 4–6. Reprinted with permission.

The Foreign Service officers predicted that the administrative officers would see them as:

1. Arrogant, snobs
2. Intellectuals
3. Cliquish
4. Resistant to change
5. Inefficient, dysfunctional
6. Vacillating and compromising
7. Effete

The administrative officers saw themselves as:

1. Decisive, guts
2. Resourceful, adaptive
3. Pragmatic
4. Service oriented
5. Able to get along
6. Receptive to change
7. Dedicated to job
8. Misunderstood
9. Useful
10. Modest! (added by the individual doing the presenting)

The administrative officers saw the Foreign Service officers as:

1. Masked, isolated
2. Resourceful, serious
3. Respected
4. Inclined to stability
5. Dedicated to job
6. Necessary
7. Externally oriented
8. Cautious
9. Rational
10. Surrounded by mystique
11. Manipulative
12. Defensive

The administrative officers predicted that the Foreign Service officers would see them as:

1. Necessary evil
2. Defensive, inflexible
3. Preoccupied with minutiae

4. Negative and bureaucratic
5. Limited perspective
6. Less cultural (educated clerks)
7. Misunderstood
8. Practical
9. Protected
10. Resourceful

After the lists were produced, the two groups met together and discussed their lists. The other group was able to ask questions with regard to their perceptions. Bennis reports that the discussion was "intense, high pitched, noisy, argumentative, good humored, and finally, several hours later, thoughtful. It appeared as if each side moved to a position where they at least understood the other side's point of view.[27]

This interdepartmental problem-solving process usually produces gratifying results. The group quickly gets into the task. While the discussion can be threatening, a great deal of humor often evolves. Checking mutual perceptions and getting feedback about a particular group's behavior is perceived as a valuable experience in and of itself. In general, the results of using this method are that (1) impressions of one another are openly discussed; (2) understandings are developed as to why a group behaves the way it does; and (3) empathy develops concerning the respective problems each department is facing.

Postscript: "That all sounds good, but you can't change ol' Mr. Smith."

In the preceding pages, an effort has been made to outline specific methods to resolve disruptive conflict. Sometimes managers will say, "Well, those methods sound OK but it would never work with my boss." The discussion then continues with a list of adjectives describing the "ol' boss." We are quickly into a game called "If it weren't for ol'. . . ." A second response, and a more thoughtful one, is that the above methodologies deal with issues and problems rationally when, in fact, many organizational problems seem to be irrational.

It is true that some people are "difficult to work with." But it is equally true that most individuals respond *positively* to administrative actions that will satisfactorily resolve interorganizational conflicts. Unfortunately, when we label individuals as "inflexible," "rigid," or "unbending" we create an immediate barrier to constructive problem solving. The absence of positive action usually accentuates the conflicts.

The perception that many organizational problems are somewhat irrational ("How could he do something like that?") is a common perspective. It

---

[27] Ibid.

is important to remember, however, that no matter how irrational a response may seem, it reflects the individual's way of coping with a stressful situation.

Individuals have many different ways of protecting themselves. They may become quiet, defensive, or withdrawn. They may even communicate in ways that seem to defy logic. However, when one understands *why* people are threatened, the rational reasons explaining their behavior become apparent. A problem-solving process will enable you to identify the nature of the threat. It will also help you identify practical actions that will reduce defensive behavior.

SUMMARY

We have discussed a number of strategies that can be utilized in successfully managing disruptive, one-to-one, intragroup, and interdepartmental conflicts. The objective of any conflict-resolving methodology should be to enable both parties to feel that they have emerged out of the conflict situation as winners. In order to accomplish this objective, careful attention should be given to one's personal approach to conflict situations. Avoiding, forcing, compromising, and smoothing are generally not as effective at satisfactorily resolving conflict as is a direct, confrontive style. A key characteristic of the confrontive style is the ability to help clarify the meaning of the messages that one is hearing. Such clarification procedures are of immense assistance in identifying the etiology of the problem. Difficult problems are best confronted by using systematic methodologies. Such systematic approaches enable clear problem identification, and the discovery of relevant solutions.

STUDY QUESTIONS

1. It has been said that "partial misunderstanding is a normal result of the communication process." Do you agree with this statement? Why or why not?

2. On the basis of your experience, what are the three most prominent reasons for organizational conflict? Can these problems be resolved from a win-win perspective? If not, how can these problems be managed?

3. Are you presently involved in a conflict situation? Analyze it on the basis of what you have learned in the past two chapters. How do you evaluate your effectiveness in managing interpersonal conflict situations?

4. Michael Korda has argued that "It is desire for power that keeps most executives working. What we are afforded is no longer a chance for

unlimited wealth, but the chance to acquire limited power, with the advantage that its satisfactions cannot be taxed and are not subject to depreciation.''* Do you agree with this statement? What implications does this statement have for being able to manage conflict within complex organizations?

ADDITIONAL READING RESOURCES

BATTEN, JOE D., *Tough-Minded Management*. New York: AMACOM, 1978.

BROTTEN, DOROTHY A., LAURA HAYMAN, and MARY NAYLOR, *Leadership for Change: A Guide For the Frustrated Nurse*. Philadelphia: J. B. Lippincott, 1978.

HERSEY, P., and K. BLANCHARD, *Management of Organizational Behavior: Utilizing Human Resources,* 3rd ed. Englewood Cliffs, N.J.: Prentice-Hall, Inc., 1977.

ROBBINS, STEPHEN, *Organizational Behavior: Concepts and Controversies*. Englewood Cliffs, N.J.: Prentice-Hall, Inc., 1979.

---

* Michael Korda, *Power: How to Get It, How to Use It* (New York: Random House, 1975), p. 12.

9 Competency: Managing Organizational Change

Strangely, the expounders of many of the great new ideas of history were frequently considered on the lunatic fringe for some or all of their lives. If one stands up and is counted, from time to time one may get knocked down. But remember this: A man flattened by an opponent can get up again. A man flattened by conformity stays down for good.
— Thomas J. Watson, Jr.,
Chairman of the Board of IBM

OVERVIEW The purpose of this chapter is to examine strategies for bringing about planned organizational change. Upon completion of this chapter the reader will be able to:

- Define three challenges confronting health administrators

- Identify the key components of rational-empirical, normative-re-educative, and power-coercive change strategies

- Define the goals of an organization development program

- Define a four-phased approach to planned change

There is one special skill that is basic to effective health administration and that is the ability to manage organizational change. This may be the most critical challenge confronting contemporary health administrators due, in part, to the dynamic political and economic forces that are shaping the health delivery system.

Many of the concepts that we have discussed in this book will help you in managing the change process. Your ability to formulate and implement a mission statement that addresses contemporary health problems is probably the initial step in competently managing change. Your skill in recruiting talented subordinates who look upon political issues as challenges rather than insurmountable difficulties is a necessary prerequisite if change is to be controlled. In addition, your commitment to building open communication systems with community leaders, consumers, and employees will not only keep you informed about emerging health problems but will give you information on which to construct policies that will keep your organization in the forefront of its field.

While innovative mission statements, competent subordinates, and open communication systems can assist you in managing change, there are specific concepts you must master if you are to be an effective change agent. In this chapter we will examine why some organizations are able to creatively manage change while others fall further and further behind their peers. We will learn about various approaches that administrators historically have taken in managing organizational change and we will study one change model that has particular relevance for human service organizations. The basic premise of this chapter is that change is an ally—not an enemy. If we initiate change thoughtfully and systematically it can help us create a more effective and efficient health delivery system.

CONTEMPORARY CHALLENGES

Perhaps the most critical issue confronting health administrators is *quality control*. The pursuit of quality medical care has always been a concern of consumers. Today, however, that concern has escalated into a demand for quality in all phases of the health delivery system. As Melvin A. Glasser has noted:

> There is mounting evidence that the consumer of health services is no longer content to leave the planning for the organization of his health services solely in the hands of the professional, doctors, hospital administrators, health insurance executives—yes, even health planners. The consumer wants in—he pays for the programs, he is the beneficiary of good contributions and the sufferer from their inadequacy, and increasingly he is insisting that his voice be heard and that he be included in the councils of those who plan for and offer health services.[1]

[1] Melvin A. Glasser, "What the Consumer Expects in Coordinated Planning for Health," in Rakich, Lougest, and O'Donovan, *Managing Health Care Organizations* (Philadelphia: Saunders, 1977), p. 13.

The insistence that medical services be of high quality is rooted in the fact that consumers are taking increased responsibility for their physical and mental well-being. It is not uncommon for dentists to be asked whether an x-ray is "really needed" or for physicians to be queried as to whether the annual physical examination is beneficial. Hospital administrators are increasingly asked why hospital procedures that last but a few minutes incur what appear to be astronomical costs. And public health officials are increasingly under fire from consumer groups for not adequately protecting the health of the community.

If there be any doubt about the seriousness with which consumers evaluate the quality of their medical care, one need only make a brief review of health legislation that has come about through the ballots citizens have cast. Medicare, Medicaid, Professional Standards Review Organization (PSRO), federal health planning legislation and a multitude of health programs have been sanctioned by voters with the hope that the health delivery system will become more effective, efficient, and humane.

One of the healthy signs of the consumer movement is an interest in broad public health problems. There is a growing recognition that the quality of our waters is being destroyed by acid rains that shower toxic chemicals onto our farmlands and into our lakes. There is concern about electrical power lines that crisscross each state like a maze of giant tripwires whose long-term effect on human health has yet to be fully comprehended. There is anxiety about the chemicals that are added to foods to make the meat tender and the beans greener as people wonder what it is they are consuming and whether years from now they will discover that it was injurious to their health. People don't want Love Canals in their backyards nor do they want the byproducts of nuclear energy plants transported through their neighborhoods. In brief, consumers are concerned about the quality of their lives. While there is a recognition that legislators, health administrators, physicians, and government officials should be protecting consumers from harm, there is a strong suspicion that the issue is much too important to be left to the deliberations in smoke-filled rooms of politicans. Therefore the consumer is more critical than ever of those who are to protect the health of our communities and the health of each citizen. As a health administrator you will not be immune from such criticism. Indeed, you many be the target of consumer frustration when it is believed that the system is not responsive to consumer needs.

A second critical issue that health administrators will confront during the remainder of this decade and probably far into the future is *cost effectiveness*. There is perhaps no issue that has stirred more criticism of the health delivery system than that of soaring costs.[2] After two decades of skyrocketing

---

[2] J. S. Rakich, B. B. Lougest, and T. R. O'Donovan, *Managing Health Care Organizations* (Philadelphia: Saunders, 1977), p. 339.

medical expenditures, both providers and consumers are alarmed. The increasing costs cannot always be explained nor can their incurrence always be justified.

The pressure to reduce costs so that they do not increase more than the consumer price index will continue to be felt. It is doubtful that expensive technology such as that represented in radiological equipment will be purchased as readily as before. Hospitals will continue to find a number of review boards which will need to be consulted prior to contracting for an expensive piece of technology. It is perhaps a sign of our times that a North Carolina hospital which wanted to purchase two x-ray machines needed to expend 160 staff hours to finish the required paperwork that weighed in at forty-seven pounds of documents.[3]

The pressure to contain costs will also come from institutional governing boards as they seek to keep their organizations solvent. There is a growing recognition that the economic resources of any institution are limited. More and more health administrators are hearing cost-conscious board members state that it is financially impossible for a hospital to be everything to everyone. While it may be possible to have the best obstetrics department in terms of personnel and equipment, it may not be possible to have the best radiology department as well. When resources are limited, difficult choices have to be made. And choices mean conflict and change.

A third issue that is creating rapid change is the growing awareness that the *purposes of hospitals and public health institutions are becoming blurred.* Hospitals are now involved in programs for the indigent, are presenting educational programs to community residents, and are emphasizing preventive medicine. Health departments have become involved in primary care as typified in childhood screening programs and the sponsorship of neighborhood health clinics. The neat distinction between hospital and public health programming no longer exists. Each perceives the other to be walking on their turf, the result of which is increased tension and suspicion about one another's motives.

The tensions between health departments and hospitals is compounded by legislation that, in some states, gives health departments the prerogative to review and approve expenditures in private and public hospitals. Unless community health departments and hospitals initiate dialogue with one another about the need for services and who should be performing them, we will see an era of increased competition and conflict between two health institutions that historically have been allies.

In summary, the external pressures for quality care at reasonable prices is causing internal changes in most health organizations. Professional groups are assuming new roles and responsibilities. Administrators have become

[3] *U.S. News and World Report,* September 22, 1980, p. 16.

acutely aware of the legal and political ramifications of their actions. Workers at all levels are increasingly held accountable for what they do, when they do it, and how it is done. As the pressures for quality programming build, it is reasonable to expect that the internal environment of hospitals and health departments will continue to change as professionals respond to the rising expectations of the public.

John Porterfield III, Director of the Joint Commission on Accreditation of Hospitals, has stated that the health care system is "at a crossroads, in time and place. Where we go from here . . . will make the difference in finding reasonable solutions to health care problems."[4] When a system is at a crossroads, decisions will be made that will fundamentally influence it for years to come. Most health organizations are making decisions *now* about future health programming, quality care problems, and cost-containment policies that will influence institutional priorities for the next decade. If sound decisons are to be made, health administrators will need to be skilled in understanding how organizations change and how the change process can be competently managed.

STRATEGIES TO BRING ABOUT CHANGE

There are three types of strategies that historically have been used to bring about organizational change:[5]

1. Rational-empirical strategies
2. Normative-re-educative strategies
3. Power-coercive strategies

A summary of the key characteristics of each change strategy can be seen in Figure 9-1.

These three strategies are not mutually exclusive for each will borrow upon the methods and techniques of the other. As we will see, rational strategies often use re-educative methods and normative strategies are often based upon data obtained through rational, data-based inquiry.

It is also important to avoid making a premature value judgment about the inherent worth of each strategy. All have strengths and limitations. Each has been successfully used dependent upon the environment in which the model has been employed.

[4] John Porterfield III, "To the Defense of the System," *Hospitals,* 48 (March 1, 1974), 49.

[5] Warren G. Bennis, Kenneth D. Benne, Robert Chin, and Kenneth E. Corey, eds., *The Planning of Change* (New York: Holt, Rinehart and Winston, 1976), pp. 44–45.

Rational-Empirical Change Strategies

The approaches to change that are termed "rational-empirical" are based upon the important assumption that people are rational and will follow their rational self-interest once it is revealed to them.[6] Therefore, if a proposed change is perceived as desirable, effective, and in line with the self-interest of the person, group, organization, or community that will be affected by the change, respondents will initiate new patterns of thought and behavior.

The chief value adhered to by proponents of the rational-empirical school is a trust in the scientific method as the predominant motivator by which to change human behavior. Therefore, most change agents utilizing this model will employ various research methods to scientifically study the organization to determine the need for change, how it should be carried out, and whether the change once initiated has improved the effectiveness of the organization.

There is obviously much to be said for any model of change that is based on empirical research. The advantages and disadvantages of moving in new directions are clearly delineated. Those who will be affected by the change know how they will be influenced by the process and often are given an opportunity to agree in advance to the proposed changes. In additon, when research has been carefully undertaken there is a base of information that can later be used to determine whether the change was beneficial.

The primary limitation of rational-empirical methods is that change is seldom a rational process. As we earlier learned, people perceive "facts" in different ways. While the benefits of fluoridation are well documented scientifically, there are people who bitterly fight state ordinances that instruct county commissioners to chemically treat their drinking water. You may have a multitude of scientific studies indicating that electrical power lines will not endanger citizen health. The resident, however, who sees the wires being routed next to their home or farm will generally find little comfort in such documents.

Another problem with rational-empirical methods is that health administrators often do not have the lead time necessary to study the change process scientifically. When the mayor of a city instructs the health commissioner to offer new programming for Hispanics, it usually is not possible to design a multiyear pilot project to compare the effects of different kinds of health programming on the well-being of Spanish-speaking people. While the rational-empirical method might be the most perfect method to bring about change, it may be the least practical method when change must be brought about quickly or when political considerations impinge upon the change process.

[6] Ibid., p. 23.

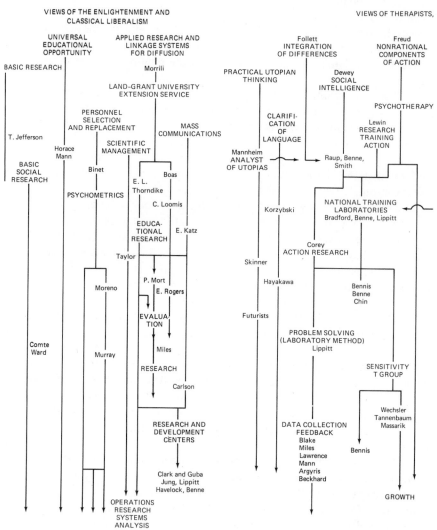

A. RATIONAL–EMPIRICAL

VIEWS OF THE ENLIGHTENMENT AND
CLASSICAL LIBERALISM

UNIVERSAL
EDUCATIONAL
OPPORTUNITY

APPLIED RESEARCH AND
LINKAGE SYSTEMS
FOR DIFFUSION

BASIC RESEARCH

Morrili

LAND-GRANT UNIVERSITY
EXTENSION SERVICE

T. Jefferson

PERSONNEL
SELECTION
AND REPLACEMENT

MASS
COMMUNICATIONS

Horace
Mann

SCIENTIFIC
MANAGEMENT

BASIC
SOCIAL
RESEARCH

Binet

Boas

PSYCHOMETRICS

E. L.
Thorndike

C. Loomis

EDUCA-
TIONAL
RESEARCH

E. Katz

Taylor

P. Mort

Moreno

E. Rogers

EVALUA-
TION

Comte
Ward

Murray

Miles

RESEARCH

Carlson

RESEARCH AND
DEVELOPMENT
CENTERS

Clark and Guba
Jung, Lippitt
Havelock, Benne

OPERATIONS
RESEARCH
SYSTEMS
ANALYSIS

B. NORMATIVE–

VIEWS OF THERAPISTS,

Follett
INTEGRATION
OF DIFFERENCES

Freud
NONRATIONAL
COMPONENTS
OF ACTION

PRACTICAL UTOPIAN
THINKING

Dewey
SOCIAL
INTELLIGENCE

CLARIFI-
CATION
OF
LANGUAGE

PSYCHOTHERAPY

Lewin
RESEARCH
TRAINING
ACTION

Mannheim
ANALYST
OF UTOPIAS

Raup, Benne,
Smith

Korzybski

NATIONAL TRAINING
LABORATORIES
Bradford, Benne, Lippitt

Skinner

Corey
ACTION RESEARCH

Hayakawa

Bennis
Benne
Chin

Futurists

PROBLEM SOLVING
(LABORATORY METHOD)
Lippitt

SENSITIVITY
T GROUP

DATA COLLECTION
FEEDBACK
Blake
Miles
Lawrence
Mann
Argyris
Beckhard

Wechsler
Tannenbaum
Massarik

Bennis

GROWTH

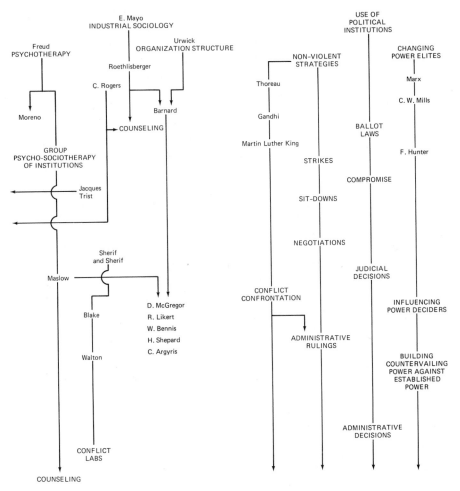

Figure 9-1 Strategies of deliberate changing. [From Warren G. Bennis, Kenneth D. Benne, Robert Chin, and Kenneth E. Corey, eds., *The Planning of Change* (New York: Holt, Rinehart and Winston, 1975), pp. 44–45. Reprinted by permission of Holt, Rinehart and Winston.]

Normative–Re-educative Change Strategies

The strategies termed "normative-re-educative" are based upon assumptions of human motivation that differ from those underlying the rational-empirical model. Proponents of normative re-educative strategies do not deny that workers can be motivated by rationality, intelligence, and the results of scientific research. They argue, however, that individuals are motivated primarily by unsatisfied needs. Employees do not passively wait for an administrator to suggest changes. Rather, employees in the pursuit of realizing their potential will initiate changes on their own. How they will subsequently function will be contingent upon the rewards and punishments they receive from their peers and from their supervisor.

There are five common elements among the family of change strategies using normative-re-educative assumptions concerning human behavior. First, each begins with the premise that the client should be directly involved in the change process. The client should help diagnose the problem and actively take part in formulating change strategies. Second, it is not assumed that organizational problems can be automatically resolved through rational problem solving or the gathering of technical information although this possibility is not ruled out. Rather, organizational problems are perceived to lie in the attitudes, values, norms, and expectations of those in the internal and external environments of the client system. Third, normative-re-educative strategies usually emphasize here-and-now learning. When clients are expected to learn new attitudes and behavior, this learning is always closely linked to specific problems that the client is experiencing in the work environment. Fourth, nonconscious elements that may be part of the problem must be brought to the surface, explored, and their impact determined. Finally, normative-re-educative strategies are largely based upon concepts in the behavioral sciences that emphasize interpersonal communication, conflict resolution, negotiation procedures, problem solving, and sensitivity training.[7]

Perhaps the most important concept underlying normative-re-educative thought is that *"people technology" is just as necessary as "thing technology" in working out desirable changes in human affairs.* Therefore, the clarification and redefinition of values is of pivotal importance in changing employee behavior. As Robert Chin and Kenneth Beene note, "By getting the values of various parts of the client system . . . openly into the arena of change and by working through value conflicts responsibly, the change agent seeks to avoid manipulation and indoctrination of the client, in the morally reprehensible meaning of these terms."[8]

A milestone in the development of the normative-re-educative approach to change was the creation of the National Training Laboratories in 1947. The National Training Laboratories have been successful in initiating various

[7] Ibid.
[8] Ibid.

client-centered approaches to change that emphasize the need to have change agents understand the values, norms, rules of conduct, hopes, and goals of those who will be affected by the change process. Among the various intervention methods that have evolved out of the National Training Laboratories are the following:

> *Personal counseling.* Normative-re-educative change agents have found that one-to-one conversations with clients is one of the most effective ways to change human behavior. When clients have an opportunity to study the need for change with a supportive counselor they are more likely to be a willing participant in the change process.
>
> *Laboratory groups.* Laboratory groups are designed to give feedback to each member about their communication style, openness, and method by which they manage conflict. Experiential learning is the primary educational method that is employed. The basic assumption underlying laboratory learning is that the potential of the average human being is rarely realized.
>
> *Training groups.* While there are many different types of training groups, a common approach is to ask five or six managers to analyze a case study of an organizational problem. Among the topics that may be discussed are (1) the *overt* and *tacit rules of behavior* impinging upon the problem (2) the *leadership styles* that increase or decrease the magnitude of the problem, (3) the *change methods* through which the problem could be addressed and (4) the specific organizational problems that will *cause* such a problem to recur. Managers often find training groups helpful for they focus on *cultural variables* that are influencing the effectiveness of their organization. For many, these cultural variables were either not known prior to the start of the training group, or their importance was not recognized.
>
> *Psychotherapy.* Psychotherapists, sometimes working within organizations or with personnel workers, have used the principles of Freud and Adler to re-educate workers and help them grow. Such efforts are prominent in mental health approaches to change and have been successfully used in educational religious, industrial, and hospital settings. The primary aim of psychotherapy is to give clients insight into their personal problems which often impinge upon their work.

Power-Coercive Change Strategies

Some approaches to change are based upon the application of power in which those with greater power will alter the behaviors of individuals who have less power. At times, change agents might seek to achieve their ends through the use of legitimate power which is derived from the position that they hold in the organization's hierarchy. When a governor releases an executive order demanding department heads to reduce their budgets by 10 percent, he or she is exercising legitimate power. The department heads might resist the reductions but, if the governor is operating within his or her authority, few will dispute the right to apply such power.

As we learned in Chapter 2 many changes in organizations come about through the use of political power. When the department heads meet informally to discuss their strategy for dealing with the governor's budget cuts, their intent will be to mass whatever power they possess in order to reverse the governor's directive. The tactics they choose will reflect how much power they collectively possess. They may use their moral power and inform the media about what proposed budget reductions will do in reducing services to the citizens of the state. Or they may inform the governor that they will resign *en masse* if the executive order is not rescinded. If the department heads have little individual or collective power they may meet to discuss tactics and quickly disband out of frustration at "not being able to do anything" about the situation.

It should be emphasized that it is not the use of power per se that distinguishes this family of change strategies from those previously discussed. A vital ingredient in all human transactions is power. Thus, those who follow the rational-empirical school of thought appeal to knowledge as a major ingredient of power. Those who adhere to normative-re-educative strategies appeal to noncognitive determinants of behavior such as resistances or supports to changing values, attitudes, and skills. Normative-re-educative change agents also have a healthy appreciation that those who will be affected by a proposed change often have considerable power to resist, accept, or modify the change being suggested.

What distinguishes power-coercive change and strategies from the others is that those who utilize them rely on economic and political sanctions to achieve their goals. Therefore, administrators who use power-coercive approaches in bringing about change usually possess a keen understanding of the rewards and sanctions that can be judiciously used to shape people's behavior. The governor might, for example, utilize legitimate power to rescind the budget reductions for those departments that are managed well and doing a respectable job. On the other hand, the governor might demand a 15 percent reduction in a department that has performed poorly during the past year.

It would be unwise to believe that all power-coercive approaches to change are undesirable or even immoral. If a particular administrative practice in the hospital poses an immediate threat to the well-being of patients, the most *efficient* solution may be a memorandum to personnel, backed by administrative authority and sanctions, to eliminate an undesirable practice. However, if the requested change is substantive in terms of altering fundamental attitudes, values, or skills it would be prudent to follow up that memorandum with some type of normative-re-educative strategy.

PREREQUISITES FOR SUCCESSFUL PLANNED CHANGE PROGRAMS

Larry E. Greiner made a substantial contribution to our understanding of the change process when he researched eighteen change programs, eleven of which were successful and seven of which were unsuccessful.[9] The objective of his research was to identify those factors that positively influence organizational change.

Greiner found that *successful change programs are usually found in organizations where top management is under considerable pressure to change.* The pressures experienced by top management in the eleven successful change programs came from outside the organization as well as from employees within the organization. The unsuccessful change programs were initiated in response to pressure originating either internally or externally, *but not both.* Greiner emphasized the probable significance of the simultaneous existence of internal and external pressures. The pressures top management experiences from one source can be rationalized as temporary and perhaps inconsequential as may happen when employee morale is low but clients consistently rate the quality of services high. Such rationalization is less likely, however, when there is poor morale *and* clients are complaining about the service they are receiving.

A second characteristic of successful change programs is that *top management makes a serious effort to find creative solutions to the identified problems.* Management in the successful change programs was convinced that some type of change was not only desirable but actually needed. They did not blame others for their problems nor did they find a scapegoat. The principle objective of the successful change programs was to identify as precisely as possible the nature of the problems the organization was experiencing and to find creative, practical solutions.

Third, successful change programs *often utilize a change agent from outside of the organization* to help diagnose organizaton problems and improve the effectiveness and efficiency of the institution. Consultants often bring new perspectives to organizational problems. Frequently they have greater knowledge about a specific problem than the client has. Generally, consultants will be less vested in a particular solution than will those who are employed within the organization. Greiner found that change agents from outside the organization did, in fact, help the organization improve its diagnosing and problem-solving abilities.

There may be times when you as a health administrator will want to use a change agent who is not employed in your organization. If so, you should carefully examine the consultant's qualifications. Perhaps most important is

[9] Larry Greiner, "Patterns of Organizational Change," *Harvard Business Review,* 1967, 45, 3 (May–June) 119–30.

the individual's *technical abilities*. The consultant should have an in-depth understanding of the problems that your organization is experiencing. If your problems are in the financial accounting system, then someone with considerable background in information and financial systems should be employed. If your problem is the turnover in personnel, then someone with an in-depth understanding of motivational processes might be turned to. The best way of assessing an individual's technical competence is to contact other organizations with whom the individual has worked. In so doing seek an honest apprisal of the individual's ability to deal with the specific problems that you are experiencing.

You will also want to learn about the change agent's *administrative ability* and skills in *interpersonal relations*. Does the consultant take care of administrative details that are part of his or her present job punctually and effortlessly, without slip-ups, flurries, or special reminders?[10] Does the consultant examine the problem from the point of view of those who are experiencing the difficulty? Does the consultant help individuals arrive at their own conclusions about what needs to be done, given adequate information to do so?

If you determine that it is in the best interests of your organization to obtain the services of an outside change agent you will want to have a written contract specifying what needs to be done, the time frame in which it should be accomplished, and the amount of reimbursement to be given for the services rendered. It is generally unwise to enter into an open-ended commitment in which no terminal date of completion is specified for the project. In addition, you may want to specify that the agreement can be terminated by either party if the relationship proves to be unsatisfactory.

Finally, Greiner found that successful change programs *test proposed solutions on a pilot basis to determine their efficacy* before initiating system-wide changes. There are several benefits that accrue from pilot studies. First, if there are doubts about whether proposed changes will actually work, the pilot study may serve to allay these doubts. If new solutions alter relationships, established work routines, or current administrative practices, there may be suspicion about the efficacy of the change program. A pilot study will either confirm those suspicions or prove that they are unfounded. Second, a pilot study will help you discover the "bugs" or problems that result once a change has been initiated. By identifying problems that emerge in the pilot study you are in a position to prevent them from recurring if the change program is to be expanded. Finally, when you undertake a pilot study it implies that you as a change agent are going about the change process in a deliberative manner. Greiner noted that in those organizations that had successful change

[10] Gerald Zaltman and Robert Duncan, *Strategies for Planned Change* (New York: John Wiley, 1977), p. 188.

programs the employees gradually became accustomed to the realization that change is a normal part of how their organization functions. Change was therefore not perceived as a threat but, rather, as an ongoing process through which management seeks to improve its services and capabilities.

One last point should be made concerning the significance of Greiner's research. It has often been said that the most successful change programs are those where there is a democratic, grass-roots commitment to change. The ideology of such an argument is that, if the employees in an organization first recognize the need to change, resistance will be minimized and the change process can be smoothly adopted.

As we will soon see, it is desirable to have grass-roots support for proposed changes. However, *Greiner's findings contradict the notion that you must have the "approval" of employees prior to initiating a successful change program.* Greiner suggests that awesome pressures, perhaps near-calamities must arise before management will consider changing their organization in substantial ways.[11] In addition, the changes must be backed by formal authority, a notion that runs counter to schools of thought that emphasize organization-wide collaboration and the absence of formal sanctions. While it is advantageous to have grass-roots support for proposed changes, it does not appear to be an immutable prerequisite in achieving substantial organizational modification and innovation.

ORGANIZATION DEVELOPMENT AND SYSTEMATIC CHANGE PROCESSES

The term *organization development* began appearing in the 1960s as a promising method by which to facilitate organizational innovation. Organization development is a systems-oriented approach to change that seeks to integrate the objectives of the organization with the talents, value, and skills of employees. The ultimate goal of organization development efforts is to increase organizational productivity and effectiveness and to do it in a way that heightens employee morale. The objectives of a typical organization development program might be as follows:

1. To increase the level of trust among organizational members
2. To increase the incidence of confrontation of organizational problems, both within groups and among groups, in contrast to "sweeping problems under the rug"
3. To create an environment in which authority of assigned role is augmented by authority based on knowledge and skill

[11] Cited in Robert A. Ullrich and George Wieland, *Organization Theory and Design* (Homewood, Illinois: Richard D. Irwin, Inc. 1980), p. 450.

4. To increase the openness of communications laterally, vertically, and diagonally
5. To increase the level of personal enthusiasm and satisfaction in the organization
6. To find synergistic solutions to problems with great frequency
7. To increase the level of self and group responsibility in planning and implementation[12]

While organization development is a relatively young school of thought it holds promise in successfully changing organizations. A survey of ten organizations using systematic development strategies—including Michigan Bell, General Electric, the city of Detroit, B. F. Goodrich Chemical Company, and ACDC Electronics—found positive results.[13] One unit of Michigan Bell noted that attendance had improved by 50 percent and productivity and efficiency were above standard figures. The city of Detroit was able to save $1.5 million with its garbage collection activity after the organization development program had been completed. The city was also able to reduce direct labor costs and saw a significant decrease in citizen complaints. The B. F. Goodrich chemical plant in Ohio was able to increase production over 300 percent as compared with earlier rates. The ACDC company obtained over a half million dollars in cost reductions, reduced turnaround time on repairs from thirty to ten days, and increased attendance from 93.5 percent to 98.2 percent.[14] In a study of the effectiveness of an organization development program in a metropolitan hospital the researcher found clearer lines of communication between hospital administrators and middle-level management personnel as reflected in fewer misunderstandings and disagreements after the organization development program had been concluded. The investigator also noted that employees had a better sense that top management was aware of the problems within their unit. Administrators were perceived to be more strongly committed to finding solutions to those problems. These perceptions helped to produce a climate of greater trust and collaboration between management and staff.[15]

The basic model that organization development practitioners commonly use involves a four-step approach to planned change as seen in Figure 9-2.

[12] Wendell French, "Organizational Development Objectives, Assumptions and Strategies," *California Management Review,* 12, no. 2 (1969), 24.

[13] W. Clay Hammer and Elle P. Hammer, "Behavior Modifications on the Bottom Line," *Organizational Dynamics,* Spring 1976, pp. 3-21.

[14] Stephen P. Robbins, *Organizational Behavior: Concepts and Controversies* (Englewood Cliffs, N.J.: Prentice-Hall, Inc., 1979), p. 389.

[15] Robert Veninga, "Organization Development: A Case Study in Communication," Ph.D. dissertation, University of Minnesota, 1972.

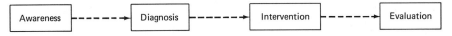

Figure 9-2 A four-step approach to planned change.

Phase 1: Awareness

In the first phase of an organization development effort, a determination is made regarding the readiness of the organization to engage in systematic planning. Three assessments are usually made, including an analysis of the life cycle of the organization, an assessment of the interest of management and staff in changing the organization, and an evaluation of the organization's environment.

Life cycle assessment   Organizations generally move through five crisis stages from growth to maturity. These stages, which are summarized in Figure 9-3, often result in stress, misunderstandings, disagreement, and conflict. Each crisis must be resolved if the organization is to grow and be viable within its competitive market.[16]

The first crisis—*leadership*—emerges after an initial period of growth. The organization has been founded and is valued by its clients. The management system used by the founders typically emphasizes practicality and efficiency. There is usually a small number of employees on the staff who know and support one another. The goals of these embryonic organizations are sharply defined as employees work diligently to establish the organization as a sound entity.

Once the organization becomes successful it undergoes a transformation. The simplified management system doesn't seem to be as efficient as it once was. The founders of the organization often find themselves spending more and more time on administrative hassles and paperwork. The work flow, which earlier was manageable, becomes unmanageable as consumers press for additional services. The organization has a difficult time meeting the increased consumer demands and this often results in disappointments and disagreements among the staff. Conflict between the harried leaders grows intense as workers blame one another for the emerging problems. Soon employees begin wondering whether anybody is in command. The inevitable question that was whispered in private is asked publicly: Who is going to lead the organization out of confusion and solve the management problems confronting the organization?

The solution to the dilemma is usually to find a new management team that is acceptable to the founders and that can pull the organization

---

[16] Larry E. Greiner, "Evolution and Revolution as Organizations Grow," *Harvard Business Review,* July-August 1972, pp. 37–46.

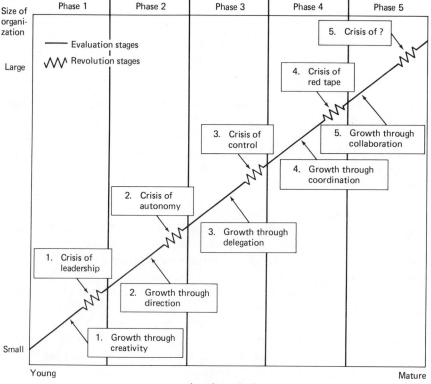

Figure 9-3 The five stages of organizational growth. [Reprinted by permission of the Harvard Business Review. An exhibit from "Evolution and Revolution as Organizations Grow" by Larry E. Greiner (*Harvard Business Review,* July-August 1972), pp. 37–46. Copyright © 1972 by the President and Fellows of Harvard College; all rights reserved.]

together.[17] Once the new management team is on board, most organizations will move into a sustained period of growth through direction.

During this subsequent stage of growth the new management team will "take most of the responsibility for institutional direction, while lower level supervisors are treated more as functional specialists than autonomous decison making managers."[18] This process is effective for a while; soon however, lower-level managers demand more *autonomy,* which is the second crisis that confront organizations as they mature.

The solution to the autonomy crisis is to delegate meaningful respon-

[17] Ibid., p. 41.
[18] Ibid., p. 43.

sibilities and tasks to staff members. The delegating of work to subordinates does seem to help the organization function more smoothly and regain its equilibrium. Nevertheless, over time, problems begin to reappear because it is difficult for top managers who were previously successful at being directive to give up responsibility. In addition, lower-level managers are generally not accustomed to making decisions for themselves, a problem that often results in poor quality products and services. As a result, numerous organizations flounder during this revolutionary period.

When management loses confidence in subordinates the organization faces a *crisis of control*. Often management will reassume the responsibilities delegated to subordinates thus creating resentment and hostility among those who had been given additional freedom. To counteract the resentment, management usually moves into a coordination stage in which some of the responsibilities are delegated but under tight control.

When management determines that it must regain control of the organization it often initiates administrative rules, regulations, procedures, and policies. Performance review mechanisms, time punch cards and machines, detailed listings of employee absences, and the initiation of grievances against employees begin to proliferate. Most of these efforts to regain control are met with resistance. Soon the organization is bogged down in the *crisis of red tape*.

When an organization is saddled with red tape it is almost impossible to innovate. The rules and regulations governing what is acceptable and unacceptable behavior stand in the way of creative thinking. However, if the organization is to move ahead, the crisis of red tape must be resolved and often it is through a new period of "growth through collaboration."

The coordination phase of growth is managed through formal systems and procedures. Managers examine the roles and policies and determine which ones are benefiting the organization and which should be eliminated. The net result is that rules are paired down to include only those that are absolutely necessary. In addition, the formal management system is evaluated—sometimes by subordinates. Administrative practices that are resented are modified. Tasks are redelegated to employees who have the best information and the most skill with which to accomplish them.

The coordination phase of collaboration comes about by increasing the effectiveness of the communication system within the organization. Staff meetings are held more frequently and substantive issues are addressed. Subordinates are asked to state their attitudes honestly and to make suggestions that might benefit the organization. Two-way feedback mechanisms are put into place. Slowly a climate of trust begins to return to the organization.

There undoubtedly is a sixth crisis that mature organizations experience. What it is, however, is uncertain, although Greiner predicted ten years ago that it would center around the "psychological saturation" of employees who grow emotionally and physically exhausted by the intensity of teamwork and the heavy pressure for innovative solutions. As we will see in the last chapter, there is evidence that supports Greiner's prediction as managers and staff members strive to cope with the stresses of their work environment.[19]

Assessing interest   A principal tenet of organization devlopment theory is that strategies for planned change must be based on an accurate assessment of "the extent and nature of the interest in change, the nature and depth of motivation to change, and the environment within which the proposed change will occur."[20] The theoretical underpinnings for this tenet are represented in Kurt Lewin's "Field Force Theory" which suggests that at any given moment the behaviors of an individual or an institution are subject to forces that promote change and forces that resist change. *No change will take place if the forces are in balance or in equilibrium.* Change takes place only when the forces to change are more heavily weighted than the forces that resist change. For example, a nurse may see a problem on the nursing station and may want to discuss the situation with her immediate supervisor; that is a force that promotes change. On the other hand, based on previous experiences with former supervisors, she fears that she might be blamed for the problem; that is a force resisting change. The nurse will not take any action unless the need to correct the problem weighs more heavily on her mind than the fear of possible retaliation. "Assessment can be viewed as the task of identifying the forces that promote change and the forces that resist it and comparing their relative strength."[21]

Before you commit yourself to engaging in a thorough systematic development effort it is prudent to determine the level of commitment of those who will be affected by the change. One method of testing the strength of the forces is to describe a problem as objectively as possible and to delineate the personal and economic resources that would be expended if the problem is to be resolved. For example, consider a chief executive officer who is meeting with the department heads of the hospital:

> We have had considerable discussion about our employee record-keeping system. I agree with those who say that it is outdated and often does not provide the information we need. To institute a computer-based information system would take approximately twelve months of detailed planning. We would need to determine data needs in each of our departments, meet with computer salespeople to determine what system best meets our needs, and then educate the staff about the new system. It will require at least biweekly meetings of this group to define our information needs and to evaluate how we should proceed. The leasing of the computer hardware will probably cost twenty to thirty thousand dollars during the first year of operation. In view of the commitment that we would have to

[19] Ibid., p. 44.
[20] Dorothy A. Brooten, Laura Hayman, and Mary Naylor, *Leadership for Change: A Guide for the Frustrated Nurse* (Philadelphia: Lippincott, 1978), p. 83.
[21] Ibid.

make to institute a new system, I am wondering whether the problem is of such a magnitude that we want to commit our resources to this issue at this time.

Such a "testing of the water" will usually provide immediate feedback on the strength of the forces to change and those that resist. The group may feel that the problem is of such a magnitude that they would willingly agree to spend the time needed to institute a sound data-based system. On the other hand, the group may throw their hands up in the air signifying that the problem "isn't so bad that we can't get along with it for a while longer."

It is important to remember that even though the forces that resist change may be greater than the forces that promote change, it is still possible to modify the organization. This is usually accomplished by strengthening the change forces by dramatically demonstrating the consequences that will follow if a change is not implemented. For example, the chief executive officer may give the department heads a sample of the types of information that each will be required to obtain from their employees in the near future. If such data is not readily available or if it would be difficult to retrieve with the present system, the department heads may begin to see the value of a computer-based system. When that happens the forces for change are beginning to counteract the forces which resist.

Assessing the environment   A manager who is serious about effecting change needs to recognize the importance of a favorable climate or "environment" for creativity and innovation. The degree to which the environment is conducive to change is contingent upon six organizational variables:

1. The primary orientation of the organization is to the future rather than the past. It is more interested in solving new and emerging problems than preserving the status quo.
2. The key leaders in the organization recognize that a problem exists that needs to be resolved. The forces for change are more powerful than the forces that resist.
3. The organization has a history of being able to change when problems occur.
4. The organization has self-evaluation mechanisms that permit it to test its operations against its goals.
5. The organization is economically prepared to undertake a planned change program. The types of expenses to be incurred include (a) staff time as employees learn new policies, procedures, and ways of doing their tasks, (b) constant assistance, (c) training materials, and (d) evaluation costs.
6. There is a willingness to experiment, to try new ideas, and to learn from the mistakes that will be made as new behaviors and policies are initiated within the organization.

While each of the above characteristics is important, special emphasis should be given to determining whether the organization has a history of being able to change when problems and challenges occur (variable 3). Some organizations are relatively low-risk operations that historically have not innovated. In analyzing why American productivity dropped during the past decade Steve S. Leuthold has noted:

> Perhaps in the organizational mode of committees, subcommittees, delegated and redelegated responsibilities, much of American industry has lost its guts, lost its nerve, lost its decisiveness, lost its willingness to take some near term risks, even if the long term payoff can be incredible. The strong captains of America's industrial past have too often evolved into the paper shuffling gray committees of the corporate industrial state where the key to survival is to protect your backside."[22]

Other organizations have a carefully calculated high-risk philosophy that recognizes that "the only stability possible is stability in motion."[23] They concur with Peter Drucker's observation that in a world buffeted by change and faced daily with new threats to its safety, the only way to conserve is by innovating.[24] These organizations, therefore, have a history of initiating new programs, learning from their mistakes, and making accurate forecasts as to how the organization should respond to new challenges and opportunities.

In assessing the environment, note whether the organization has a low-risk or high-risk approach to change. Low-risk organizations will be wary of change, may resist it, and will usually be suspicious of the motives of a change agent. High-risk organizations will see change as inevitable, desirable, and a prerequisite for survival in a competitive world.

In summary, before an organization development effort is initiated, the change agent should make a preliminary assessment of the organization. The assessment should include a subjective analysis of the organization's readiness to change and whether the environment is conducive to change. It is also helpful to view the organization as being at some point on a historical continuum (birth to maturity) and to determine the types of problems it might be experiencing given its point of development.

Phase 2: Diagnosis

While the awareness stage usually represents a subjective and preliminary analysis of the organization, the diagnosis phase is designed to retrieve objective information. The primary purpose of the diagnosis is to collect data on which to base subsequent interventions.

[22] Steve S. Leuthold, "Captains of U.S. Industry Forsake Growth to Avoid Risks," *Minneapolis Star,* July 11, 1980, p. 6A.

[23] John Gardner, *Self-Renewal* (New York: Harper & Row, 1963), p. 7.

[24] From Peter Drucker, *Landmarks of Tomorrow,* cited ibid., p. 7.

The process of data collection serves three important functions:

1. Data collection, if performed carefully, can reduce the degree to which change is haphazard and relatively unplanned by creating a realistic information base for organizational diagnosis. It often leads to an increased awareness of the areas in which organizational behavior could be fruitfully and effectively changed.

2. Out of what is termed *pluralistic ignorance,* people often assume that their observations of the way the organization is functioning are unique, even when in fact these observations may be widely shared by others. One way of overcoming this gap in knowledge is through data collection. Revealing these commonly held perceptions often provides an impetus toward organizational problem solving. It may provide a focus around which organization members can come to understand how other people feel about their job and about the ways in which the organization is functioning. People may become able, perhaps for the first time, to share with each other their perceptions, feelings, ideas, and other information bearing on organizational performance. Information obtained from one person or from one group can be linked systematically to that from other individuals or groups, and hence may provide a much fuller understanding of the current status of the organization and the available avenues for potential change.

3. Data collection, as the initial step in a change effort, has the effect of involving people at many levels in the organization in the assessment and diagnostic activities which are traditionally the domain of top management and are often conducted in a cautious, semisecretive manner.[25]

There are a number of tools that you as a manager can use in making a diagnosis of the organization. Among the most common are (1) survey questionnaires, (2) interviews, (3) organizational sensing, (4) the organization "mirror," and (5) self-generated scales.

Survey questionnaires   An efficient method of obtaining information is the survey questionnaire, which is designed to obtain specific kinds of information. The questions are often very specific and structured and usually require a simple checked response. Such questionnaires produce considerable data. However, unless the questionnaire has been thoughtfully designed the results may prove to be of limited use. Many change agents, therefore, prefer to pretest questionnaires with a small group of individuals in order to make certain that the survey is sensitive to the types of problems that the organization is experiencing.

You may find it useful to design your own questionnaire. The advantage of doing so is that you can ask the type of questions that will focus on specific characteristics of your organization. There is some evidence that such questionnaires are the most useful since they limit themselves to specific organiza-

[25] Newton Margulies and John Wallace, *Organizational Change* (Glenview, Ill.: Scott, Foresman, 1973), pp. 22–23.

tional problems.[26] However, they often suffer from poor construction. Unless the manager has had experience with test construction it is likely that the questions may be shaded by the perceptions of the manager and may, in fact, not generate useful information.

Fortunately, for the manager who does not want to spend time constructing questionnaires, there are a number that have been designed and tested for validity. The Position Analysis Questionnaire designed by E. J. McCormick and his colleagues provides information about specific positions within organizations.[27] It will give you information on (1) the job context or setting (for example, unpleasant or hazardous settings, noise), (2) the interpersonal relationships found in the job (communication, contact with others), (3) the amount of information input that is required to do the job (visual, perceptual), (4) the factors in work output (machine or manual control, body activity, dexterity and handling skills required), and (5) the mediation methods involved (decision making, information processing).

W. W. Tornow and P. R. Pinto developed a similar position analysis for managers.[28] The instrument measures the degree to which managers engage in various activities such as planning, coordination, control, consulting, approval of financial expenditures, direction, supervision, and so forth. One objective of the analysis is to determine what aspects of managerial work may be causing organizational problems.

These two survey instruments are primarily concerned with the *structural* and *procedural* aspects of a position. Their basic purpose is to measure what is required on the job in terms of time, skill, effort, and activities as well as to obtain a description of the setting in which the activities take place.[29] There are, however, other instruments that are more *process* oriented.

J. R. Hackman and G. R. Oldham have designed a Job Diagnostic Survey that examines work satisfaction according to the following variables: (1) the type of activities performed and skills needed and the amount of personal identity with the task, (2) the significance of the task, (3) the degree of job autonomy, and (4) the amount of feedback about performance. Included in the questionnaire are a number of psychological indicators that have to do with the *meaningfulness* of work including some assessment of the affective reactions to the job overall and its subparts.[30]

---

[26] J. K. Fordyce and R. Weil, *Managing with People* (Reading, Mass.: Addison-Wesley, 1971).

[27] E. J. McCormick, P. R. Jeanneret, and R. C. Mecham, "A Study of Job Characteristics on Job Dimensions as Based on the Position Analysis Questionnaires (PAQ)," *Journal of Applied Psychology,* 56 (1972), 346–60.

[28] W. W. Tornow and P. R. Pinto, "The Development of a Managerial Job Taxonomy: A System for Describing, Classifying and Evaluating Executive Positions," *Journal of Applied Psychology,* 61 (1976), 419–28.

[29] Terrence Mitchell, *People in Organizations* (New York: McGraw-Hill, 1978), p. 387.

[30] Ibid.

A comprehensive diagnostic instrument was developed by Rensis Likert.[31] The instrument examines leadership style of management and provides information on interpersonal, motivational, and small-group issues. Employees are requested to assess the types of leadership patterns that are used in the organization. Managers are requested to describe the highest- and lowest-producing departments. The types of management practices found generally fall into four patterns: (1) *exploitive-authoritative,* typified by low trust and no participation; (2) *benevolent-authoritative,* typified by condescension and token participation; (3) *consultative,* in which management asks for advice yet retains decision-making prerogatives; and (4) *participative,* typified by complete confidence in subordinates and democratic decision-making methods.[32] When administrators use Likert's instrument they are in a position to understand how they are perceived by others within the organization and to determine whether the leadership patterns are conducive to optimal productivity and morale.

Interviews   Some managers will follow survey questionnaires with in-depth interviews with selected personnel. At times the interviews will be structured and require the respondents to provide detailed descriptive information. At other times managers will prefer unstructured conversation that allows respondents to express themselves freely on whatever seems pertinent.

The success of an interview is usually dependent upon the following factors:

Are the purposes of the interview understood by the respondent?

Does the interviewer have a clear focus on the types of information that are needed from the respondent?

Is the respondent convinced that his or her responses will be held in confidence?

Does the respondent trust the interviewer?

Has adequate time been allotted for the interview?

The primary advantage of face-to-face conversation is that respondents have the opportunity to share information that probably would not be recorded on an objective survey instrument. The primary disadvantage is that the responses are subject to interpretation bias.

Organizational sensing   The primary purpose of organizational sensing is to retrieve information from key employees concerning organizational performance. A common method used by organization development practi-

[31] Rensis Likert, *The Human Organization* (New York: McGraw-Hill, 1967).
[32] Mitchell, *People in Organizations,* p. 308.

tioners is to select a stratified sample of employees who have the most knowledge about an emerging organizational problem. The sample often includes representatives from the executive ranks, mid-level managers, and/or rank-and-file employees. These individuals are brought together and the symptoms of the problem as reflected in statistics on employee turnover, absenteeism, grievances, union disputes, or complaints from patients/clients are displayed. The change agent will assist the group in understanding the possible meanings of the statistics and formulate a *problem statement* which is the identification of some issue that is keeping the organization from being optimally productive. Once the problem statement has been formulated the group is asked to define solutions as well as methods through which the solutions can be implemented.

The organization mirror   This method is particularly useful when one department is having difficulty with another department in the same institution. The purpose of the method is to unfreeze the communication channels between two groups who are in conflict with one another. Usually the change agent will first obtain agreement from the respective department heads to initiate a process through which the differences between the units can be identified. Once agreement has been reached on the department head level, each unit is requested to write out a composite *personality profile* of the other unit. This profile is completed by answering questions, such as the following:

To what extent does the _____ department produce quality services (or products, as the case may be)?

To what extent are the employees of the _____ department committed to the goals of the total organization?

What are the most significant problems within the _____ department?

To what extent is the department aware of these problems and willing to do something about them?

What are the most serious difficulties we experience in working with the _____ department?

If we could change one thing within the _____ department it would be _____ .

Each of the questions should be fully answered and then distributed to the members of the other unit. The two departments are subsequently brought together to share their perceptions, to correct erroneous perceptions, and to discuss ways that the two units could work more closely with one another. When departments have large numbers of employees it is often helpful to do this exercise with a small group of individuals who are representative of their unit. A detailed example of how this method has been used in mediating conflicts can be found on pp. 245–247.

Self-generated scales   At times it may be helpful to have a department evaluate itself through criteria determined by the department members themselves. This is commonly undertaken by having the members list what they believe are the characteristics of an outstanding organization. These characteristics are listed on a blackboard and prioritized. Most groups find this exercise relatively easy to undertake and will create lists of between fifteen and thirty-five characteristics, some of which are common to most work groups while others reflect the particular functions the department members happen to perform.

After the exercise is completed the group will have generated a scaled list of criteria. Alongside each criterion should appear a continuum scaled from 1 to 10, with 10 signifying the greatest possible effectiveness. The members of the group, working alone, are asked to rate their department on the agreed upon criteria. These anonymous individual evaluations are compiled into a group composite evaluation. At the completion of the exercise the group will have an accurate assessment as to how they evaluate their unit's effectiveness. An example of a self-generated scale is found in Figure 9-4.

The advantage of self-generated scales is that defensiveness is minimized

Characteristics of an effective group	Most effective 10	9	8	7	6	5	4	3	Least effective 2	1
1. Clearly defined goals		x								
2. Open communication							x			
3. Feelings openly expressed							x			
4. Information sharing						x				
5. Activities well planned						x				
6. Highly motivated members							x			
7. Conflicts openly resolved						x				
8. Minimal dysfunctional interperson hostility						x				
9. High participation						x				
10. High technical skills						x				
11. Availability of information							x			
12. Technical leadership		x								
13. Work of individuals well coordinated						x				

Figure 9-4 An example of a self-generated scaling instrument. [From *Organizational Change: Techniques and Applications* by Newton Margulies and John Wallace. Copyright 1973 by Scott, Foresman & Company. Reprinted by permission.]

as the group members begin talking with one another about the characteristics of an effective organization. After the exercise has been completed the *group* has diagnosed its own problems rather than a consultant or even top management stepping in to do the evaluation. This is a significant characteristic of this technique as group members take responsibility for evaluating their effectiveness and bringing about changes that they perceive to be beneficial.

In summary, the diagnosis stage of an organization development effort is designed to identify the types of problems the organization is experiencing. Ideally the diagnoses should be data based. *The more objective the inquiry, the greater the probability that organizational members will accept the results of the survey.* The need to undertake an objective diagnosis is one of the basic principles emanating from rational-empirical strategies for change. This principle should not be forgotten by any practicing health administrator for the likelihood that meaningful interventions can take place will be contingent upon whether there has been an objective and dispassionate analysis of organizational issues and problems.

Phase 3: Intervention

Kurt Lewin's *unfreezing-changing-refreezing* model provides a helpful vehicle for understanding how change actually takes place within people and within organizations.[33] Lewin suggested that behavior is determined by the composite effect of a complex set of contemporaneous forces impinging upon an individual. There are *driving forces* acting upon people, driving them towards new attitudes and behaviors. Likewise there are *restraining forces* that restrict deviations and perpetuate the status quo.

Take, for example, the case of Mary Martinson, a secretary who shares an office with four other secretary-clerks. Within this work group there is a strong belief that no one should volunteer for extra work, even if all tasks have been completed prior to the end of the day. Usually the secretaries feign busyness for an hour or two rather than ask their supervisor for additional work.

Mary has silently gone along with this practice although she would prefer to be busy on work-related matters for the entire day. The driving forces that would cause her to ask for additional assignments are, however, offset by more powerful restraining forces. Mary knows that if she volunteered for additional work she would be ostracized from the group. She therefore says nothing and goes along with the group's expectations. The forces to change are not as powerful as the forces that restrain.

Lewin suggested that if you are to unfreeze the quasi-stationary

[33] Kurt Lewin, *Field Theory in Social Science* (New York: Harper & Row, 1951).

equilibrium within an individual, group, or organization you must do one of three things: (1) increase the forces driving the individual, group, or organization to change, (2) decrease the restraining forces, or (3) accomplish some combination of the first two.

You can increase driving forces by using positive or negative incentives. For example, Mary Martinson's supervisor may sense that the five secretaries loaf through the last hour of each day. She might inform the secretaries of impending layoffs that can be avoided only by an increase in their productivity. Or she might use an incentive payment scheme by which output is correlated with yearly merit salary increases. The success of either of these approaches is not guaranteed. While the secretaries may fear that their present level of productivity may result in unemployment they may also believe that if they yield to these pressures they will encourage their supervisor to seek further changes in the same autocratic manner. They may also fear that if they increase their productivity it might cost one of them her job ("What if it turns out that four of us can do all the work?"). The supervisor's attempt to change the behavior of her subordinates might actually produce additional restraining forces inadvertently.

A supervisor who is sensitive to the fear that might be aroused may need to heighten the driving forces in order to lessen the restraining pressures. This could be accomplished by reassuring the secretaries that none will lose their jobs if productivity increased. Showing them the salary increases that could potentially be given might also help ("It is possible for each of you to be making fifty dollars more per month if we meet this year's goals"). The supervisor may also choose to work more closely with the group, to give additional reinforcement when tasks are done well, and generally seek to build the cohesiveness of the unit. If she does so, the positive forces for change will be strengthened and the restraining forces will be diminished.

As a general rule it is more desirable to increase the driving forces while decreasing the restraining forces than *only* to increase the driving forces or *only* to decrease the restraining forces. For example, if you delegate a tough, challenging task to a subordinate you might increase the driving forces by saying, "I can think of no one in this organization who could do a better job on this project than you." But you may also need to diminish the restraining forces, particularly if there is a risk of failure. By indicating that you realize it is a high-risk project in which success is not guaranteed and by indicating your support as problems are encountered, you are taking steps to diminish the power of the restraining forces.

Once employees have become motivated to change, they are ready to be provided with new patterns of behavior. This process is most likely to occur through *identification* and/or *internalization*.

Identification occurs "when one or more models are provided in the environment, models from whom individuals can learn new behavior patterns by identifying with them and trying to become like them.''[34] If Mary Martinson is a respected and valued member of the secretarial group, her willingness to follow the suggestions of the supervisor might unfreeze the restraining attitudes of the other secretaries.

Internalization occurs when employees determine that the new behaviors contain more positive rewards than negative sanctions. If the secretarial group realizes that it is more rewarding to work a solid eight-hour day than to feign busyness they will adopt behaviors that will make the group more productive. Likewise, if the promise of fifty dollars more per month is a motivator, the restraining forces will be diminished.

As employees practice new behaviors there is a high probability that refreezing will occur. As Edgar Schein has noted, when new behavior is internalized while being learned this has "automatically facilitated refreezing because it has been fitted naturally into the individual's personality."[35] To make certain that refreezing of newly learned behaviors occurs it is important to give positive reinforcement, either on a continuous or intermittent schedule. If continuous reinforcement is given, the individual can be expected to learn new behaviors quickly. However, it should also be noted that if reinforcement is suddenly stopped, the new behaviors would probably be extinguished quickly. Therefore, if you want fast learning, give continuous reinforcement. But if you want the changes to be permanent, switch to intermittent reinforcement.

As a practicing health administrator there will be times when you are convinced that a change needs to be made within your organization, only to find that your change efforts meet with resistance. When you bump headlong into a situation where beliefs, attitudes, and behaviors are frozen like chunks of northern Minnesota ice, you may want to remember the following principles of change that evolve out of Kurt Lewin's theory: (1) Have your change target clearly in focus; (2) anticipate resistance to proposed change; (3) to diminish resistance to change, encourage direct participation in the change process; and (4) reinforce newly learned behaviors.

Principle 1: Have your change target clearly in focus.

As Figure 9–5 suggests, the change target may be jobs, relationships, or organizational policy.[36] If patient education activities are not being coordinated in an effective manner, a hospital administrator may consider

[34] Paul Hersey and Kenneth Blanchard, *Management of Organizational Behavior* (Englewood Cliffs, N.J.: Prentice-Hall, Inc., 1969), p. 162.

[35] Edgar H. Schein, "Management Development as a Process of Influence," in *Behavioral Concepts in Management,* ed. David R. Hampton (Belmont, Calif.: Dickenson, 1968), p. 112.

[36] Mitchell, *People in Organizations,* p. 385.

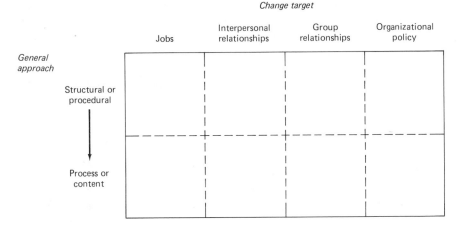

Change target

Figure 9-5 A classification of change strategies. [From Terrence R. Mitchell, *People in Organizations: Understanding Their Behavior* (New York: McGraw-Hill, 1978), p. 384.]

employing a patient educator on a full-time basis. This would represent a change in someone's *job*. There may be *relationship* problems within the organization as exemplified in tensions between nurses, physicians, and allied health personnel as to who has primary responsibility for coordinating patient education activities. If these relationships are clarified by redefining formal position descriptions this would represent a change in *policy*.

In addition to determining whether your changes will be primarily in jobs, relationships, or policy it is important to determine whether your primary aim is a structural or a process change. *Structural changes* are represented in technological innovations (such as new equipment or changing the design of a task), social-structural changes (for example, in lines of authority or communications), or procedural changes (in rules or regulations). Structural changes imply that some aspect of the organization will be modified in an attempt to bring about greater effectiveness, satisfaction, and adaptability.[37] *Process* changes are primarily concerned with interpersonal attitudes and feelings and are often the result of humanistic concerns. For example, instead of introducing a new form that would help make the hospital transcriber more efficient, the supervisor may choose to find ways to make the job of being a transcriber more interesting and challenging. Rather than transfer or even terminate employment of quarreling employees (a structural technique) management might suggest a confrontation meeting between the antagonists in an effort to resolve the difficulty (a process technique).

If the diagnosis of the organization has been thorough, there should be a sound understanding as to whether jobs, interpersonal or group relationships,

[37] Ibid., p. 384.

and/or organizational policy needs to be altered. You should also be able to make a preliminary judgment as to whether structural or process changes need to be made. As indicated by the dotted lines in Figure 9-5, the boundaries between change targets are not alway clear and distinct. A change in organizational policy may be reflected in changes in relationships and possibly changes in job function. In addition, there may be times where you will want to alter both structure and process variables. The key point, however, is to keep your target clearly in focus.

Principle 2: Anticipate resistance to proposed change.

When an organization plans for the future it is natural for some members to perceive change as a threat. Although an organization itself was originally an innovation, it is equally true that most organizations are innovation resistant. As Donald Klein notes, "It has been suggested that just as individuals have their defenses to ward off threats, maintain integrity, and protect themselves against the unwarranted intrusions of others' demands, so do social systems seek ways in which to defend themselves against ill considered and overly precipitous innovations."[38]

It is important that you as a change agent see resistance as a natural part of the change process. Resistance is, in fact, a healthy phenomenon. As Jerry Rubin notes: "By resisting, actively or passively, an organization is communicating a message—it is providing data. In a very real sense, an organization is telling us something about 'who it is'—its major resources and limitations, its attitudes toward outsiders and change, its important internal norms and values, and the nature of its relationship to other systems in the environment."[39] Thus any resistance should be viewed as an opportunity for insight into the various conditions that should be considered when selecting and shaping intervention strategies.

There are three major sources of resistance to change: (1) uncertainty about the causes and effects of change, (2) threats to power and influence, and (3) awareness of weaknesses in proposed changes.

Uncertainty about the causes and effects of change   When change is proposed, the first question that employees want answered is "Why are they doing this?" Implicit in that question is a feeling that, if something is not going well, it may reflect adversely on the employees. If the change is imposed

[38] Donald Klein, "Some Notes on the Dynamics of Resistance to Change," in *The Planning of Change*, eds. W. Bennis, K. Benne, R. Chin, and K. Corey (New York: Holt, Rinehart & Winston, 1976), p. 502.
[39] Cited in Zaltman and Duncan, *Strategies*, p. 62.

on personal grounds ("That is the way I want things done"), it is often interpreted as a sign that subordinates have not done their jobs properly.[40]

When employees feel threatened by a change they may look for a "hidden agenda," that is, the true reason why a change is being suggested rather than the reason that has been articulated. Therefore it is not uncommon for rumors to quickly infiltrate the organization about the "real reason" behind a new policy or procedure.

The second question that employees ask when a change is proposed is "How will this change affect me?" If a health commissioner suggests, for example, that the organization initiate a flextime program, employees will evaluate the suggestion in terms of what the change will do to their personal well-being. This is an important point for top managers to remember. *While you may want to make a change for the good of the total system, employees will evaluate the change primarily in personal terms.* Therefore, in giving the reasons for a proposed change, it is important to discuss not only how this will help the system ("We are hopeful that flextime will help us become more productive by diminishing tardiness") but also to describe how employees will benefit from the change ("Each of you will have a lot more freedom in determining when you want to begin and end your work day").

In brief, if resistance is to be minimized there should be a straightfoward description of the reasons that have led to the change as well as a description of the benefits that will occur to both the organization and to its membership.

Threats to power and influence   Perhaps the most important source of resistance comes when an individual's base of power is threatened. This is exemplified in the problems that result when two or more organizations merge. It has been well documented that when a merger takes place managers fear that they will lose control over decision making and have less power with which to influence events. In a recent study of hospital mergers, Robert Duncan and his associates found that the fears of reduced power and influence are, in fact, justified. After merger, managers indicated that they had a significant reduction in influence on anywhere from eight to fifteen of some twenty decision-making areas.[41] Their power to influence key decisions had been shifted to the centralized corporate staff.

As one would expect, change is acceptable when it heightens influence and is usually unacceptable when it diminshed influence. Therefore, if possible, point out to those being asked to change how their status will be increased by a proposed change rather than decreased. In those instances where power *is* being diminished, it is helpful to provide a full explanation of the reasons

[40] James A. F. Stoner, *Management* (Englewood Cliffs, N.J.: Prentice-Hall, Inc., 1978), p. 378.
[41] Cited in Zaltman and Duncan, *Strategies,* p. 75.

necessitating the change. While such explanations will not totally eradicate resistance, they may serve to diminish resistance, providing the explanations are defensible on their own merits.

It is also important when bringing about a change to be aware of the attitudes and perceptions of those who are *indirectly* affected by the change. Often, out of fear that they will be treated the same way, departments that are only tangentially involved will keep a keen eye on how you manage a department whose power is being diminished. To counteract such fears it is important to emphasize by your actions that your primary concern is the good of the total organization, not simply one of its parts. Communicate your intentions forthrightly, answer questions that may arise, and be willing to change your approach if conditions necessitate a reexamination of what you are undertaking.

Awareness of weaknesses in the proposed changes   Earlier we noted that resistance can be a healthy phenomena. This is particularly true when individuals resist change because they are aware of the potential problems that have been overlooked by the change agent. For example, a hospital administrator concerned by excessive rates of tardiness and absenteeism might advocate flextime as a way to help employees become more productive. Most department heads who supervise clerks and technicians might readily agree to the change. However, the head of the hospital's maintenance department may disagree, citing the fact that most of the institution's maintenance programs have been carefully scheduled to fit into prescribed time periods so as to minimize disruptions in patient care. Such an objection should be evaluated on its own merit. If the objections are valid, the proposed change should be altered. If they lack validity, the incentives may have to be strengthened in order to create an environment where change can occur.

In summary, it is important to see resistance as a natural part of the change process. The individual who resists change may appear to be unbending, unreasonable, and even irrational. Nevertheless such a person has something of value to communicate about the nature of the system that you are seeking to influence. "It is important," states Donald Klein, "for those seeking change to consider the costs of ignoring, overriding, or dismissing as irrational those who emerge as their opponents. To ignore that which is being defended may mean that the planned change itself is flawed; it may also mean that the process of change becomes transformed into a conflict situation in which forces struggle in opposition and in which energies become increasingly devoted to winning rather than to solving the original problem."[42] Therefore the more you as a change agent can view the situation with a sympathetic understanding of what the resister is seeking to protect, the better you will be able to shape your change strategies in order to overcome the resistance.

[42] Donald Klein, "Some Notes on the Dynamics of Resistance to Change: The Defenders Role," in Bennis et al., *Planning of Change,* p. 122.

Principle 3: To diminish resistance to change, encourage direct participation in the change process.

If there is one cardinal principle of change theory it is that resistance is reduced when individuals "take part in the fact-finding and the diagnosing of needed changes and in the formulating and reality-testing of goals and programs of change."[43]

Ideally those who will be affected by a change should be involved from the beginning in the change process. They should have an awareness that there is a problem (Phase 1), be involved in the design of an instrument which will objectvely define the problem (Phase 2), develop intervention strategies (Phase 3), and finally, evaluate the effectiveness of the change program (Phase 4).

There usually is little resistance to the suggestion that a problem be discussed, although there may be varying perceptions about the severity of the issue. Likewise, most do not perceive an instrument such as a survey questionnaire to be a threat providing that they have input into the design of the instrument or, in the case of a standardized instrument, believe that it will be used objectively. You are more likely to feel resistance, however, after the problem has been defined and you begin to search for solutions. Individuals often cease to be creative and fall back on positions that protect their power and stabilize their influence. George M. Prince, after studying the creative-resistance behaviors of people, summarized the difficulty as follows:

> Free speculation and disciplined reaction to it is of urgent importance, for there is a relentless gravity-like force working against speculation. This force is dangerous especially because it is so easily justified as realistic thinking. It is a well-kept secret that people in general are determined enemies of free speculation. Each of us pays convincing lip service to his willingness—even eagerness—to consider new thoughts and ideas. But a thousand (recording) tapes, such as we have made, make liars of us all. People use remarkable ingenuity to make clear by tone, nonverbal slights, tuning out, supposedly helpful criticisms, false issues, and outright negativity, that they are not only against ideas and change but also against those who propose them. We humans eventually try to protect ourselves *even from our new ideas.*[44]

In helping a group find solutions to an identified problem it is helpful to recognize that creative problem solving usually evolves out of a six-stage process.[45]

---

[43] Ibid., p. 334.

[44] George M. Prince, *The Practice of Creativity* (New York: Harper & Row, 1970), p. 9.

[45] Adapted from Joseph L. Massi and John Douglas, *Managing: A Contemporary Introduction* (Englewood Cliffs, New Jersey, Prentice-Hall, Inc., 1977), pp. 336–37.

1. The familiarizing stage The purpose of this stage is to help group members understand the magnitude of an issue that will probably necessitate some change in jobs, relationships, or organizational policy. The participants should learn the basic facts of the problem by reviewing the information accumulated in the diagnosis phase.

The familiarizing stage of group problem solving involves hard work as participants immerse themselves in all aspects of an issue. Not only should they review data, but they should interview others who are directly or indirectly involved in the problem. The degree to which creative solutions will be discovered will be positively correlated with the group's ability to undertake a *thorough* assessment of the nature of the problem and its impact on organizational performance.

2. The mulling over stage Creative solutions usually do not spring out of the consciousness overnight. Therefore it is unwise to press for creative solutions soon after the group has defined the problem. It is helpful to separate Stages 1 and 2 by several working days to give participants an opportunity to mull over the issue and begin speculating about possible solutions.

3. The speculating stage If the problem requires some real breakthrough in thinking, it is important for group members to shake off inhibiting forces that tend to restrict thought to past conscious patterns. In other words, participants must be willing to allow the "wealth of subconscious elements to break through the barriers" of their consciousness.[46] *Deliberation must always be accomplished, therefore, with speculation,* even though some thoughts may appear to be unworkable, impracticable, or even irrelevant. At the completion of this stage the group should have produced a number of ideas that, if implemented, would address problems discovered in the diagnosis stage.

4. The gestation stage Once creative ideas have been identified, it is wise for the group to step back for a period of time to refresh the mind. The first three stages involve a great deal of thought and concentration. It is helpful again to let several working days pass prior to moving into the implementation stage of group problem solving.

5. The insight stage After a group has thought creatively about a problem and has evolved a number of ideas, there usually is a short period in which an original idea comes forward that represents the best possible solution to a given organizational problem. The key "is to be receptive to the new idea and be able to recognize it as a breakthrough. While many individuals

[46] Ibid., p. 336.

have had the same insight the creative person will be the one who can recognize its significance and interpret that significance to the group."[47]

6. The testing stage   In the final stage the group tries out the new idea to see if it is truly effective in bringing about a desired change. It is wise to obtain a consensus from the group about how much time should elapse before a decision is made as to the effectiveness of the change. Skeptics of a proposed solution will argue that the evaluation should take place relatively soon, while proponents will want to give the solution ample opportunity to prove its effectiveness. One way out of this dilemma is to have an ongoing evaluation program in which group members periodically assess whether or not the change is beneficial on the basis of predetermined criteria.

In summary, the more you can assist employees in understanding the scope of a problem and the more you can enlist their help in generating solutions to the difficulty, the greater the probability that subsequent change will be embraced rather than resisted.

Principle 4: Reinforce newly learned behaviors.

The need to give adequate reinforcement cannot be overemphasized if newly learned attitudes, skills, and behaviors are to be permanently in place. Employees will cease to use new skills unless they are rewarded. The reward does not need to be given continuously, but it does need to be given intermittently.

If you are undertaking a planned change program you should, once the change has been initiated, review the types of reinforcement being given in shaping the change process. There are three prerequisites for effective reinforcement which should be kept clearly in focus.[48] First, reinforcement contingencies should be clear and unambigious. The dispensers and the recipients of the reinforcements should be clear as to what behaviors lead to what outcomes. They need to know which behaviors are perceived positively and will lead to some reward and which behaviors are perceived negatively. From this perspective members will tend to see the applications of reinforcement theory not as a manipulative procedure but as a means through which workers can gain a measure of control over their work environment. "When the outcomes for given behaviors are clear and unequivocal, the person is operating in a known environment, one which he can control if he wishes, by choosing to perform behaviors that will produce desired outcomes."[49]

A second prerequisite for effective reinforcement is that reinforcing

---

[47] Ibid., p. 337.

[48] Margulies and Wallace, *Organizational Change*, pp. 44–63.

[49] Ibid., p. 57.

events should be sufficiently varied. As we learned in our discussion of motivation, workers respond in their own unique way to specific motivators. Some will be motivated to change if they know that they will receive additional financial remuneration; others will change if they receive greater respect and are given additional opportunities to achieve. There are many motivators including increased pay, rest periods, vacation time, social recognition, increased space, increased privacy, more responsibility, and increased opportunity for affiliating with other workers. Managers have at their disposal a relatively rich mix of reinforcements that can be applied given the values and needs of those who will be affected by a change.

A third prerequisite is that reinforcements should be presented in sufficient number and strength. It is important for members of an organization to feel that reinforcements are not so scarce as to convince them that the obtainment of them is exceedingly improbable. For example, if a health commissioner continually rejected the recommendations made by the executive committee, the committee members would soon become discouraged because no reinforcements are being given that would cause them to move ahead. Conversely, if reinforcements are too easy to obtain, their reinforcing value is likely to be diminished over time.

There is no ironclad rule that states how often a reinforcement should be given. Suffice it to say, however, that when a change agent sees newly learned skills being substituted with old routines, some type of reinforcement is necessary. If none is given, the worker will continue to go back to the old ways of doing things for they usually represent less investment in energy and involvement.

In summary, the intervention stage of organization development involves the unfreezing of old attitudes, skills, and behaviors and the refreezing of new ones. For change to be most effective it is important that you as a change agent have a clear focus on what is to be changed, whether it be jobs, relations, or policies, and whether the changes be structural or process oriented. Second, be prepared for resistance to suggested change. Listen to the resistance; learn from it; increase the driving forces and decrease the restraining forces. Third, keep in mind the time-honored axiom that resistance to change is diminished when affected individuals are involved in the change process. Finally, give adequate reinforcement so that newly learned attitudes, skills, and behaviors will continue to be effectively used.

Phase 4: Evaluation

It is an unfortunate fact that most organization development programs have not made a serious effort to evaluate the effectiveness of the change efforts. "It is sad but true," state Newton Margulies and John Wallace, "that the history of change technology has followed the familiar pattern of enthusiastic endorsement by the partisans of this or that approach with little empirical support for the often far-reaching and sometimes downright extravagant claims of effectiveness."[50]

Fortunately this situation is being reversed as change agents recognize that the evaluation process is an indispensable part of the development process. As a manager you will want to monitor the change process by asking two probing questions:

1. Did the intervention resolve the organizational problems that were identified in the diagnoses?
2. Did the intervention result in any unanticipated problems that require action?

If you made an objective diagnosis you should have base-line information that can be used to determine the impact of the interventions. For example, let us assume that you used a Likert survey (see p. 273) in diagnosing the leadership practices of middle-management personnel. From that study you should have learned whether the middle managers are exploitive-authoritative (pattern 1), benevolent-authoritative (pattern 2), consultative (pattern 3), or participative (pattern 4) in their leadership style. Let us assume that that survey indicated that the composite ranking was 2.5—that is, the middle-level managers were between being benevolently authoritative and consultative—and that a management development program was initiated to move to a participative leadership style. At three-month intervals follow-up surveys could be undertaken, using the same measuring instrument, that would indicate whether the management development program was having an impact on the organization. The results should be shared with the middle-level managers, and their implications assimilated.

It is also important in the evaluation process to determine what problems have resulted when an intervention program has been initiated. It is an ironic fact of organizational life that when you solve one problem others are often created. For example, as the middle-level managers move towards a participative style of supervision, it is likely that the productivity and morale of their subordinates will improve. However, there may be some subordinates who prefer the old autocratic styles of supervision rather than a new pattern that demands more participation from them. If this problem results from the change process, it should be dealt with by (1) diagnosing the severity of the difficulty, (2) creatively planning how to intervene, and (3) evaluating—again—the effectiveness of the intervention.

[50] Ibid., p. 14.

Postscript: The Value of Crises

In examining strategies for bringing about planned organizational change, we noted that the environment in which health organizations exist is dynamic and ever changing. New regulations, changing patterns of financial support, emerging community health problems, and changing opportunities to resolve those problems often create a crisis atmosphere in which systematic *planned* change may be difficult to achieve. Nevertheless, all organizational theorists are agreed on one central point: *Crisis can be the impetus for needed organizational growth.* It is somewhat ironic that an organization's crises are often the pillars upon which new structures, programs, and policies are built. Oftentimes a crisis forces management to consider alternatives that had previously been unthinkable and to design blueprints for the future that hold creative promise. While a crisis in itself does not necessarily generate good ideas, the uncertainty and anxiety generated by a crisis makes the membership of an organization eager to adopt new structures that promise to relieve the anxiety.[51]

Although emerging problems can produce conditions that promote organizational change, it should be remembered that whether change actually takes place will be largely determined by the will of those who take on the necessary risks that come in designing new programs and innovative ways of operating. "I think we are in constant danger—not from technology, but from losing our nerve," said Dr. Herbert A. Simon, Associate Dean of Carnegie Mellon University's Graduate School of Industrial Administration. "When Columbus came to this continent, he could come in hope of fulfilling his goals—and ignorance of the plague and syphilis he was bringing to the Indians. We don't have that ignorance anymore. We know a lot about the germs we are bringing with us and we tend to become overawed by the responsibility for these waves of consequences of any actions that we take."[52]

Nevertheless while the consequences of our actions may cause us to study our innovations carefully, they must not keep us from venturing into the unknown which is inherent in newness. Lincoln stated the issue succinctly: "The dogmas of the quiet past are inadequate to the stormy present. The occasion is piled high with difficulty and we must rise to the occasion. As our case is new, so we must think anew and act anew."[53]

SUMMARY

The purpose of this chapter was to examine the concept of organizational change. We learned that there are rational-imperical, normative–re-educative, and power-coerceive change strategies. Each of these strategies has

[51] Bennis et al., *Planning of Change,* p. 522.
[52] Quoted in J. S. Morgan, *Managing Change* (New York: McGraw-Hill, 1972), p. 61.
[53] Ibid., p. 167.

strengths and limitations. We examined a four-step model that is commonly used to bring about organizational change. If this model is to succeed, (1) the change target must be clearly identified, (2) resistance to proposed change will need to be understood and overcome, (3) those who will be influenced by the proposed change should be included in the formulation and testing of new goals and programs, and (4) appropriate reinforcement should be given to those who are learning new behaviors.

STUDY QUESTIONS

1. At the beginning of this chapter we noted three challenges confronting health organizations. What additional challenges will confront health administrators during the next five to ten years?

2. Have you changed any significant values, attitudes, or behaviors during the past five years? What were the "driving forces" that brought about the changes and what were the "restraining forces"?

3. Select an organization with which you are familiar and analyze it according to Larry Greiner's "Five Stages of Organizational Growth" (Figure 9-3). What stage of crisis/growth is the organization in? Give reasons for your answer. Can you predict what will be the next crisis confronting this organization?

ADDITIONAL READING RESOURCES

FLAHERTY, JOHN E., *Managing Change: Today's Challenge to Management.* New York: Nellen Publishing Co., 1979.

FRENCH, W. L., AND C. H. BELL, *Organization Development.* Englewood Cliffs, N.J.: Prentice-Hall, Inc., 1978.

HEATWOLE, KATHLEEN B., and CHARLES L. BREINDEL, "A Political Paradigm for the Health Care Administrator," *Health Care Management Review* 5, no. 4 (Fall 1980), 67-74.

METZGER, NORMAN, "Overcoming Resistance to Change," *Health Services Manager,* 13, no. 8 (August 1980), 3-5.

PORTER-O'GRADY, TIMOTHY, and ROYCE D. HARRELL, "Transitional Management: Planned Change in a Rural Hospital," *Health Care Management Review* 5, no. 3 (Summer 1980), 46-49.

SCHERMERHORN, JOHN R., JR., "The Health Care Manager's Role in Promoting Change," *Health Care Management Review,* 4, no. 1 (Winter 1979), 1-3.

SPRADLEY, BARBARA WALTON, "Managing Change Creatively," *Journal of Nursing Administration,* 10, no. 5 (May 1980), 32-37.

10 Competency: Managing Occupational Stress and Job Burnout

It's not the big issues that grind you down; it's the little daily insults that do violence to your spirit.

—Anonymous

OVERVIEW The purpose of this chapter is to describe the relationship between work and health. Upon completion of the chapter the reader will be able to:

- Differentiate "eustress" and "distress"

- Describe the stress response

- Define the determinants of stress within the occupational setting

- List major studies that demonstrate a positive correlation between various work environments and coronary heart disease

- Differentiate Type A behavior from Type B

- Define the stages of occupational burnout

- List strategies that can be employed in preventing disabling occupational stress

Jere E. Yates, an authority in the relationship of work and health, states: "Chronic stress is the major health problem facing managers in America today."[1] Empirical studies support his observation. In a study of over 100 occupations the position of "manager/administrator" was judged to be one of the most stressful vocations anyone can enter.[2]

The purpose of this chapter is to determine how work influences health. Specifically we will explore the concept of occupational stress. We will learn that there is "positive stress" which heightens productivity and well-being and there is "negative stress" which threatens not only our effectiveness but our very lives. We will review some of the most important studies on occupational health and we will delineate strategies that administrators can employ in keeping themselves—and their organization—in optimal health. The underlying premise of this chapter is perhaps best summarized in a comment made by William E. Channing: "Health is a working man's fortune and he ought to watch over it more than the capitalist over his largest investment."[3]

THE NATURE OF STRESS

During the past five years professional journals have highlighted the fact that human service work is highly stressful.[4] We know for example, that the hospital is one of the most stressful of all work environments. When the National Institute for Occupational Safety and Health studied the relative incidence of mental health disorders in 130 major occupational categories they found that 7 of the top 27 occupations related to health care operations—health technologists, licensed practical nurses, clinical laboratory technicians, nursing aides, health aides, dental assistants, and registered nurses.[5] If the list of health care occupations were to include those not involved exclusively in patient care (secretaries, laborers, telephone operators, and so forth) 15 of the top 27 occupations with the highest incidence of mental disorders would come from hospitals.

[1] Jere E. Yates, *Managing Stress* (New York: AMACOM, 1979), p. 3.

[2] "How to Deal with Stress on the Job," *U.S. News and World Report,* March 13, 1978, p. 80.

[3] Quoted in John R. Phillips and George E. Allen, "Industrial Health Education: A Model," *Health Values, Achieving High Level Wellness,* 3 (1979), 95–98.

[4] See for example Steven H. Applebaum, "Managerial/Organizational Stress," *Health Care Management Review,* 5, no. 1 (Winter 1980), 7–15; Gary L. Calhoun, "Hospitals are High-Stress Employers," *Hospitals,* June 16, 1980, pp. 28–33; Ayala Pines and Dista Kafry, "Occupational Tedium in the Social Services," *Social Work,* 23, no. 6 (November 1978), 499–507; Seymour Shubin, "Burnout: The Professional Hazard You Face in Nursing," *Nursing 78,* 8, no. 7 (July 1978), pp. 22–27; and Robert Veninga, "Administrator Burnout: Causes and Cures," *Hospital Progress,* February 1979, pp. 48–53.

[5] M. J. Colligan, "Occupational Incidence Rates of Mental Health Disorders," *Journal of Human Stress,* 3 (September 1977), 34.

It should not be surprising that hospitals are high-stress institutions for it has been aptly demonstrated that responsibility for people (patients and/or staff members) causes considerably more stress than does responsibility for things.[6] In addition, the health care team is influenced by a great number and diversity of professional occupations whose interprofessional conflicts in goals, orientation, and purpose greatly enhance the possibility of organizational conflict and stress.[7]

Stress Defined

The concept of stress was first formulated by Hans Selye in 1936. He defined stress as "the nonspecific response of the body to any demand."[8] Subsequent scholars have distinguished three aspects of the stress model.[9] A *stressor* is anything that an individual perceives as a threat. It may be a sharp rebuttal from a supervisor, a colleague whose personality is ingratiating, or a recognition that important deadlines are at hand. Such stressors produce a *state of stress* in which the individual's homeostasis (well-being) is disrupted. Finally there is the *stress response*. Physiologically this may include an altered heart rate, increased secretion of gastric juices, and muscular tension. Psychologically the stress response may include worry, anxiety, guilt, and tension.

Individuals proceed through a three-stage process when under stress. In the first stage there is the *mobilization of resources* in order to confront the threat. Consider Marcia Cooper, a nurse in a coronary care unit. The change of shifts has occurred and Marcia has reviewed each patient's chart. Suddenly the monitor alarm sounds noting that a patient is in cardiac distress. Immediately and almost unconsciously the nurse mobilizes herself for action. Quickly she examines the monitor and notes that the patient's heart is fibrilating. She checks the patient's blood pressure, noting that his breathing is irregular and that his fingernails have turned blue. She calls out instructions to a colleague to start the defibrilator. The patient is shocked at a predetermined voltage. The heart rate becomes regular. The breathing cycle gradually improves. Soon the patient's life is out of danger.

Like anyone under stress, Marcia was keenly aware of her feelings, thoughts, and actions—what is called the behavior aspects of the stress response. However, hidden from view, a host of endocrine and autonomic nervous system functions were taking place. A dramatic biochemical change took place in Marcia's physiological state. Messages raced from the

[6] Calhoun, "Hospitals Are High-Stress Employers," p. 171.

[7] R. Schulz and A. C. Johnson, "Conflict in Hospitals," *Hospital Administration in Canada,* 16 (Summer 1971), 36.

[8] Hans Selye, "A Syndrome Produced by Diverse Nocuous Agents," *Nature* (London), 138 (1936), 32.

[9] James P. Spradley and Mark Phillips, "Culture and Stress: A Quantitative Analysis," *American Anthropologist,* 74, no. 3 (June 1972), 519.

hypothalamus which is a tiny bundle of nerve cells at the center of the brain. The message that the hypothalamus received was essentially, "There is a threat; mobilize for action." Instantly physiological responses could be detected. The tiny capillaries under the skin shut down permitting more blood to flow to vital organs. The blood vessels constricted while the muscles became tense. The pituitary gland sent out two hormones that moved through the blood stream to stimulate the thyroid and adrenal glands. One of the basic functions of the thyroid hormones is to increase the energy supply which one needs to physically cope with the stressful event. The adrenal gland sends some thirty additional hormones to nearly every organ of the body. This automatic stress response causes the pulse rate to shoot up and the blood pressure to soar. The stomach and intestines suspend their function of digesting food. The senses, particularly hearing and smell, become more acute. Hundreds of other physical changes occurred without Marcia even being aware of the process.[10]

In the second stage of the stress response there is a *sharp increase in energy consumption*. The alarm reaction that occurs when there is a threat burns up considerable energy. That is why, after a stressful day, workers will feel exhausted even though they undertook little physical labor. Dr. Selye suggests that the body has a finite amount of adaptation energy that can be tapped to mobilize against a threat. After burning up the amount of energy that is available, the body needs time to recover and to replenish the supply. When stress continues for long periods of time most of the adaption energy will be consumed. That is why *unrelieved stress* is the chief culprit in dissipating an individual's mental and physical well-being.

Finally, after the stress event has ended, the body returns to a *state of equilibrium*. Two hours later Marcia Cooper was in the coffee shop visiting with other nurses. She felt tired but relaxed. During the next few days her body would build up the supply of adaptation energy. In fact, even before she went off her shift she could have competently handled other stressful events. By having relatively stable periods in which our bodies can restore our adaptation energy we are able to meet and manage new stressful situations.

Eustress versus Distress

In 1936 when Selye published his first work on stress he believed that the effects of stress were inevitably harmful. Today, however, Selye suggests that stress is impossible to avoid. A well-deserved promotion can cause as much stress as can a harmful dispute within the office. Therefore Selye has

[10] For a more detailed explanation of the stress reponse see Jean Tache, Hans Selye, and Stacey B. Day, eds., *Cancer, Stress and Death* (New York: Plenum Medical Book Company, 1979); and Robert L. Veninga and James P. Spradley, *The Work-Stress Connection: How to Cope with Job Burnout* (Boston: Little, Brown and Company, 1981).

differentiated two types of stress, eustress and distress. Eustress (the Greek prefix *eu* means "good") is a powerful positive force that adds excitement and challenge to our lives. Distress, on the other hand, occurs when there is unrelieved tension. A government official might enjoy and feel exhilarated by testifying to a joint House-Senate legislative committee (eustress). However, if the official is called up to return for hour upon hour of grueling testimony, the eustress could turn to distress. This is particularly true if the official perceives that he has been ineffective. Figure 10-1 represents a description of how eustress leads to happiness, health, and longevity. You will note that the contributors to eustress are represented in physical activity-inactivity, mental activity-inactivity, sound nutrition, and meaningful relationships. Figure 10-2 represents a similar description for distress which leads to grief, disease, and premature death.

Personality Factors and Stress

Not everyone responds to stressful situations in the same way. What is stressful to one person may seem inconsequential to another. One worker, when learning that she will be transferred to another job, becomes depressed at the thought of leaving friends and well-established work routines. Another worker, when appraised of a transfer, will take it as a matter of course,

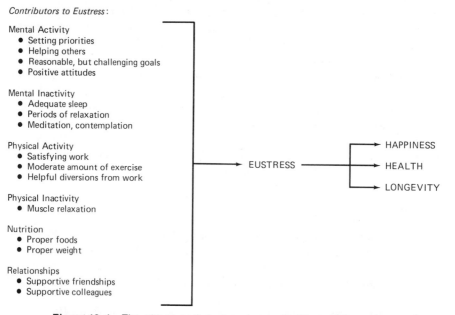

Contributors to Eustress:

Mental Activity
- Setting priorities
- Helping others
- Reasonable, but challenging goals
- Positive attitudes

Mental Inactivity
- Adequate sleep
- Periods of relaxation
- Meditation, contemplation

Physical Activity
- Satisfying work
- Moderate amount of exercise
- Helpful diversions from work

Physical Inactivity
- Muscle relaxation

Nutrition
- Proper foods
- Proper weight

Relationships
- Supportive friendships
- Supportive colleagues

EUSTRESS → HAPPINESS, HEALTH, LONGEVITY

Figure 10-1   The stress path to happiness, health, and longevity. [Modified from Donald R. Morse and M. Laurence Furst, *Stress for Success: A Holistic Approach to Stress and Its Management* (New York: Van Nostrand Reinhold Company, 1979) p. 5. Reprinted by permission of Van Nostrand Reinhold Company.]

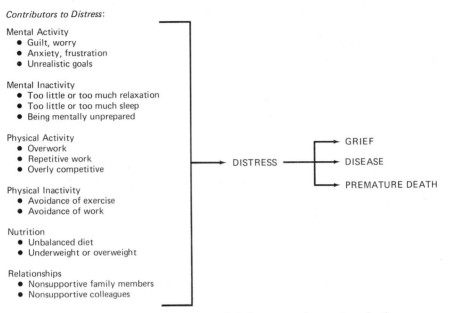

Contributors to Distress:

Mental Activity
- Guilt, worry
- Anxiety, frustration
- Unrealistic goals

Mental Inactivity
- Too little or too much relaxation
- Too little or too much sleep
- Being mentally unprepared

Physical Activity
- Overwork
- Repetitive work
- Overly competitive

Physical Inactivity
- Avoidance of exercise
- Avoidance of work

Nutrition
- Unbalanced diet
- Underweight or overweight

Relationships
- Nonsupportive family members
- Nonsupportive colleagues

DISTRESS

GRIEF

DISEASE

PREMATURE DEATH

Figure 10-2 The stress path to grief, disease, and premature death. [Modified from Donald R. Morse and M. Laurence Furst, *Stress for Success: A Holistic Approach to Stress and Its Management* (New York: Van Nostrand Reinhold Company, 1979), p. 5. Reprinted by permission of Van Nostrand Reinhold Company.]

perhaps shrugging her shoulders, and saying, "I might even like it better in the new department."

Figure 10-3 illustrates how three individuals might have three very different threshold points as well as three different elastic limits. You will note that person C can tolerate a greater amount of stress than can either A or B before encountering the *yield point,* which is seen in a slight change from "normal behavior." The symptoms of having reached the yield point might be reflected in increased nervousness, inability to concentrate, and fatigued expressions. Equally critical is the *elastic limit.* From an engineering perspective this is the point at which a stretched steel spring would show deformation. When stretched too far the spring will not return naturally to its original shape. So it is with you and me. "As long as the stressors are not intense enough to push us to our elastic limit, we thrive on stress. The yield point is a kind of early warning device that indicates we are close to our limit which is also called our *stress threshold.* Only a slight increase in stress is needed to take us from the yield point to the elastic limit."[11] As long as we are functioning within our elastic limits the stress load will not be too great. However, once the stress continues beyond the elastic limit we eventually reach the *rupture point* and experience seriously maladjustive behavior.

[11] Yates, *Managing Stress,* pp. 23–24.

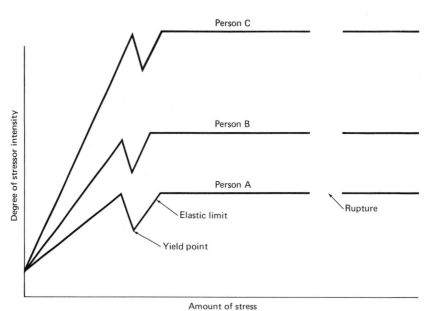

Person C

Person B

Person A

Elastic limit

Rupture

Yield point

Degree of stressor intensity

Amount of stress

Yield Point = mild change from "normal" behavior
Elastic Limit = severe change in "normal" behavior
Rupture = serious maladjustive behavior (nervous breakdown)

Figure 10-3 Elastic limits. [Reprinted by permission of the publisher, *Managing Stress: A Business Person's Guide* by Jere E. Yates (New York: AMACOM, a division of American Management Associations, 1979), p. 23. All rights reserved.]

Every person has a unique elastic limit. Likewise each of us has a different recovery time. In Figure 10-4 we note two different rates of recovery. Person B's threshold (that is, the amount of stress that can be endured) is almost twice that of person A. Equally significant is that B's recover is much more rapid. Person A feels the impact of a great amount of stress for longer periods as can be seen by the gradual slope of the recovery rate line as opposed to the steeper slope of B's recovery rate line. Consequently B can tolerate more stress within a set amount of time and can recover faster than A. Science has yet to determine why some people can bounce back faster than others from stressful situations but we do know heredity and past experiences are a major part of the explanation.[12]

In summary, whenever a demand is placed upon us stress is created. When those demands are enjoyable we are in a state of eustress. However when tension is unrelieved, resulting in lower and lower levels of adaptation energy, we are in a state of distress. Everyone responds to stressful situations differently as reflected in our levels of elasticity and in the amount of time it takes us to recover once the stressful situation has passed.

[12] Ibid., p. 26.

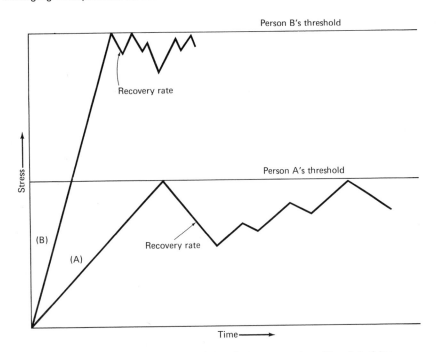

Figure 10-4 Stress thresholds and recovery rates. [Reprinted by permission of the publisher, *Managing Stress: A Business Person's Guide* by Jere E. Yates (New York: AMACOM, a division of American Management Associations, 1979), p. 26. All rights reserved.]

DETERMINANTS OF STRESS: OCCUPATIONAL FACTORS

Figure 10–5 represents a model of stress at work. We want to examine the key variables of this model for it will help us understand how unrelieved tension can lead to the onset of disease and poor mental health. Let us begin by examining five sources of stress found in working environments.

Factors Intrinsic to a Job

A great deal of research has explored the relationship between working conditions and physical and mental well-being. Much of the work has centered on *quantitative and qualitative overload*. Researchers defined quantitative overload as "having too much to do" while qualitative overload means that the work is perceived to be "too difficult."

In 1960, J. G. Miller theorized that "work overload" in most systems leads to breakdown, whether we are dealing with single biological cells or individuals within organizations.[13] This hypothesis has been verified, most

[13] J. G. Miller, "Information Input Overload and Psychopathology," *American Journal of Psychiatry,* 8 (1960), 116.

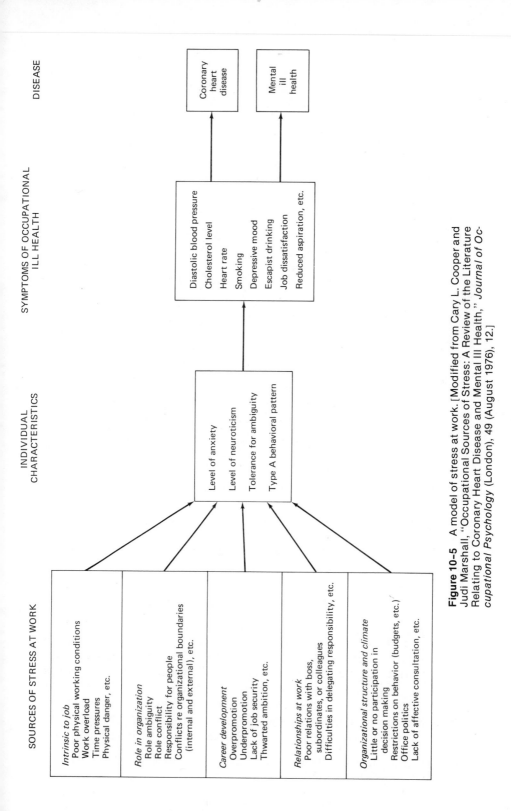

Figure 10-5 A model of stress at work. [Modified from Cary L. Cooper and Judi Marshall, "Occupational Sources of Stress: A Review of the Literature Relating to Coronary Heart Disease and Mental Ill Health," *Journal of Occupational Psychology* (London), 49 (August 1976), 12.]

notably in a study by Russek and Zohman of one hundred young coronary patients. The researchers found that 25 percent of these patients had been working at two jobs prior to the discovery of their coronary problems while an additional 45 percent had worked at jobs that required (due to work overload) sixty or more hours per week. The researcher noted that prolonged emotional strain preceded the heart attack in 91 percent of the cases.[14] In an investigation of mortality rates of men in California, Breslow and Buell found that workers in light industry under the age of forty-five who were on the job more than forty-eight hours per week had twice the risk from coronary heart disease as compared with individuals working forty or fewer hours per week.[15]

Qualitative work overload also takes its toll on workers. When demands are made on workers that are perceived to be "too high" or "unrealistic" workers often blame themselves ("I'm not up to the job") resulting in lower self-esteem. It is interesting to note that when workers believe that the standards are too high their cholesterol levels increase as observed in accountants seeking to meet deadlines and medical students performing in medical examinations.[16] This finding is significant because certain types of cholesterol are believed to be an important risk factor in the occurrence of coronary heart disease.

In brief, quantitative and qualitative work overload is one important source of stress in contemporary work environments. Among the visible effects are job dissatisfaction, increased job tension, lower self-esteem, high cholesterol levels, increased heart rate, increased smoking,[17] escapist drinking, absenteeism from work, and low motivation to work.[18] The significance of this research for administrators becomes clear when it is recognized that 45 percent of the executives in this country work all day, in the evening, and on weekends, and that a further 37 percent keep weekends free but work extra hours in the evenings.[19] In many organizations this type of behavior has become the norm to which most administrative officers feel they must adhere.

---

[14] H. I. Russek and B. L. Zohman, "Relative Significance of Hereditary Diet, and Occupational Stress in CHD of Young Adults," *American Journal of Medicine,* 235 (1958), 266–76.

[15] L. Breslow and P. Buell, "Mortality from Coronary Heart Disease and Physical Activity of Work in California," *Journal of Chronic Disease,* 11 (1960), 615–26.

[16] Cary L. Cooper and Judi Marshal, "Sources of Managerial and White Collar Stress," in *Stress at Work,* ed. C. L. Cooper and R. Payne (New York: John Wiley, 1978), p. 85. The author is indebted to C. L. Cooper for his research into work, stress, and health. One of the most thorough reviews of the research on work and health can be found in *Stress at Work.*

[17] J. R. French and R. D. Caplan, "Psychosocial Factors in Coronary Heart Disease," *Industrial Medicine,* 39 (1979), 383–97.

[18] B. L. Margolis, W. H. Kores, and R. Quinn, "Job Stress: An Untested Occupational Hazard," *Journal of Occupational Medicine,* 16, no. 10 (1974), 654–61.

[19] Cooper and Marshall, "Sources of Managerial and White Collar Stress," p. 85.

Role in the Organization

A great deal of research has focused attention on the stress that results from one's role within an organization. Specifically researchers have examined role ambiguity, role conflict, and role responsibilities.

Role ambiguity takes place when workers have inadequate information about what is expected of them. Usually this implies that work objectives are not clear nor is the scope and responsibility of the job delineated. Earlier we noted that role confusion usually results in conflict. In addition, role ambiguity may have an adverse impact on a worker's health. Researchers are generally agreed that role ambiguity is correlated with lower job satisfaction, high job-related tension, greater sense of futility, and lower self-confidence.[20] Role ambiguity is also correlated with lower motivation to work and a greater intention to leave one's job.[21] One can correctly conclude from these studies that if you have talented subordinates whom you want to retain as employees it is prudent to have explicit position descriptions in order to minimize role ambiguity.

Role conflict is also an important potential stress in contemporary organizations. Such conflicts exists when an "individual in a particular work role is torn by conflicting job demands or doing things he/she really does not want to do or does not think are a part of the job specification."[22]

Most workers feel role conflict when they are caught between the demands of two different groups. Most notably this occurs in mid-level management positions where managers frequently complain that they are caught between the directives of top management and the expectations of subordinates. As might be expected, the more role conflict exists, the more the individual will experience stress and dissatisfaction. In addition, there is a correlation between role conflict and the onset of coronary heart disease, particularly when the role conflict continues over a protracted period of time.[23]

The nature of a worker's *responsibilities* also creates occupational tension. It has been found for example that foremen (high role conflict work) are seven times as likely to develop ulcers as shop floor workers.[24]

Must of the research on the relationship of work responsibilities and heart disease has sought to differentiate "responsibility for people" and "responsibility for things." Since health administrators and health practitioners are more directly involved in being responsible for people as opposed to inanimate objectives, the research has special significance. Generally, if you have responsibility for people you are likely to be under considerably

[20] Ibid., pp. 85–86.

[21] Ibid.

[22] Ibid.

[23] Margolis, Kores, and Quinn, "Job Stress," pp. 654–61.

[24] G. Pincherle, "Fitness for Work," *Proceedings of the Royal Society of Medicine,* 65, no. 4 (1972), 321–24.

more stress than if you are only dealing with things. In a study of 1,200 managers who were sent by their companies for an annual physical examination the researchers found that there was evidence of physical stress linked to age and level of responsibility.[25] The older and more responsive the executive, the greater the probability that there would be coronary heart disease risk factors or symptoms present. It could be argued that the relationship between age and stress-related illness could be explained by the fact that, as the executive gets older, factors other than increased responsibility might be a mitigating factor for the heart disease (for example, a recognition of reaching a career plateau or an awareness of approaching retirement). However, French and Caplan found that responsibility for people does, in fact, play an important role in heightening stress, particularly for managerial and professional workers. Their studies indicate that "responsibility for people was significantly related to heavy smoking, diastolic blood pressure and serum cholesterol levels—the more the individual had responsibility for 'things' as opposed to 'people' the lower were each of these CHD risk factors."[26]

Career Development

It has been suggested that there are two major clusters of potential stressors that can be identified in the area of career development:

1. Lack of job security; fear of obsolescence; fear of early retirement
2. Status incongruity; under or over promotion; frustration at having reached one's career ceiling.[27]

An important personal issue for most administrators is career progression. Most hope that the future is going to be better than the past—a hope that is translated into a desire for a better position, higher salary, higher status, and new work challenges.

In the early years of one's career such hopes are usually achieved. However, at middle age and often at middle-management levels, careers become more problematic. Most executives find their progress slowed if not actually stopped. There are fewer job positions offered, basically because there are fewer good jobs available. The individual may feel locked into a position and may sense that the old way of doing things is no longer being rewarded with additional responsibilities and increased pay. Compounding

[25] John Sweetland, *Occupational Stress and Productivity* (Scarsdale, N.Y.: Work In America Institute, 1979), p. 2.

[26] Cited in Cooper and Marshall, "Sources of Managerial and White Collar Stress," p. 88.

[27] J. Erikson, D. Edwards, and E. K. Gunderson, "Status Congruency and Mental Health," *Psychological Reports,* 33 (1973), 395–401.

the situation is the addition of fresh young recruits, some of whom may leap-frog the middle-aged manager into better positions.

The fear of being demoted or being "put on the shelf" is very strong for those who sense that they have reached their career ceiling. Most workers inevitably suffer some erosion of status before they finally retire. When executives find that their fears are coming true they may blame themselves for not being more aggressive or they may take out their frustration on the organization which they perceive did not give them "a fair shake."

An important inquiry into the relationship of career development to psychological health indicators was undertaken by the U.S. Navy's Neuropsychiatric Unit.[28] The researchers found that sound mental health was positively correlated with opportunities for advancement. As would be expected, dissatisfaction increased as the advancement rates were restrained. Individuals who were less successful in regard to advancement perceived that they had a great deal of stress in their lives.

Relationships at Work

The quality of one's working relationships will have a great deal to do with work satisfaction. If you have colleagues who are supportive and understanding of your point of view and who contribute to your success, it is likely that you will have positive perceptions of your work environment. It has been suggested that good relationships between members of a work group are a central factor in both individual and organizational health.[29] Unfortunately, however, there has been little empirical research undertaken on how working relationships influence occupational stress. One exception to this has been studies on supervisor-subordinate relationships. V. Buck has demonstrated that if you work for a supervisor who has low "consideration" for you, it is likely that you will experience a high level of job tension. In Buck's study, workers under stress reported that their supervisor did not give them helpful criticism, frequently "pulled rank," and "took advantage of them." Buck concluded that behavior of such supervisors greatly contributed to feelings of job pressure.[30]

Organizational Structures and Climate

The fifth potential source of managerial stress comes about from organizational norms that threaten an individual's freedom, autonomy, and identity. Specifically, workers become stressed when they have little or no

[28] Cooper and Marshall, "Sources of Managerial and White Collar Stress," p. 88.
[29] Chris Argyris, *Personality and Organization: The Conflict between System and the Individual* (New York: Harper and Row, 1957), p. 10.
[30] V. Buck, *Working Under Pressure* (London: Staples Press, 1972), p. 68.

participation in the decision-making process, have little sense of belonging, are seldom consulted before a policy is implemented, receive incomplete and at times inaccurate communications from supervisors, and are subject to petty office policies ("Everybody's desk must be cleaned up before going home").

Of the above stressors lack of participation appears to be most significant. It has been repeatedly established that when workers have an opportunity to participate in the decision-making processes of the organization they have greater job satisfaction, a lower incidence of job-related feelings of threat, and higher self-esteem.[31] Conversely, nonparticipation in decisions is correlated with overall poor physical health, escapist drinking, depressed mood, low self-esteem, low life satisfaction, low job satisfaction, low motivation to work, intention to leave job, and absenteeism from work.[32]

In summary, organizational stress emanates from the job itself, the role one has in the organization, career mobility, relationships among co-workers, and the structure and climate of the organization. There are, of course, additional stressors such as salary inequities, authority problems, and regulatory pressures. However, if you want to define the types of occupational stresses that workers most frequently acknowledge, concentrate on the five areas that we have explored.

DETERMINANTS OF STRESS: PSYCHOLOGICAL FACTORS

The work of cardiologists Meyer Friedman and Ray H. Rosenman has made an enormous contribution to our understanding of the relationships among psychological variables, stress, and the onset of coronary heart disease.[33] Friedman and Rosenman have identified two types of personalities which they defined as "Type A" and "Type B."

Type A personalities have a chronic struggle with time. They are always seeking to finish massive amounts of work in the shortest possible time. They are innately competitive and aggressive and frequently have some sort of underlying hostility lying just below the surface waiting to be provoked.

Type B personalities also strive for things worth having. However they are less likely to feel "under pressure." They want to meet deadlines, but if they don't it is not perceived to be a personal failure. Type B personalities have the capacity to play and enjoy simple pleasures in life. When they engage in recreation it is to have fun, not to demonstrate their superiority. Type B personalities know how to relax and can do so without feeling guilty. A summary of some of the key characteristics of Type A and Type B behavior patterns can be found in Figure 10–6.

[31] Margolis, Kores, and Quinn, "Job Stress," pp. 654–61.

[32] Ibid.

[33] Meyer Friedman and Ray H. Rosenman, *Type A Behavior and Your Heart* (New York: Fawcett Crest, 1974).

You possess Type A behavior patterns:

1. If you always move, walk, and eat rapidly.

2. If you feel an impatience with the rate at which most events take place.

3. If you become unduly irritated or even enraged when a car ahead of you in your lane runs at a pace you consider too slow; if you find it anguishing to wait in a line or to wait your turn to be seated in a restaurant.

4. If you find it always difficult to refrain from talking about or bringing the theme of any conversation around to those subjects which especially interest you, and when unable to accomplish this maneuver, you pretend to listen but really remain preoccupied with your own thoughts.

5. If you almost always feel vaguely guilty when you relax and do absolutely nothing for several hours to several days.

6. If you no longer observe the more important or interesting or lovely objects that you encounter in your milieu.

7. If you do not have any time to spare to become the things worth being because you are so preoccupied with getting the things worth having.

You possess Type B behavior patterns:

1. If you are completely free of *all* the habits and exhibit none of the traits we have listed that harass the severely afflicted Type A person.

2. If you never suffer from a sense of time urgency with its accompanying impatience.

3. If when you play you do so to find fun and relaxation, not to exhibit your superiority at any cost.

4. If you can relax without guilt, just as you can work without agitation.

Figure 10-6   Type A and Type B behavior. [From Meyer Friedman and Ray H. Rosenman, *Type A Behavior and Your Heart* (New York: Fawcett Crest, 1974), pp. 100–102.]

It is believed that approximately half of the American population consists of Type A personalities due to the socioeconomic system that consistently rewards many of the values implicit in this type of behavior.[34] Most of us have some mixture of A and B traits, but researchers suggest that one is usually dominant. You can determine the extent to which you have Type A behavior by filling out the questionnaire in Figure 10-7.

The primary health significance of Friedman and Rosenman's research is that the chances of having coronary heart disease dramatically increase for individuals who exhibit Type A behavior. Specifically, Type A men aged 39–49 and 50–59 had 6.5 times and 1.9 times respectively the incidence of coronary heart disease as comparable Type B men.[35] In brief, the stress that individuals bring upon themselves through their personality traits can be a forerunner of debilitating coronary problems.

Additional studies have lent credibility to the premise that personality

[34] Yates, *Managing Stress,* pp. 64–65.
[35] Ibid., p. 67.

SYMPTOMS OF TYPE A BEHAVIOR

Rating

1. To what extent do you hurry the ends of a sentence or explosively accentuate key words even when there is no real need to do so? ____

2. To what extent do you always move, walk, and eat rapidly? ____

3. To what extent do you feel impatient with the rate at which most events progress and openly exhibit your impatience to others? ____

4. To what extent do you strive to think or do two or more things simultaneously? ____

5. To what extent do you always find it difficult to listen to those who don't especially interest you? ____

6. To what extent do you always feel vaguely guilty when you relax and do absolutely nothing for several hours to several days? ____

7. To what extent do you no longer observe the more important or interesting or lovely objects in your environment? ____

8. To what extent do you attempt to schedule more and more activities in less and less time? ____

9. If you meet another severely afflicted Type A person, to what extent do you find yourself compelled to challenge him instead of feeling compassion for him? ____

10. To what extent do you resort to certain characteristic gestures or nervous tics? ____

11. To what extent do you believe that your success is due in good part to your ability to get things done faster than anyone else, and are you afraid to stop doing everything faster and faster? ____

12. To what extent are you increasingly committed to evaluating in numerical terms not only your own behavior but also the behavior of others? ____

Total Score ____

Instructions: On a scale of 0–10 with 10 being extremely high and 0 being extremely low rate yourself. Consider 5 to be an "average" person's response to each question. Add up your ratings. If you score higher than 60 it is likely that you have a Type A personality. You might want a co-worker to confirm your score.

Figure 10-7 Questionnaire to determine Type A behavior. [Reprinted by permission of the publisher, *Managing Stress: A Business Person's Guide* by Jere E. Yates (New York: AMACOM, a division of American Management Associations, 1979), p. 67. All rights reserved.]

variables influence levels of stress and subsequently physical and mental well-being. One of the most intriguing studies was undertaken by G. R. Gernill and W. I. Heister who set out to investigate the relationship between "Machiavellianism" and job strain, job satisfaction, positional mobility, and perceived opportunities for formal control. Machiavellianism is defined as a tendency to manipulate and persuade others, to initiate and control in group situations, and generally to be a "winner"—all symptoms of Type A behavior. High Machiavellian scorers were, overall, much less happy in their jobs. They exhibited considerably more job strain then did low scorers and they feel that they had fewer opportunities to exert control over their work environment.[36]

It is important to monitor work routines and work habits. If you are a Type A individual, it would be to your advantage to modify your behavior. Modification does not imply that one should give up goal directive and competitive behavior. But modification does imply that periodically you should pull back, regain your adaptive energy, and pause to enjoy *being* as much as doing. By so doing you will place yourself at lower risk in terms of heart disease; equally important you will become more effective in realizing your goals due to the fact that your mental and physical energy has been replenished.

THE STRESS RESPONSE: OCCUPATIONAL BURNOUT

In the preceding paragraphs we learned that stress emanates from both organizational and personal considerations. We have seen that unrelieved tension can have an adverse affect on both the individual and the organization. But how does stress actually take its toll on one's health? How does stress erode positive feelings about our work and our careers?

During the past twelve years Dr. James Spradley, an urban anthropologist, and I have been investigating job stress. Initially Dr. Spradley focused on Peace Corp volunteers[37] and fishermen working on the shores of British Columbia, Canada.[38] My work began with an investigation of stress associated with health administration, particularly the stress felt by mid-level managers working within urban hospitals.[39] Since that time we have turned to other occupations—more than one hundred in all. We have talked with nurses, college professors, service station attendants, veterinarians, window washers, public health workers, psychologists, housewives, social workers, probation officers, and publishers, to name only a few of the other fields. We found that intense occupational stress, while more prevalent in some occupations, affects all of them.

We had a single purpose in our investigations and that was to get beneath the surface of everyday jobs. We wanted to probe the feelings that people have about their work and how those attitudes impinge on how they

---

[36] G. R. Gernill and W. J. Heister, "Machiavellianism as a Factor in Managerial Job Strain, Job Satisfaction and Upward Mobility," *Academy of Management Journal,* 15, no. 1 (1972), 51–62.

[37] Spradley and Phillips, "Culture and Stress: A Quantitative Analysis."

[38] James P. Spradley, *Guests Never Leave Hungry: The Autobiography of a Kwakiutl Indian* (New Haven: Yale University Press, 1969).

[39] Robert Veninga, "A Case Study in Organization Development: The Role of Communication," Ph.D. dissertation, University of Minnesota, Minneapolis, 1972.

view their lives and the lives of family members. We looked for the hidden meanings that work takes for all of us. We sought to discover why some people suffer intense stress, while others, doing essentially the same tasks, remain free of most of the stress symptoms. In addition to anthropological field work that involved on-the-job observations, we conducted in-depth interviews and asked workers to fill out open-ended questionnaires. Our basic goal was to identify the cultural patterns associated with work in our society. Specifically, we wanted to identify the range of job pressures, trace their consequences, and find out how people managed stress on the job.

One of the conclusions of our research is that workers can "burn out" on their jobs. We define job burnout as a debilitating psychological condition brought about by *unrelieved* work stress, resulting in:

1. Depleted energy reserves
2. Lowered resistance to illness
3. Increased dissatisfaction and pessimism
4. Increased absenteeism and inefficiency at work

There are several key concepts in the above definition. The first is *unrelieved stress*. Most everyone experiences stress in their work. For some it may be the stress that comes from trying to balance a budget that is already bent out of shape by unexpected expenditures. For others it may emanate from the tension of working in an emergency room or surgical suite. For others it may come from standing in the same two- or three-foot area for eight hours a day, packaging tiny computer parts that come down an assembly line. Each of these situations places special demands on workers—a stress to which they must respond.

Most of the time, workers can cope with these stressors. They take a vacation or a long weekend and find that when they return they are better able to cope with those aspects of their job that seem to grind them down. Or they develop strong social support systems with colleagues. They may bowl together or go to a football game or two. They may even help one another when the work demands become too great. In brief, they have successfully adapted to a stressful work environment.

A problem emerges, however, when the stress is not relieved. The tension goes on day after day, month after month, and perhaps year after year. And, when workers do not help one another, when there is no hope of reducing the tensions, when there is little possibility of being promoted out of a dead-end job, when the worker suddenly realizes that the situation is not likely to change for the better, the worker becomes aware that his or her *energy reserves are severely depleted.*

When workers shared with us their perceptions of being burned out they usually spoke of exhaustion, weariness, and loss of enthusiasm. They complained of feeling "bone tired." Frequently they noted that they were so preoccupied with their work problems that their sleep patterns were disrupted.

As the stress continues, there is *lowered resistance to illness.* Dr. Carroll Brodskey, a physician at the University of California Medical School in San Francisco, studied the way in which work stress led to illness in prison guards and teachers. He found that two-thirds of those he studied suffered from diseases such as ulcers, hypertension, arthritis, and mental problems—most commonly depression.[40]

The exact manner in which work stress lowers one's resistance to illness and contributes to disease is not fully known. Yet numerous scientific studies have demonstrated that stress is implicated in many serious illnesses. One of the best-known studies, which surveyed NASA personnel working on space flights, demonstrated a causal relationship between coronary artery disease and stressful jobs.[41]

Unrelieved stress also leads to *dissatisfaction and pessimism.* Again and again we found that as workers live with unrelieved stress the jobs that they once enjoyed turned sour. The head of personnel in a large organization who recognized his own symptoms of job stress stated: "I started noticing a definite change in how I felt about my job. Like staff meetings. I used to eagerly look forward to them but now I dread them like the plague. I'm just too tired to put up with the hassles."[42]

Finally, job burnout leads to an increase in *absenteeism and inefficiency at work.* The Laboratory of Clinical Stress Research at Sweden's renowned Caroline Institute has estimated that one-third of the working days lost to sickness in industrialized nations are attributable to stress-connected diseases.[43] As burnout sets in even those days spent in work become less productive as workers take longer coffee breaks, take longer to accomplish tasks, make more mistakes, and put off tasks that require immediate attention. The financial costs of such actions are high. The U.S. Clearinghouse for Mental Health Information recently reported that U.S. industry has experienced a $17 billion annual decrease in its productive capacity over the past few years due to stress-induced mental dysfunctions. Other studies estimate even greater losses (at least $60 billion) arising from stress-induced physical illness.[44]

---

[40] Carroll M. Brodsky, "Long-Term Work Stress in Teachers and Prison Guards," *Journal of Occupational Medicine,* 19, no. 2 (February 1977), 133–38.

[41] J. R. P. French and R. D. Caplan, "Organizational Stress and Individual Stress" in *The Failure of Success,* ed. A. J. Marrow (New York: AMACOM, 1975), pp. 30–66.

[42] Veninga and Spradley, *The Work/Stress Connection,* p. 10.

[43] Jim Hampton, "Stress—the Enemy Within," *National Observer,* February 8, 1975, p. 8.

[44] Applebaum, "Managerial/Organizational Stress," p. 8.

Stages of Burnout[45]

Like the human life cycle, job burnout goes through distinct stages. It begins when one is under continuous stress resulting in lower and lower energy reserves. This can take place within a few weeks after one has taken a new and demanding job or after ten or fifteen years of work on an old job.

We found that burnout progresses through five stages, each more serious than the last. However, we learned that no two people experience these stages of burnout in exactly the same way. One worker may stay in the earliest stage of burnout for many years, then rapidly progress to a later crisis stage. Another may quickly move through each stage, then recover and remain free of burnout symptoms. While we were able to identify certain symptons in each stage, wide variations existed. One person may have mild tension headaches in an early stage while another person may not have headaches at all. It is for this reason that it is important to have a broad picture of the stages of burnout, recognizing that the symptoms may differ from one person to another.

Stage 1: Job contentment Most workers begin their jobs with enthusiasm and a desire to succeed. They often enjoy the exhilarating stress of learning new things, meeting new people, and providing their competence. Consider Bobby McDonald who vividly remembers the first day after his promotion to vice-president of a large firm. "I went to my office for the first time. It was really beautiful. The staff had put a beautiful plant on my desk wishing me luck. The president came by and shook my hand and told me how much he was looking forward to working with me. He left the office and I felt a big smile come over my face. I thought to myself, 'All the hard work was worth it.'"

If this first stage continues, workers often report that they are perfectly matched with their jobs. What stress they experience gives meaning to their work and adds to their sense of fulfillment. They usually report that "work is my love; I'd rather do it than anything else."

Two important developments take place in this stage. The first is that, in spite of the individual's enthusiasm, even enjoyable stress will use up important adaptation energy. Although the psychological bills may not come due for months or even years to come, unless the worker has learned to replenish valuable adaptation energy, he or she may later feel the effects of having too little energy to do the necessary tasks.

The second important development during the first stage is that habits of

---

[45] In *The Work/Stress Connection* Dr. James Spradley and I have used different wording to convey the meaning of these five stages to the general public. The stages as defined with slightly altered concepts are (1) honeymoon, (2) energy shortage, (3) chronic symptoms, (4) crises, and (5) hitting the wall.

dealing with stress are being established. If the individual develops adequate coping mechanisms, the job contentment stage can go on for years. If sound coping mechanisms are not implemented the burnout process may begin in earnest.[46]

Stage 2: Job disappointment   The first tangible sign that the burnout process has begun takes place in this stage. Generally, workers indicate a sense of disappointment in how things are turning out for them in their jobs. There usually is little bitterness, only a quiet resignation that the job did not turn out to be all that one had hoped. A typical comment was expressed by an attorney who had joined a law firm a year earlier: "Well, I thought it was going to work out better than it has. But I suppose I was a little naive. Not many clients appreciate what you do for them and most of your colleagues don't care."[47] It is interesting that those who have entered this second stage are often amused by those who still charge around with the idealism that is often seen in stage 1. When a young, idealistic law student took an internship in his law firm, the same attorney smiled and muttered to himself, "He'll get over it."[48]

In this stage workers often complained about being "overloaded." "There's just too much to do in too little time," said a public health nutritionist. A head nurse commented: "I'm always rushed and never can give the kind of patient care that I would like. And then there are the meetings. My God, the meetings never seem to stop. And they are so unproductive."

The feeling that we are overworked is a common feeling shared by many individuals. In a nationwide study conducted by the Labor Department, 42 percent of the respondents said that they never seemed to have enough time to get everything done on their jobs.[49]

The feeling of being overworked is particularly acute in the human services. "There is so much need," stated a welfare case worker, "that I could continue working around the clock and still not take care of all the problems." As Harry Wasserman has noted, stress is particularly experienced by the human service worker who continually faces emergency situations in which he can be "overwhelmed by the cumulative impact, perhaps the cumulative terror of a large number of cases—by the human suffering, deprivation, disorder, ignorance, hostility, and cruelty he must face as a part of his everyday work situation."[50] One of the surprises we had in our research

---

[46] Veninga and Spradley, *The Work/Stress Connection,* pp. 55–56.

[47] Ibid., p. 61.

[48] Ibid., p. 62.

[49] Robert P. Quinn and Graham L. Staines, *The 1977 Quality of Employment Survey* (Ann Arbor: Survey Research Center, University of Michigan, 1979), p. 88.

[50] Harry Wasserman, "Early Careers of Professional Social Workers in a Public Child Welfare Agency," *Social Work,* 15 (July 1970), 96.

was learning how frequently nurses reported that they dream about their patients. Obviously, even while sleeping, they are still on the job.

Perhaps the primary characteristic of individuals in the second stage of burnout is their sense of mental fatigue. General fatigue is the body's first line of defense against too much stress. It's hardly any wonder, therefore, that workers who had been living with unrelieved stress for months and even years told us that they had "learned to wake up tired."

When we confronted feelings of exhaustion we would often ask harassed workers why they didn't take time off in order to recoup their energy reserves. One health administrator stated: "Oh no. I couldn't take time off now. There is simply too much to do."

It is interesting to note that 64 percent of the workers in this country indicate that they do not have a lot of energy left over when they get off of work. More than one out of four state that they become tired in what they considered to be a short period of time. When asked if they would rather have a 10 percent pay raise or work fewer hours per week, 37 percent indicated that they would rather have a shorter work week. Even in a period of double-digit inflation, nearly one in five indicated that they would opt for less tiring work over a 10 percent raise in pay.[51]

Stage 3: Job disillusionment Two factors seem to differentiate individuals from the second and third stage of burnout. The first is the tone of the conversation. In the second stage, the workers speak matter of factly about their work situation. They may complain about how overloaded they are, but it is seldom in anger. In the third stage, however, the burnout victim is angry and resentful. The person resembles a volcano, always on the verge of eruption.

Not only are they angry, but burned out workers in this stage frequently distance themselves from their clients. In Christina Maslach's pioneering work on burnout victims she noted that derogatory terms are frequently used to describe clients. "They're all just animals" or "They come out from under the rocks" were comments she heard while undertaking her research. She also noted that clients were often referred to in abstract terms such as "the poor" or "my case load" or "my docket."[52] Seymour Schubin in investigating burnout of nurses saw a similar distancing. A supervisor noted: "The main sign of burnout that I've noticed in ICU personnel is that they become more *technical*; their primary concerns are the *machines*—not the *patients*. When you ask them how their patients are doing, their first comment is that the machines are okay or the signs are okay, but they don't refer directly to the patients. For example, they might say, 'Well, his blood pressure's good' or 'His sinus rhythm is good,' but they never state directly how the patient says

[51] Quinn and Staines, *Quality of Employment Survey,* p. 51.

[52] Christina Maslach, "Burned Out," *Human Behavior,* September 1976, pp. 16–17.

he's feeling or how he might actually look. It's never a central answer. It's more peripheral. They won't answer about the whole patient, but rather about one system at a time—his kidneys or heart or blood pressure."[53]

In stage 3, relationships between co-workers often become severely strained. As Herbert J. Freudenberger notes:

> The burn-out candidate finds it just too difficult to hold in feelings. He or she either is, or feels, so overburdened that the slightest occurrence can set them off . . . a word, a felt slight, a small disappointment, not to mention an outright tirade, criticism, or abuse. With the anger such an individual feels, there may also be a suspicious attitude, a paranoia that evolves. The burn-out victim begins to feel that just about everyone is out to screw him—and this can include his own brothers and sisters on the staff."[54]

Maslach notes that the burned out victim not only may be angry with colleagues but will even begin to believe that the clients somehow deserve any problems they have. As one psychiatric nurse reported to Maslach: "Sometimes you can't help but feel, 'Damn it, they want to be there, and they're fuckers, so let them stay there.' You really put them down. . . . "[55]

In the later part of this stage we found that burned out workers would frequently begin to treat their work "as a job." They put in their hours. They tried to avoid all conflict situations. But they didn't arrive at work one minute early and they certainly didn't stay any longer than what was absolutely necessary.

The health problems in this third stage were indicative of the toll that stress had taken. A U.S. Air Force officer, talking about his stressful job, said: "I become almost physically ill. My body aches like I have a viral illness. I get tension headaches and am nauseated." A finance officer in a bank said: "About three o'clock almost every day I'd need an aspirin; my head would pound. And after a meeting my head would throb."[56] Maslach found that burnout often led to a deterioration of physical well-being including exhaustion, more frequent sickness, insomnia, ulcers, and migraine headaches.[57] In coping with these problems workers frequently turned to tranquilizers, drugs, and alcohol—all solutions that have the potential for being abused. It is a sobering fact that in a given year 599 million diazepam (Valium) tablets are consumed in the United States.[58]

---

[53] Shubin, "Burnout," p. 25.

[54] Herbert J. Freudenberger, "The Staff Burn-out Syndrome in Alternative Institutions," *Psychotherapy Theory: Research and Practice,* 12, no. 1 (Spring 1975), 53.

[55] Maslach, *Burned Out,* p. 16.

[56] Veninga and Spradley, *The Work/Stress Connection,* p. 87.

[57] Maslach, *Burned Out,* p. 19.

[58] Applebaum, "Managerial/Organizational Stress," p. 8.

Stage 4: Job despair   A frequent word used by individuals in the fourth stage of burnout is the word "trapped." Frequently this word was used by professional workers. A public health dentist said: "I have gone to school for nine years. My education cost me over fifty thousand dollars. How can I walk away from that investment?" The lines of tension were deeply etched into his face. As we talked, it was evident that he perceived himself to be as dead-ended in his career as a man on an assembly line who has little hope for advancement.

One of the questions we asked in our written questionnaires was, "How would you feel if you had to continue your present job for the rest of your life?" A social worker said, "Horrible. I would feel pinned down; locked into a position where there would be very little sense of achievement." A dental hygienist responded, "Totally defeated. There would be little to look forward to." A clergyman under extreme criticism from his congregation said, "The thought of staying in my job for the rest of my life is nothing less than a nightmare."

When workers give up hope and are in a stage of crisis, they find that their burnout symptoms become even more critical. The chronic acid stomach is now a bleeding peptic ulcer. The tension headaches are exasperated by chronic backaches, high blood pressure, and difficulty in sleeping. Perhaps most importantly, burned out individuals become obsessed with their problems. Dramatic evidence of this is seen in Brodsky's study of teachers and prison guards.[59] The subjects had very few waking moments when their thoughts were not back on the job. They thought about work as they were driving home and as they watched TV. Falling asleep became difficult because of their preoccupation, going over and over the argument with the principal, the fear of a prisoner's threats, the responsibilities that were before them. Increasingly, they became aware that "this job is bad for me, the problem isn't going to go away."[60]

Unfortunately, when he is in a crisis stage the burned out victim begins to doubt himself and his competence. The wife of a young attorney who failed his bar exam for the third time told us: "Ron has really changed; he's so down I can't even get him to talk about it. He hasn't told anyone at the office that he failed the exam. It's like nothing has happened on the outside, but underneath that's all he thinks about. He doubts that he has any ability at all."

Stage 5: Work redefined   We can see a clear progression during the first stages of job burnout. In the first stage individuals are satisfied with their work, even exhilarated about it. They use their energy in constructive ways as they seek to do their job in a competent manner. Some will form sound work

[59] Brodsky, "Long-Term Work Stress," p. 135.
[60] Ibid., p. 135.

and rest routines that will keep them from burning out. Others, however, soon begin to feel that the job isn't all that they had hoped and the first indication of job dissatisfaction is apparent. They will complain in the second stage of how overloaded they are and note their tiredness in trying to meet needs of clients or deadlines imposed by their supervisor. In the third stage the worker becomes angry at the real imagined injustices that they are experiencing. They often seek to cope by distancing and detaching themselves from colleagues and the people they are to be serving. They frequently become physically ill. In the fourth stage the worker feels trapped; the burnout symptoms become acute, often resulting in serious physiological and psychological problems.

In stage 5 the worker redefines the job. Some are forced out of their job for their health no longer permits them to work. The results are often tragic, particularly for those who would like to return to work but are not able to due to health. Others resign their positions and angrily denounce colleagues as they leave their employer for the last time. Frequently they do not understand the complex psychological and organizational factors that have caused their stress. Often they take a similar job in another organization and become burn-out repeaters.

Other workers come to grips with the fact that they have burned out and that their attitudes are destructive not only to themselves but to family members and their employer. They want to change. They want to become more productive and they want to recapture the positive feelings about work that they once had. But most of all they want to recapture their health and mental well-being.

In the following section we will learn specific strategies to avoid job burnout. What works for one person may not work for another. Nevertheless we want to define some of the most effective strategies that individuals use to keep mentally and physically healthy.

STRATEGIES FOR PREVENTING OCCUPATIONAL BURNOUT

One of the goals of our research was to identify individuals who had re-covered from burnout and to learn of the strategies that they employed to regain their physical and mental health. Regardless of which strategy they followed, we noted that those who recovered had a keen understanding of the interrelationship of work and health.

Becoming Conscious of the Consequences of Work Stress

The beginning point in recovering from job burnout is to be aware of how work influences your health. Unfortunately, because our interactions with stress go on almost continuously they become routines that slip into the less-conscious recesses of our minds. Take for example a thirty-two-year-old college professor who had become very bitter about the teaching profession. Over the years he had grown accustomed to the fact that his schedule was so full that it left little time for exercise and relaxation. In helping him become aware of the stress he was experiencing we asked him to write a "log" of all the major events that took place at work in a given week. When he handed us the log he commented: "I can't believe all the things that happened last week. I met with sixteen students, most of whom wanted to talk at length about their problems. I taught for a total of sixteen hours. The dean told me that unless I get some things published I probably wouldn't have my contract renewed—which really disturbed me. I gave two speeches for the college last week and attended four committee meetings. And, as my wife pointed out, I was out four out of the five evenings to a professional meeting or doing business for the school."

After reviewing the many demands on his time the college professor paused and said: "No wonder I feel the way I do. No mortal could do a good job on all those things." The beginning of his recovery was marked with a determination to get his stressful life under control. He talked over this job description with the head of the department, who agreed that his advising load was too heavy. He began to set priorities, something he always had difficulty doing but which now gave him a sense of accomplishment at the end of a workweek. But perhaps most importantly he came upon a particularly important perception about himself: "For years I have lived less than healthy. It's not that I have been sick—it's just that I have not been healthy."

The feeling that "I'm not totally healthy" is a common perception of individuals who become aware of the effects of work stress on their lives. In a recent study by the State Department of Mental Health in California only one-third of the adults surveyed indicated that they were in top health either physically or emotionally.[61] Fortunately many are becoming aware of not being in top shape, sometimes with the help of their employer. The New York Life Extension Institute conducts 40,000 health examinations annually and has found that psychological stress signs are becoming epidemic when compared with similar data collected in 1958. The observable signs included early retirement, alcohol consumption, sleeping difficulties, neurotic competition, and other problems. When employees become aware at the time of their physical examination of what job stress is doing to their well-being a strong motivator emerges helping them alter their work and health behavior.[62]

One of the benefits that comes when individuals recognize the consequences of work stress in their lives is that they tend to feel less guilty about their feelings. The pervasive attitude of burned out individuals frequently is, "I am to blame. . . . Something is wrong with me for feeling exhausted, for getting sick, for having headaches, for not keeping up at work, for failing to

---

[61] "Most Californians Don't Feel Healthy," *Minneapolis Star,* June 18, 1980, p. 10A.
[62] Sweetland, *Occupational Stress,* p. 2.

handle the conflicts at home." The litany goes on and on, but the theme is always the same: "I am the one at fault for my problems."

Dr. Maslach has noted that guilt is a common reaction of workers under stress and at times the guilt is reinforced by colleagues.

> By turning the heat on themselves, helping professionals begin to make more self-deprecatory remarks, to question their suitability for this line of work, and in general to lose those qualities which are essential for a helping professional, namely self-confidence, sense of humor, and a balanced perspective. The alleged personal flaws of helping professionals do not go unnoticed by critics who are willing to argue whether the matter involves a lack of ability, a motivational deficit, or a character defect. "He's a cold fish," "She hasn't got a brain in her head," "You have to be crazy to be a psychiatrist," "What can you expect from cops, since they are all sadistic types to begin with," so goes the diagnostic analysis.[63]

When you begin to feel guilty and blame yourself, the possibility for recovery is diminished. As Dr. Herbert Adler, Associate Professor of Psychiatry at Hahneman Medical College in Philadelphia, states, "When it [guilt] runs amok inside, it can—quite literally—paralyze us, making us totally unable to function as human beings."[64]

The starting point in recovery from job burnout is to examine the points of stress in your work life. Explain your job to a friend and hear yourself describe the demands that are made on your time. You may want to write down all the difficult and taxing situations you experience in a given workday. You may be surprised at the number of stressful work situations you encounter as well as the intensity of them. A busy writer and consultant told us: "I used to just plow into my work without much thought. It didn't occur to me that some things might be more stressful than others. Then I began analyzing it with my wife and discovered something I hadn't realized. My major stress came from bringing work home every night, thinking I may work if I feel up to it or maybe I won't. But at least it will be there if I decide to work. But here's what happens. On those nights I decide to work, I have trouble sleeping and the work I do isn't very good. But here's the real catch: If I don't work I feel guilty all evening and I still have trouble sleeping!"[65] Once this writer's consciousness was raised about this conflict he made one minor, yet significant change in his work routine: Two nights of the week he would bring work home; the others he defined as "my recuperation period." This brought him just enough relief to bring his life back on keel. His leisure evenings became more enjoyable and his work evenings more productive.

[63] Christina Maslach, "Burnout: A Social Psychological Analysis," paper presented to the American Psychological Association, San Francisco, August 1977, p. 3.
[64] Lester Davis, "The Many Faces of Guilt," *Family Health,* July 1977, p. 22.
[65] Veninga and Spradley, *The Work/Stress Connection,* p. 119.

Developing Space from Work

In *Every Employee a Manager,* M. Scott Meyers suggests that it is not uncommon to encounter "overcommitment to the job." When an individual is overcommitted he is deprived of a well-rounded life.

> [He] rarely has enough energy and time left over from his company duties to attend to his personal and professional growth, his family and community responsibilities. . . . The more engaged he becomes in the pursuit of meaningful goals on the job, the more tunnel visioned he becomes and the more disengaged he becomes from involvement with the members of his family, and hence, the less opportunity he has to experience goal setting within family and community units. Moreover, his family's familiarity with his vocational role is usually so fragmentary that it offers little opportunity for them to experience his achievements vicariously.[66]

The solution to being "overcommitted" at work is to develop space from work. The concept of "space" emerges from the writings of Kahlil Gibran, who suggested that whenever one becomes totally absorbed in one entity other aspects of life are negated.[67] Gibran suggests that if individuals are to discover their creative potential they must enter into many realms of human existence. Any person, movement, activity, or working situation that demands an investment of one's total psychological energy slowly diminishes one's ability to creatively relate to other aspects of life that bring meaning and fulfillment.

The development of space from work might be defined as a willingness to become involved in the issues and problems confronting other disciplines. Individuals who become overcommitted to their narrow area of interest slowly shrink into a highly discipline-oriented existence. Over time, such individuals find it difficult to relate to any discipline other than their own.

We found many instances where health professionals were able to cope with their stressful work environments by broadening their interests. A public health nurse, for example, found relief by serving on the board of directors of a Development Achievement Center, an organization for mentally retarded children. A hospital administrator, caught in the cross fire between a powerful board of trustees and an equally powerful medical staff, became a member of the Citizen's League and chaired an consumer committee looking into mass transportation for his community. He discovered new friends and came to look forward to their weekly Tuesday morning breakfast meetings as a needed breather from the continuous pressures he was experiencing within his hospital. A welfare case worker, besieged by a high case load, was able to get permission to be away from the office one afternoon a week in order to attend

[66] M. Scott Meyers, *Every Employee a Manager* (New York: McGraw-Hill, 1970), p. 40.
[67] Kahlil Gibran, *The Prophet* (New York: Knopf, 1923), pp. 15–16.

two courses at the University of Minnesota. That one afternoon away from the pain and suffering of her clients gave her just enough relief to be able to continue working in a stressful environment.

The development of interests outside of work should include a regular exercise program. Dr. George Williams, Director of the Institute of Health Research in San Francisco, believes that exercise is one of the most effective ways of counteracting work stress. He suggests that exercise works as a stress inoculation, not only relieving the pressure after the end of a hectic day, but making it possible for you to deal more effectively with the stress the next day.[68]

The research on exercising is now beginning to appear and its significance for the health of workers is being documented. Scientists studied a group of workers at Exxon's physical fitness lab in New York and found that after only six months of exercise, their workers had an increased capacity for work. Most reported they felt less tired at the end of a work day.[69] Dr. John Greist of the University of Wisconsin tested the value of jogging as a treatment for depression, one of the major symptoms of burnout. He divided depressed patients into two groups. One underwent psychotherapy, the other began jogging. At the end of ten weeks those who exercised showed more improvement than those undergoing psychotherapy.[70] A Soviet factory introduced a running program for its employees and absenteeism due to sickness dropped dramatically. Days lost went from 436 per year to 42.[71] It has been found, furthermore, that regular exercise may be helpful in preventing coronary heart disease.

Exercise does not have to be competitive in order to achieve the above results. An ideal workout should last about one-half hour using the first five or six minutes to slowly build the pulse rate with warm-up exercises followed by vigorous exercise for about eighteen minutes and then five minutes of cooling down exercise. The warm-up is necessary to prevent a sudden taxing of the heart and other muscles while the cool-down exercise prevents pooling of the blood in the musculature, which can result in dizziness or faintness. Such an exercise routine should be undertaken three or four times a week.[72]

If you do not want to jog consider a brisk walking program. Dr. Arthur Leon and his associates have found that individuals who engage in ninety minutes of walking a day for sixteen weeks (a) lose excess fat and weight, (b) gain muscle, which offsets some, but not much of the lost weight in fat, (c)

[68] "How to Deal with Stress on the Job," pp. 80–81.
[69] James F. Fixx, *The Complete Book of Running* (New York: Random House, 1977), p. 28.
[70] Cited ibid., p. 16.
[71] Ibid., p. 6.
[72] Herbert Weinberg, "Role of Heartbeat Reveals a Great Deal about Physical Condition," *Minneapolis Tribune,* September 30, 1979, p. 8A.

change their appetite so that they don't hunger for more food than they need, and perhaps (d) improve their body's ability to clear cholesterol deposits out of the linings of arteries.[73]

In initiating an exercise program it is important to build up gradually to vigorous activity. In Leon's study the subjects began with only fifteen-minute walks. If there are pains, cramps, or other ill effects, back off the exercise program. To be on the safe side have a complete physical examination.

The importance of developing a sound exercise program cannot be overemphasized. It was very rare that we found anyone in the third or fourth stage of burnout who was exercising on a regular basis. Conversely, practically all those suffering from the more serious burnout symptoms were living sedentary lives, often eating, smoking, and drinking in an effort to cope with their work stress.

Setting Challenging Yet Realistic Goals

When under stress most individuals have difficulty prioritizing their tasks. "I never know what I am going to get hit with when I walk in the office at the beginning of the day," said a supervisor of fourteen social workers. "At the end of the day I find that I have responded to most everybody's request, but when I ask what I have accomplished, I sometimes really don't know."

Individuals who are able to prevent job burnout have a keen understanding of the importance of setting priorities. Several types of goal problems seem to affect burned out workers. First, they often have *too many goals*. An executive wearied from grueling fourteen-hour workdays aptly summarized the problem: "I simply do not know how to delegate. I try to do everything myself and of course there is no problem that I don't try to solve. After awhile it just grinds you down."

Some workers are *uncertain about their goals* and this too leads to dissatisfaction. The supervisor of the fourteen social workers is a case in point. She conscientiously responds when there is a complaint from clients, she quickly meets with staff members if they have a problem, and she is always the first to volunteer to serve on any agency committee. However, when we asked, "What is it that you are specifically trying to accomplish in this agency?" there was a blank stare. Although she was very busy, she could not verbalize how her work was going to lead to the achievement of any predetermined goal.

It is not only possible to have too many goals but to have *overly high expectations* about realizing them in a short period of time. Darrell Sifford has noted that stress comes when you "peek at reality and see a discrepancy be-

---

[73] Cited in Gordon Slovut, "A Brisk Walk away from Fat," *Minneapolis Star,* October 15, 1979, p. 7B.

tween your high expectations and what's actually happening to you."[74] Borrowing from one of the fundamental principles in the PERT process, we have found it helpful to ask managers to list their goals and then establish three types of deadlines: (1) a minimum deadline reflecting the shortest amount of time it will take to achieve the goal, (2) a maximum deadline, and (3) the "best estimate" deadline. This exercise helps managers to think realistically about the amount of time it will take to finish a task and consequently helps them avoid the feeling of panic that emerges when an unrealistic deadline has been set.

Finally, it is important to have in your list of work goals at least one that has personal meaning for you. In working over goal statements of managers we often ask them to identify one goal that has intrinsic meaning. As they look over their goal statements we look for the grin and the "fire in the eyes" as they come across one that has a great deal of meaning. "If I don't accomplish anything else this year," said a nursing executive, "I'm going to make certain that the board understands why it is that turnover in this hospital is so great." If there isn't at least one goal that has strong personal meaning, the probability increases that the worker's commitment to the job will slowly but very definitely erode.

Developing Social Support

A number of studies have produced strong evidence indicating the importance of the work group to an employee's mental health.[75] As we earlier noted, the "human relations" approach to the workplace emphasized the role of social relationships in achieving a satisfying and rewarding work environment. There is new evidence that the individual's work group may provide effective social support which not only permits workers to cope with stress on the job, but also diminishes the threat of coronary heart disease.[76]

We viewed many situations where colleagues eagerly sought to help one another cope with job pressures. Some of the most helpful social support systems we found were in nursing units. We met three nurses who work in pediatric oncology unit who have breakfast with one another every Monday morning. "We sit and talk about our weekends, but we also talk about our patients. We work in a tough environment. There are kids with terminal diseases, parents who are extremely worried, and colleagues who demand that we be mentally sharp. But sometimes we don't feel sharp and sometimes we

---

[74] Darrell Sifford, "Some Methods of Coping with Stress," *Philadelphia Inquirer,* April 4, 1978, p. 22.

[75] See, for example, Chris Argyris, *Interpersonal Competence and Organizational Effectiveness* (London: Tavistock, 1962).

[76] Cary L. Cooper and John Crump, "Prevention and Coping with Occupational Stress," *Journal of Occupational Medicine,* 20, no. 6 (1978), 48.

just don't feel that we can cope with all the suffering. So one day we decided that we would meet once a week and see if we couldn't assist one another."[77]

The idea of having one really good friend whom you can contact when the going gets rough has been pioneered by Alcoholics Anonymous. Local A.A. groups usually have a "buddy system" in which every member has the name and telephone number of someone whom they can call twenty-four hours a day. Many recovered alcoholics have had a buddy who threw them a life preserver when they were about to go under for the third time. We all need psychological life preservers when the pressures of work are churning around us. A good friend is about the best insurance policy one can have.

Practicing Relaxation Techniques

The stress response goes through three processes: mobilization in preparation to meet a demand, energy consumption, and then a return to equilibrium. This last stage is when relaxation naturally occurs and our body restores itself. There are a number of ways we can accentuate the restoration process.

Planning ahead   It may seem strange to think of planning as a relaxation activity, but for many people the very act of planning for the future is therapeutic. An individual who thinks about forthcoming events and the potential stressors that may arise is seemingly in a better position to make a proactive adaptive response than the individual who rushes headlong and blindly from one life event to the next.

The most important time period in the workday may be the last thirty minutes. One executive noted: "When it's 4:00 p.m. my secretary knows that I will not take any more calls. Nor will I see anyone else. I clean up my desk and I think about the following day and what I want to accomplish. Then I take out a small three-by-five card and write down what I hope to accomplish in the morning and I put it on top of my calendar. That's the first thing I see when I arrive at work and it keeps me focused on what I want to accomplish. When I leave the office I feel that I am in control of my work life."

Relaxing at work   One of the best ways to diminish the tension is to creatively use coffee and lunch breaks to restore your mental energy. Unfortunately the contemporary coffee break often increases rather than decreases our tension. It is known, for example, that only 250 mg. of caffeine can cause you to exhibit the same symptoms as people who are suffering from clinical anxiety.[78] The average cup of coffee contains at least 100 mg. of caffeine and

[77] Veninga and Spradley, *The Work/Stress Connection,* pp. 347–48.
[78] Yates, *Managing Stress,* p. 123.

as much as 150 mg. Tea and cola drinks also contain caffeine, though in lesser amounts than coffee.

Not only do workers consume stimulants during their breaks but they often smoke. Nicotine initially acts as a stimulant and only sometime later does it have a depressant effect on one's nervous system. When the first puff of smoke is consumed smokers may be psychologically relaxing, but their heart rates are actually climbing. With their coffee and cigarettes people often eat junk foods that have a lot of fat and sugar. While such foods may taste good they have little nutritional value and are potentially harmful because they contribute to higher levels of cholesterol and fatty deposits in the bloodstream.[79]

You may want to take brisk walks during the lunch hour rather than consume coffee. If you have one hour off you may even want to begin a regular exercise program including jogging, swimming, or biking. A recent study undertaken at the Eltra Corporation's Converse Rubber Company indicates that relaxation breaks in which workers are given the opportunity to exercise instead of the traditional coffee break tended to improve workers overall health and helped them get greater satisfaction from their jobs. At the end of the study the researchers reported that those who took a relaxation break had a greater drop in blood pressures, headaches, and sleep problems as well as improvement in their job satisfaction as compared with those who continued to take the standard coffee break.[80]

Taking a vacation   The restoration of one's adaptation energy often comes about quickly while taking a vacation. However unless the vacation has been carefully planned, it can be equally as taxing as the stressful work environment.

What appears to be important in reducing stress is to have (a) an understanding of the type of vacation that brings you the most relief and (b) a recognition of how much time you need to fully recover from the tensions within the work environment.

Some respondents in our survey indicated that they enjoy driving to the northern Minnesota woods on a Thursday afternoon for a three-day weekend. But others indicated that fighting traffic and rushing up a freeway in order to beat their neighbors to one of the few unreserved spots at a campsite is too much like the treadmill they feel they are on at work. For a vacation to be renewing it is important that it be planned around an activity that will help you to regain your energy. For one person this might be hunting, fishing, or camping. For another it might be spending a long weekend with close friends.

It is equally important to know how much time you need to adequately recover your adaptation energy. Some executives told us that they prefer short mini-vacations. Often they felt uptight if they were away from the office for

[79] Ibid., p. 124.
[80] Ibid.

more than a few days. But others stated that they needed a full three or four weeks to finally feel that they have been renewed. There is some evidence that if an individual is highly involved in her work a three-week-vacation may be needed. Yates has noted that during the first week most executives are thinking about problems they have at work. During the second week they genuinely relax, but during the third week their thoughts return to the office. "Thus, if you haven't taken three weeks," he notes, "you wouldn't have had the one week of pure vacation."[81]

Meditating Meditation is not simply a matter of thinking about some concept, religious or otherwise. Rather it is an exercise in which you seek to alter your state of consciousness. Concentration is central to the process. When meditating properly there is almost a temporary shutdown of the information processing within the brain. The primary attribute of meditation is that you can induce a relaxation response whenever you are confronted with a particularly stressful situation.

There have been a number of studies completed on various approaches to meditation including studies on transcendental meditation, yoga, biofeedback, and autogenic training. Researchers are fairly well agreed that many benefits accrue to an individual who meditates. Usually oxygen consumption decreases as does the respiratory rate. The heart rate decreases, but the alpha brain waves, which signify a more relaxed state, increase. Blood pressure also decreases as does the muscle tension. All of these changes are associated with *de*stressing and *un*stressing the body.[82] In a study undertaken by D. R. Frew, meditating was positively correlated with better performance, increased job satisfaction, and reduced turnover.[83] While there are many meditation modalities, one that holds particular promise in reducing stress was developed by Herbert Benson in Havard's Thorndike Memorial Laboratory.[84] The technique is summarized in Figure 10-8.

Knowing When a Job Is Hopeless

One of the frequent questions we encountered was, "How do I know when I should quit and get a different job?" Unfortunately the stress of a tension-filled work environment can cloud one's judgment which may result in one of two extreme decisions.

On the one hand we found workers who quit their jobs impulsively, prematurely, and with a great deal of anger. Oftentimes they had not adequately explored the ways through which they could creatively manage their

---

[81] Ibid., pp. 109–10.

[82] Ibid., p. 125.

[83] D. R. Frew, "Transcendental Meditation and Productivity," *Academy of Management Journal,* 17, (1974), 262–68.

[84] Herbert Benson with Miriam Z. Klipper, *The Relaxation Response* (New York: Morrow, 1975).

1. Sit quietly in a comfortable position.

2. Close your eyes.

3. Deeply relax all your muscles, beginning at your feet and progressing up to your face. Keep them relaxed.

4. Breathe through your nose. Become aware of your breathing. As you breathe out, say the word "one" silently to yourself. For example, breathe in . . . out, "one"; in . . . out, "one"; and so on. Breathe easily and naturally.

5. Continue for 10 or 20 minutes. You may open your eyes to check the time, but do not use an alarm. When you finish, sit quietly for several minutes, at first with your eyes closed and later with your eyes open. Do not stand up for a few minutes.

6. Do not worry about whether you are successful in achieving a deep level of relaxation. Maintain a passive attitude and permit relaxation to occur at its own pace. When distracting thoughts occur, try to ignore them by not dwelling on them and return to repeating "one." With practice, the response should come with little effort. Practice the technique once or twice daily, but not within two hours after any meal, since the digestive processess seem to interfere with the elicitation of the Relaxation Response.

Figure 10-8 The relaxation response. [From *The Relaxation Response* by Herbert Benson, M.D. with Miriam Z. Klipper. Copyright 1975 by William Morrow & Company, Inc. By permission of publishers.]

stress. On the other hand, we interviewed individuals who continued to hang on to their job with the hope that somehow, someday it was going to get better. Oftentimes it didn't get better and many of these workers became increasingly disillusioned and bitter about their working life.

How do you know when a job is hopeless and on what basis should you make a judgment about whether it's time to move on to another place of employment? From our research we sifted out three major indicators of a hopeless job. Any one of these may be a signal that there is a mismatch between you and your job. If several of these indicators occur in your job, or if one becomes extremely serious, you probably should consider other job possibilities.

1. A hopeless job has a destructive influence on your personal life. In a thought-provoking article in the *Harvard Business Review,* Fernando Bartolome and Paul A. Lee Evans note that work spills over into our private lives in both positive and negative ways.[85] When an executive is enjoying his or her work, when it is found to be exhilarating and challenging, the executive probably returns home feeling good about life. Such individuals are enjoyable to be with. However, there is also "negative emotional spillover" in which the executive brings the problems of work to the home. As one executive's wife in the Bartolome and Evans study noted: "Yes, his mind is often on other things. Yes, he often worries and it *does* disturb the family life. When he is like that he can't stand the noise of the children. . . . He can't stand the fact

[85] Fernando Bartolome and Paul A. Lee Evans, "Must Success Cost So Much?" *Harvard Business Review,* March–April 1980, p. 139.

the children are tired. In general we have dinner together so he can be with them. And obviously they chatter, they spill things, they tease each other—and he blows his top. He is tense and uptight—it's disturbing; I can't stand it. I have to try to mediate between them and cool things down. The only thing is to finish everything as soon as possible and get everyone quickly off to bed." Another wife said: "My husband is not one of those men who vents all his frustrations on his family. One cannot reproach him for being aggressive or for beating his wife. Instead he closes up like a shell. Total closure. The time he thinks he spends here isn't spent here."[86]

After interviewing over 2,000 managers over a five-year time period the researchers concluded:

> When negative emotions spill over, managers often express dissatisfaction with their life styles and complain of wanting more time for private life. But because their minds are numbed by tension, these people cannot use even their available time in a fulfilling way. Some report needing a double martini just to summon the energy to switch on the television. Many read the newspapers, not because they're interested in world events, but to escape into personal privacy. Some mooch around in the basement or the garden as a way of getting through the day. Again and again the spouse of the executives they interviewed said: "I don't really mind the amount of work he has to do. That is, if he is happy in his work. What I resent is the unhappiness that he brings home."[87]

If your job is having a destructive influence on your personal and family life and if that has been going on for months or perhaps years, it may be one indicator that it is time to look for a different job.

2. A hopeless job seriously impairs your health. A serious health problem may be a strong indicator that your attempts to cope with problems at work have not been successful. This is particularly true if you are experiencing health problems related to stress such as chronic ulcers, migraine headaches, dangerously high blood pressure, or coronary problems.

Every individual has a unique tolerance for different degrees of impaired health. Some workers will not believe that their job is hopeless even though work stress brings on heavy drinking, a coronary attack, and a bleeding ulcer. Even while laying in an intensive care unit of a hospital they may chafe to get back to work. We believe it is important to place a high premium on optional health and to recognize that mild symptoms can foreshadow more serious problems. If you stay on a job that impairs your health, you run the real risk of losing both your health and your job. By quitting one you may save the other.

3. A hopeless job has insufficient rewards. Most executives work for more than their salary and fringe benefits. We often are not aware, however,

[86] Ibid., p. 139.
[87] Ibid., p. 139.

of the importance of the nonmaterial benefits of our work. Three of these appear to be particularly important in a healthy work environment.

The first nonmonetary reward is the nature of the work itself. If you like the tasks which you are doing and if your workload is reasonable, you probably look forward to most days at work. However if your work provides little intrinsic payoff and if you don't believe in what you're doing, it could mean a mismatch has occurred.

We talked with a number of individuals who were very skillful in staff work and, because of their skills, were promoted to management positions. For some, the adjustments were minor as they quickly learned and enjoyed their new responsibilities. Others, however, yearned for their old jobs. For them, the sooner they could return to do what they felt they did best, the sooner they would be able to bring their work frustrations under control.

A second nonmonetary reward is represented in our relationships at work. "We have a close group at the office," said one worker. "We help each other move; if someone's sick you know everyone will visit and pitch in to do their work; we're a family and everyone really cares." Friends at work can make many frustrating jobs tolerable particularly if colleagues are eager to help one another. On the other hand, if your job offers no friendships, that may be a sign that you should begin to look for a better working environment.

Finally, a strong nonmonetary reward can be the relationship between supervisor and subordinates. When the relationship is effective there is a willingness to share responsibilities, to solve problems, and to give support to one another. If it is ineffective, valuable adapative energy is consumed—not on task-related issues, but in coping with abrasive personalities.

As you examine your job, ask yourself about the nonmonetary rewards that you receive. It may give you an indication as to whether you should continue to work for your employer. If you determine that the job is hopeless keep your decision to yourself or share it only with close friends away from work. Consider all your options before leaving; don't make a decision in haste. Then, before announcing your intent to resign, quietly begin searching for a new position. Don't let yourself get caught by a feeling of panic. Eventually you will find a working environment that is more conducive to your mental and physical well-being.

Addressing the Problems Associated with Shift Work

There is little doubt that shift work creates serious problems for workers. One of the most extensive studies on shift work was undertaken by the Stanford Research Institute on 12,000 nurses and 12,000 food processors. The researchers examined dispensary logs and personnel records in order to compile health and safety information. The results of this study indicated that nurses and food processors who work rotating shifts had significantly more dispensary visits and recordable accidents (almost twice as many) than did those workers on fixed shifts. Individuals who worked day shifts had the fewest health and safety problems, followed by afternoon and evening fixed-shift workers. Those who worked rotating shifts showed a significantly higher incidence of the following problems than did fixed shift workers: digestive trouble, chest pains, wheezing, nervousness, inadequate sleep patterns, colds, fatigue, less satisfactory domestic and social life, alcohol consumption, use of stimulants, and use of sleep-enhancing medications.[88]

Two specific responses can be made by administrators to the problems associated with rotating shifts. The first is to permit employees to choose the shift they would prefer working and to allow them to stay on that shift on a permanent or semipermanent basis. The physiological and psychological problems appear to be most acute for workers whose shifts are rotated frequently—for example, the nurse who changes shifts every two weeks. Apparently our systems are such that a change in sleep and work patterns every few weeks disrupts our circadian biological rhythms.[89]

The second suggestion in coping with the stresses associated with shift work is to reimburse such workers at a substantially higher rate of pay than they would receive during the daytime. Increasingly this is being done in various parts of the country. Unfortunately there has not been any research completed that would indicate whether higher rates of pay serve to decrease the stress levels of those who work on night shifts. There is, however, self-reported evidence that nurses are more willing to work such shifts if there are adequate economic incentives for so doing.[90]

Adopt Flexible Working Schedules

One of the most encouraging developments in Western society in reducing debilitating stress has been the advent of flextime. The flextime movement began in 1965 when a woman economist in Germany, Christel Kammerer, recommended it as a way to bring women into the job market. In 1967, Messerschmitt-Bolkow-Blohm, the "deutsche Boeing," found that many of its employees were arriving at work worn out from fighting rush-hour traffic. Management gingerly experimented and permitted 2,000 workers to go off the rigid eight-to-five schedule and to chose their own hours. Two years later, because of highly favorable reaction to the experiment, all 12,000 of its

[88] Michael J. Smith, Michael J. Colligan, and Joseph J. Hurrell, *A Review of Psychological Stress Research for the National Institute for Occupational Safety and Health, 1971 to 1976* (Cincinnati: Behavior and Motivational Factors Branch, National Institute for Occupational Safety and Health, 1978), pp. 10–12.

[89] A summary of the research on shift work and circadian biological rhythms can be found in Lenart Levi, "Occupational Mental Health: Its Monitoring, Protection and Promotion," *Journal of Occupational Medicine*, 21, no. 1 (January 1971), 28–30.

[90] "Pact Aimed at Luring Nurses to Night Shift," *Minneapolis Tribune*, July 1, 1980, p. 6B.

employees were given the opportunity to go on flextime. Quickly the concept spread in Europe and then in the United States. In 1977, 13 percent of all U.S. companies were using flexible hours. Within a few years the number is anticipated to reach 17 percent, representing more than 8 million workers.[91]

The basic structure of flextime is known as the "bandwidth" and usually runs from 7:30 A.M. to 6:30 P.M. for daytime workers. Inside this bandwidth are core times when you have to be on the job—usually from 9:30 to 11:30 A.M. and 2:00 to 3:30 P.M.— and the rest is flextime. How employees schedule their hours is pretty much a personal choice, providing that the worker puts in the required time.

The objective of flextime is to "reduce the strangle hold that the clock has on you. It can help you do such things as get the kids off to school, avoid peak rush hours on the highways, . . . keep a dental appointment at lunch, or arrange a game of tennis before or after work."[92] In brief, it permits you to gain control over your day.

There are some drawbacks to flextime such as management difficulties in scheduling everyone's working hours and in not always being able to give employees their first scheduling preference for hours to be worked. A survey by the Administrative Management Society also noted that accommodating employees whose output is the input for others can be a problem. And flextime is sometimes not conducive to an organization where an entire staff must, because of the nature of the tasks, begin their workday simultaneously.

Nevertheless the advantages appear to far outweigh the disadvantages. The American Management Association reports that worker morale improves in 97 percent of the organizations who use flexible time. It is believed, although not yet empirically substantiated, that flextime has a positive impact on worker productivity. It is perhaps fitting tribute to the concept that only 2 percent of the organizations who have implemented flextime work schedules have gone back to the rigid time structure used in former years.[93]

Building a Healthier Organization

More and more organizations recognize that they have a responsibility in keeping employees healthy. In a survey of 130 of the largest companies in the United States there was a growing recognition of the value of employer-sponsored physical fitness programs. Thirty-four of the 130 companies had fitness programs and 8 percent of these were established in the 1970s. Seventy percent of the 130 firms stated that their fitness programs improved the health of employees and reduced absenteeism and increased mental alertness.[94] One

[91] Alvin Toffler, "The Third Wave," *Playboy,* January 1980, p. 152.
[92] Sylvia Porter, *Minneapolis Tribune,* July 12, 1978, p. 14A.
[93] Toffler, "Third Wave," p. 152.
[94] "Health Education in Industry: The Key to a Vigorous Work Force," *Occupational Health and Safety,* April 1980, p. 2.

sign of the increased interest is the fact that the American Association of Fitness Directors in Business and Industry has only three dozen members when it was formed in 1975. Currently the membership is more than 1,200. Today almost every company with an established fitness program is expanding it.[95]

The motivation for initiating fitness programs within organizations has been primarily a "gut feel" on the part of administrators that such programs would increase productivity, diminish absenteeism, heighten morale, and build a healthy work force. The research evidence is now beginning to document such changes. Dispensary visits for various health problems diminished when opportunities for exercise were given to employees.[96] Workers are less ill and consequently miss work on fewer occasions and have fewer accidents when engaged in a regular exercise program. In a study of 259 NASA workers who participated in a three-times-a-week exercise program, half indicated that their job performance was higher and that they had a better attitude towards their work. Almost all said they felt better.[97]

Physical fitness programs and facilities vary widely. Some companies have only a small exercise room or running track while others have exercise and sport complexes that rival private clubs and colleges. Most employees work out on their own time but some employers give employees time off for such exercise.[98] Some organizations are so convinced of the positive effects of exercising that they pay their employees for taking part in an established fitness program. The Hospital Corporation of America, based in Nashville, Tennessee, pays exercisers by the mile—16 cents for runners and walkers, 5 cents for bicyclists, and 64 cents for swimmers.

There are arguments against establishing physical fitness programs but most have proven to be invalid. One such argument is that "We can't afford it." This argument is often heard in human service organizations whose budgets seem to preclude an investment in health programming. However, many organizations find that it takes relatively little cost to begin a fitness program. Prudential Insurance Company uses the roof of its Houston office for a quarter-mile jogging track. The Boeing Company at its 747 plant in Everett, Washington, permits runners to use a maze of tunnels beneath its building. In Dallas, the Forney Engineering Company has made an arrangement with a nearby school for swimming.[99] Inexpensive lockers and showers in a basement or storeroom are enough for a perfectly good exercise program.

A second argument against fitness programs is that "Time off for exer-

[95] "As Companies Jump on Fitness Bandwagon," *U.S. News and World Report,* January 28, 1980, p. 42.

[96] "Employees as Health Educators: A Reality at Kimberly Clark," *Occupational Health and Safety,* April 1980, p. 24.

[97] *Building a Healthier Company* (Chicago: Blue Cross Association, 1979).

[98] "As Companies Jump on Fitness Bandwagon," p. 42.

[99] Ibid.

cise will reduce productivity.'' The evidence does not support the assertion. The NASA study mentioned earlier demonstrates that fit employees work harder and may be more productive. However, if there is a strong feeling that workers should not be given time off for exercise it is still possible to develop an exercise program that employees can take part in before or after work, or during the noon hour.

The third argument that is commonly heard is that ''We might be liable for injuries or heart attacks.'' This is probably the most frequent concern that is raised by executives. However, as Blue Cross and Blue Shield note, everything an organization does involves some liability including ''the annual dinner to pass our service pins.'' The risks of an exercise program are minimal. At the Aerobics Activity Center in Dallas, over 3,000 people have logged over 1,300,000 miles since 1971. Only two problems have occurred and no deaths.[100]

How do you initiate a physical fitness program in your hospital or health agency? You should have a leader—someone who will take an interest in establishing a sound program. Sometimes someone from the YMCA or YWCA, a health club employee, a university physical education expert, or a high school coach could be employed on an hourly basis to set up the program. If you want to learn the experiences of other organizations you may want to write for the booklet ''Building a Healthier Company'' from the President's Council on Physical Fitness and Sports, 400 6th Avenue S.W., Suite 3030, Washington D.C. 20201.

Maintain Your Vitality!

The goal of this book has been to help you become a consciously competent health administrator. We have examined many concepts and explored many ideas. However if you are to be consciously competent you will need to continue to learn, to grow, and to feel the excitement that comes when you have grasped a new subject and learned a new skill. ''Only birth can conquer death,'' says Joseph Campbell. ''Within the soul, within the body social, there must be—if we are to experience long survival—a continuous 'recurrence of birth' to nullify the unremitting recurrence of death.''[101]

Commencement speakers frequently admonish their audiences saying, ''This should be a beginning for you, not an ending. Don't stop learning!'' John Gardner says that in spite of the good advice a high proportion of graduates will pay little heed to it for by the ''time they are middle-aged they are absolutely mummified. . . . Many young people have stopped learning in the religious or spiritual dimensions of their lives long before they graduate from college. Some settle into rigid and unchanging political and economic

[100] *Building a Healthier Company.*
[101] Joseph Campbell, *The Hero with a Thousand Faces* (New York: Pantheon, Bollingen Series XVII, 1948), p. 16.

views by the time they are twenty-five or thirty. By their mid-thirties most will have stopped acquiring new skills or new attitudes in any central aspect of their lives."[102]

To stay alert, young in spirit, and ever inquisitive is to avoid occupational burnout. Equally important if the challenges of availability, accessibility, prevention, and high quality care at affordable costs are to be successfully met, health administrators such as yourself will need to think anew, act anew, and learn to creatively address the challenging problems that are before us. There is little room for those who are apathetic. As Gardner perceptively notes: "Men who believe in nothing change nothing for the better. They renew nothing and heal no one, least of all themselves. Anyone who understands our situation at all knows that we are in little danger of falling back through lack of material strength. If we falter, it will be a failure of heart and spirit."[103]

SUMMARY

This chapter has sought to examine the relationship between work and health. We learned that there are organizational as well as psychological determinants of stress. Among the important occupational factors causing stress are factors intrinsic to a job (quantitative and qualitative overload), role ambiguity and conflict, ineffective working relationships, and the inability to participate in the decision making process. We noted that unrelieved stress is the fundamental cause of job burnout, resulting in depleted energy reserves, lowered resistance to illness, increased dissatisfaction and pessimism, and increased absenteeism and inefficiency at work. Burnout can progress through five stages, each of which has a definite effect on mental health and physical well-being. Various strategies that can be used to lower stress and recapture one's vitality were discussed in this chapter. Among the strategies were the ability to understand the consequences of work stress, the ability to develop space from work, the creation of challenging goals, developing flexible working hours, and understanding when a job is hopeless. Finally, we observed that many organizations are taking an active role in promoting the health of employees. The research evidence suggests that such programs have a positive effect on employee health and may improve job performance.

STUDY QUESTIONS

1. Do you agree with Jere E. Yate's observation that "Chronic stress is a major health problem facing managers in America today"? Explain your answer.

[102] John Gardner, *Self-Renewal* (New York: Harper & Row, 1965), p. 15.
[103] Ibid., p. xiii.

2. What was the most stressful environment in which you have worked? How did you cope? If you were to be reemployed in that organization, and if it is a highly stressful work environment, what would you do differently in better managing your job?

3. One of your subordinates appears to be the victim of unrelieved job stress. You note the symptoms: chronic tiredness, frequent illness, and poor judgment. List specific strategies you would consider taking in assisting this employee.

ADDITIONAL READING RESOURCES

"As Companies Jump on Fitness Bandwagon," *U.S. News and World Report,* January 23, 1980, p. 42.

COOPER, CARY L., and JUDI MARSHALL, "Occupational Sources of Stress: A Review of the Literature Relating to Coronary Heart Disease and Mental Ill Health," *Journal of Occupational Psychology* (London), 49 (August 1976), 12.

COOPER, CARY L. and R. PAYNE, *Stress at Work.* New York: John Wiley, 1978.

LaROCCO, JAMES M., JAMES S. HOUSE, and JOHN R. P. FRENCH, JR., "Social Support, Occupational Stress, and Health," *Journal of Health and Social Behavior,* 21, no. 3 (September 1980), 202–18.

MASLACH, CHRISTINA, "Burned Out," *Human Behavior,* September 1976, pp. 16–17.

SWEETLAND, JOHN, *Occupational Stress and Productivity.* Scarsdale, N.Y.: Work in America Institute, 1979.

Index

Psychological noise, 99
Psychology Today, 10
Psychotherapy:
    compared to jogging, 318
    and organizational change, 259
Public health organizations:
    causes of conflict in, 197
    changing purposes of, 253
    effect of changing cultural values on, 20
    governing boards, 189
    new challenges for, 2–3
    role confusion in, 202
    traditions, 19
Punishment, 129, 130

Quality control, 251–52

Railroad industry, 12
Rating scales, for performance appraisal, 138,
    140–41 *fig.*
Rational-empirical change strategies, 255
Rationalization, 6
Reagan, Ronald, 77
Recruitment, 106–16
    screening, 109–14
    searching, 106–9
    selecting, 114–16
    and time management, 58
Red-crossing technique, 225–26
Redding, W. Charles, 216
Red tape crisis, 267
Reeser, Clayton, 39, 119
Referent power, 40, 42, 45
Reflective observation, 157
Reinforcement theory, 129–32
Relational management style, 155–56
Relationships, as change target, 278–79
Relaxation techniques, 321–23
Report writing, and time management, 57
Resignations, 85
Responsibility:
    delegating, 69–79
    and self-management of time, 63
    as stressor, 300–301
Responsiveness, and competence, 8, 15
Restraining forces, 276–77
Revenue and expense budget, 46
Revolution:
    to adapt to environmental demands, 51–52
    in health system, 2
Reward power, 40, 42, 45
Rewards:
    for group performance, 186
    insufficient, 325–26
    and operant conditioning theory, 129–31
    and performance, 121–23
    role in performance appraisal, 148–50
Risk taking:
    assessing organizational propensity for, 270
    attitudes in groups, 160
Risky shifts, 160
Robbins, Stephen P., 39
Rogers, Carl, 95, 96, 100, 102
Role ambiguity, 300
Role behavior, and conflict, 198–218
Role conflict, 300
Role confusion, 200–205, 300
Role description, 203
Role fulfillment, 212–18
Role prescription, 203, 204–5
Role security, 205–12
Roosevelt, Franklin D., 167
Rosenman, Ray H., 303–4
Rotating shifts, 326–27
Rubin, Irwin, 157

Rubin, Jerry, 280
Rumors, 36–37
Russek, H. I., 299
Russell, Bertrand, 39

Safety needs, 212
Salaries:
    avoiding discrimination in, 108
    of men and women compared, 10
    negotiating with applicant, 115–16
    and work satisfaction, 115
Sampling, 177 *fn.*
Scapegoating, 6
Schein, Edgar, 278
Schubin, Seymour, 311
Scientific Management, 64
Scott, Walter D., 136
Screening, and recruitment, 109–14
Search committee, 191
Searching, recruitment stage, 106–9
Seachore, Stanley, 185
Secondary tension, 172
Selecting, and recruitment, 114–16
Self-actualization, 212
Self-awareness, 96–97
Self-concept:
    and communication, 86–89
    effect of feedback on, 217
Self-disclosure, 95–96
Self-esteem, 299
Self-fulfilling prophecy, 87–88
Self-generated scales, 275–76
Self-management, 56–79
    defining objectives, 65–69
    delegating, 69–79
    importance of, 56
    and time management, 56–65
Self-respect, 240–41
Selye, Hans, 292, 293
Sense Relaxation (Gunther), 97
Sex discrimination:
    in nursing, 3
    in salary levels, 10
Shift work, 326–27
Sifford, Darrell, 319
Similarity errors, 148
Simon, Herbert A., 288
Simulation, 177 *fn.*
Skinner, B. F., 129–30, 135
Sloan, Alfred P., 58
Smith, Donald, 2–3
Smoothing, 227–28, 231
Social support:
    to avoid job burnout, 320–21
    group norms, 168–72
Soviet Union, 189, 318
Span-of-control principle, 25, 28
Sponsors, 43
Spontaneous orientation, 210
Spradley, James P., 20, 306
Standard Oil Company, 132
Standards, and competence, 4
Standing committees, 60
Stanford Research Institute, 326
Status differences, 91–92
Stereotyping, 90
Stevens, Leonard A., 99
Stogdill, R. M., 167
Stoner, James A. F., 48, 106
Strategy orientation, 207, 210
Stress (*see also* Occupational stress; Job burnout)
    defined, 292–93
    and personality factors, 294–97
    unrelieved, 307
Stressor, 292
Stress response, 292–93
Stress threshold, 295

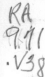